Child and Adolescent
Health and Health Care Quality

MEASURING WHAT MATTERS

Committee on Pediatric Health and Health Care Quality Measures

Board on Children, Youth, and Families

Board on Health Care Services

INSTITUTE OF MEDICINE *AND*
NATIONAL RESEARCH COUNCIL
OF THE NATIONAL ACADEMIES

THE NATIONAL ACADEMIES PRESS
Washington, D.C.
www.nap.edu

THE NATIONAL ACADEMIES PRESS   500 Fifth Street, N.W.   Washington, DC 20001

NOTICE: The project that is the subject of this report was approved by the Governing Board of the National Research Council, whose members are drawn from the councils of the National Academy of Sciences, the National Academy of Engineering, and the Institute of Medicine. The members of the committee responsible for the report were chosen for their special competences and with regard for appropriate balance.

This study was supported by Contract No. HHSP23320042-509X1 between the National Academy of Sciences and the Department of Health and Human Services. Any opinions, findings, conclusions, or recommendations expressed in this publication are those of the author(s) and do not necessarily reflect the view of the organizations or agencies that provided support for this project.

International Standard Book Number-13: 978-0-309-18623-0
International Standard Book Number-10: 0-309-18623-4

Additional copies of this report are available from the National Academies Press, 500 Fifth Street, N.W., Lockbox 285, Washington, DC 20055; (800) 624-6242 or (202) 334-3313 (in the Washington metropolitan area); Internet, http://www.nap.edu.

For more information about the Institute of Medicine, visit the IOM home page at: **www.iom.edu.**

The serpent has been a symbol of long life, healing, and knowledge among almost all cultures and religions since the beginning of recorded history. The serpent adopted as a logotype by the Institute of Medicine is a relief carving from ancient Greece, now held by the Staatliche Museen in Berlin.

Suggested citation: IOM (Institute of Medicine). 2011. *Child and Adolescent Health and Health Care Quality: Measuring What Matters*. Washington, DC: The National Academies Press.

THE NATIONAL ACADEMIES
Advisers to the Nation on Science, Engineering, and Medicine

The **National Academy of Sciences** is a private, nonprofit, self-perpetuating society of distinguished scholars engaged in scientific and engineering research, dedicated to the furtherance of science and technology and to their use for the general welfare. Upon the authority of the charter granted to it by the Congress in 1863, the Academy has a mandate that requires it to advise the federal government on scientific and technical matters. Dr. Ralph J. Cicerone is president of the National Academy of Sciences.

The **National Academy of Engineering** was established in 1964, under the charter of the National Academy of Sciences, as a parallel organization of outstanding engineers. It is autonomous in its administration and in the selection of its members, sharing with the National Academy of Sciences the responsibility for advising the federal government. The National Academy of Engineering also sponsors engineering programs aimed at meeting national needs, encourages education and research, and recognizes the superior achievements of engineers. Dr. Charles M. Vest is president of the National Academy of Engineering.

The **Institute of Medicine** was established in 1970 by the National Academy of Sciences to secure the services of eminent members of appropriate professions in the examination of policy matters pertaining to the health of the public. The Institute acts under the responsibility given to the National Academy of Sciences by its congressional charter to be an adviser to the federal government and, upon its own initiative, to identify issues of medical care, research, and education. Dr. Harvey V. Fineberg is president of the Institute of Medicine.

The **National Research Council** was organized by the National Academy of Sciences in 1916 to associate the broad community of science and technology with the Academy's purposes of furthering knowledge and advising the federal government. Functioning in accordance with general policies determined by the Academy, the Council has become the principal operating agency of both the National Academy of Sciences and the National Academy of Engineering in providing services to the government, the public, and the scientific and engineering communities. The Council is administered jointly by both Academies and the Institute of Medicine. Dr. Ralph J. Cicerone and Dr. Charles M. Vest are chair and vice chair, respectively, of the National Research Council.

www.national-academies.org

v

ALAN R. WEIL, Executive Director, National Academy for State Health Policy
ALAN M. ZASLAVSKY, Professor of Health Care Policy (Statistics), Department of Health Care Policy, Harvard Medical School

Study Staff

ROSEMARY CHALK, *Study Director*
PATTI SIMON, *Program Officer*
CHELSEA BODNAR, *Fellow* (January to April 2010)
YEONWOO LEBOVITZ, *Research Associate* (from November 2010)
WENDY KEENAN, *Program Associate*
JULIENNE PALBUSA, *Research Assistant*
PAMELLA ATAYI, *Senior Program Assistant*

Reviewers

This report has been reviewed in draft form by individuals chosen for their diverse perspectives and technical expertise, in accordance with procedures approved by the National Research Council's Report Review Committee. The purpose of this independent review is to provide candid and critical comments that will assist the institution in making its published report as sound as possible and to ensure that the report meets institutional standards for objectivity, evidence, and responsiveness to the study charge. The review comments and draft manuscript remain confidential to protect the integrity of the deliberative process. We wish to thank the following individuals for their review of this report:

Anne Beal, Aetna Foundation

Mary Byrne, Stone Foundation and Columbia University School of Nursing

Elena Fuentes-Afflick, Departments of Pediatrics and Epidemiology, University of California, San Francisco

Darcy Gruttadaro, National Alliance on Mental Illness Child & Adolescent Action Center

Kelly J. Kelleher, Office of Clinical Sciences, Columbus Children's Research Institute, Ohio State University College of Medicine and Public Health

Jonathan Klein, American Academy of Pediatrics and Julius B. Richmond Center of Excellence

Milton Kotelchuck, MGH Center for Child and Adolescent Health Policy, MassGeneral Hospital for Children, and Harvard Medical School

Rita Mangione-Smith, University of Washington Center for Child Health, Behavior, and Development, Seattle Children's Hospital Research Institute

Karen A. Matthews, Pittsburgh Mind-Body Center, Department of Psychiatry, University of Pittsburgh School of Medicine

Wilhelmine Miller, NORC at the University of Chicago

Michael Msall, Developmental and Behavioral Pediatrics, University of Chicago

Edward B. Perrin, Department of Health Services, University of Washington

Sandeep Wadhwa, 3M Health Information Systems

Deborah Klein Walker, Abt Associates Inc.

C. Jason Wang, Department of Pediatrics, Boston University School of Medicine, and Department of Community Health Sciences, Boston University School of Public Health, Boston Medical Center

Although the reviewers listed above have provided many constructive comments and suggestions, they were not asked to endorse the conclusions or recommendations nor did they see the final draft of the report before its release. The review of this report was overseen by **Paul J. Wallace,** The Permanente Federation and Kaiser Permanente, and **Nancy E. Adler,** Departments of Psychiatry and Pediatrics, and Center for Health and Community, University of California, San Francisco. Appointed by the National Research Council and Institute of Medicine, they were responsible for making certain that an independent examination of this report was carried out in accordance with institutional procedures and that all review comments were carefully considered. Responsibility for the final content of this report rests entirely with the authoring committee and the institution.

Preface

As the nation has invested in and made new commitments to programs offering health care services to children, child health advocates, policy makers, families, and the media have raised questions arise regarding the evidence to support claims that these efforts have led to improvements in the overall health status of children and adolescents or to a substantial increase in access to appropriate health care services for these populations. For those who use various categories of health care services, questions arise regarding the presumed impact on processes and outcomes of care. Even as recent legislation has enabled the expansion of child and adolescent health care services, concern persists as to whether significant gaps in access to these services exist and whether these gaps can be filled through a redirection of resources to meet the health care needs of particular populations.

All of these issues serve as the backdrop for the work of a committee convened by the Institute of Medicine (IOM) in fall 2009 to begin a year-long study of current national data systems pertaining to child and adolescent health status, health care access, and quality of care. The committee's creation was one of the outgrowths of the reauthorization of the Children's Health Insurance Program, enacted by the Congress in 2009. As it passed this important legislation, the Congress asked: "How can we know that our programmatic efforts are having the intended impact on the health of the nation's children?"

Embedded in this question are concerns about health care outcomes and eventual summative evaluations of the overall health of the nation's children and adolescents, but also concerns about the ability to monitor, evaluate, and manage an expanding array of programs and services for these populations. The committee was asked to assess both the state and the science of child and adolescent health and health care quality measurement, as well as the capacity of existing data systems (particularly at the federal level) to track and evaluate programs and services intended to serve the health care needs of these populations, including the analytical capacity of federal and state agencies that use these data for these purposes.

The 16-member committee formed by the IOM to address these issues comprised an array of experts from the fields of clinical pediatrics, health services research, health program evaluation and policy analysis, and the statistical and epidemiological sciences. The committee's work was augmented by the expert assistance of four consultants—Patricia MacTaggart, Gerry Fairbrother, Jessica McAuliffe, and Lisa Simpson—whose work greatly facilitated dealing with specific issues related to child health and health care quality measurement.

The committee is especially grateful for the assistance received from the staff of the IOM and the National Research Council, specifically from the Board on Children, Youth, and Families, whose director, Rosemary Chalk, served as principal study director for this study. Ms. Chalk is herself a widely known specialist on policy issues surrounding the health of children and is one of the most expert leaders of the processes through which a study of this kind takes place under the aegis of the National Academies. She was assisted by Patti Simon, program officer at the IOM, who was a mainstay in the committee's communications and in the drafting of key chapters of the report. Other IOM staff who played key roles in assisting the committee were Pamella Atayi, senior program assistant; Wendy Keenan, program associate; and Julienne Marie Palbusa, research assistant. The committee is grateful for the work of each of these individuals.

In the course of this study, the committee concluded that the nation is fortunate to have a wide array of data sources and frequent analyses addressing the health and health care quality of children and adolescents, each providing a partial set of observations and benchmarks with which to answer some of the above questions of concern to the Congress and the American people. However, the patchwork of clinical information systems, periodic sample surveys, registries, and vital and health statistics reported by state and federal agencies does not facilitate the determination of reliable and valid indicators of either health status or health care access and quality for the nation's youth as a whole. The committee's survey of existing data sets and methods for their analysis revealed the need for a national core set of salient measures (some of which may require new data definitions and approaches to collection). These measures need to be collected in every jurisdiction; analyzed using a standard methodological approach; and made available to the nation in a form that will enable policy makers, health care administrators and providers, and the general public to assess the health status and access to quality care of children and adolescents and to determine whether and to what extent programs funded to provide health care services for these populations are achieving their goals. It is the committee's hope that its recommendations and the logic underlying them will resonate with those whose efforts will be critical to answering this call in the coming years. Surely having a national data set of this kind will do much to sharpen the nation's focus and resolve to do what is necessary to ensure the health of its greatest resource—its youth.

Gordon H. DeFriese
Chair
Committee on Pediatric Health and
Health Care Quality Measures

Acknowledgments

Beyond the hard work of the committee and project staff, this report reflects contributions from various other individuals and groups that we want to acknowledge.

The committee greatly benefited from the opportunity for discussion with the individuals who made presentations at and attended the committee's workshops and meetings (see Appendix B). The committee is thankful for the useful contributions of these many individuals.

This study was sponsored by the U.S. Department of Health and Human Services, the Centers for Medicare and Medicaid Services, and the Agency for Healthcare Research and Quality. We wish to thank Barbara Dailey, Denise Dougherty, Marsha Lillie-Blanton, and Cindy Mann for their support.

We would like to thank those who wrote papers that were invaluable to the committee's discussions: Christina Bethell, Gerry Fairbrother (with colleagues Jessica McAuliffe and Rachel Sebastian), Patricia MacTaggart, and Paul Newacheck. Thank you also to Brett Brown, whom we commissioned to provide a technical review of the report, and Michael A. Stoto, who provided guidance on report drafts. Together, their insight and expertise added to the quality of the evidence presented. Additionally, Rona Briere and Alisa Decatur are to be credited for the superb editorial assistance they provided in preparing the final report.

Contents

APPENDIXES[1]

---

[1] Only Appendixes A-E are printed in this volume. The other appendixes are included on the CD in the back of the report or online. Go to http://www.nap.edu/catalog.php?record_id=13084.

Summary

Monitoring the status of the health of the nation's children and adolescents is important because health matters both in and of itself—as a measure of a society's values and capabilities—and as a direct determinant of adult health, productivity, and longevity. The health of children and adolescents in the United States is influenced by multiple factors, including biology, behavior, and social and physical environments. It also is influenced by the availability, use, and quality of health care services, especially for those with life-threatening conditions or special health care needs that require frequent interactions with health care providers. Therefore, understanding the health status of children and adolescents is closely intertwined with understanding the quality of the health care they receive.

Conceptually sound and reliable health and health care measures for children and adolescents can be used to assess the effects of disease or injury on health; identify vulnerable children in clinical settings and vulnerable population subgroups in health plans or geographic regions; measure the effects of medical care, policy, and social programs; set targets for improving health care; and improve health outcomes. Despite the presence of multiple data sets and measures, however, the United States currently has no robust national information system that can provide timely, comprehensive, and valid and reliable indicators of health and health care quality for children and adolescents.

Progress has been made in selected areas to improve measures of health and health care quality for younger populations, and interest is growing in developing standardized measures that could yield the information needed in these areas. What is needed now is a comprehensive strategy that can make better use of existing data, offer a basis for integrating or linking different data sources, develop new data sources and data collection methods for difficult-to-measure indicators and difficult-to-reach populations, and put a system in place for continuously improving the measures and the measurement system.

STUDY CHARGE

This study responds to a mandate in the Children's Health Insurance Program Reauthorization Act (CHIPRA) of 2009 for a study by the National Academies "on the extent and quality of efforts to measure child health status and the quality of health care for children across the age span and in relation to preventive care, treatments for acute conditions, and treatments aimed at ameliorating or correcting physical, mental, and developmental conditions in children." To this end, the Institute of Medicine (IOM) and the National Research Council (NRC) of the National Academies were engaged under contract with the U.S. Department of Health and Human Services (HHS) to conduct an 18-month study "to identify key advances in the development of pediatric health and health care quality measures, examine the capacity of existing federal data sets to support these measures, and consider related research activities focused on the development of new measures to address current gaps." The IOM and NRC subsequently formed the Committee on Pediatric Health and Health Care Quality Measures to conduct this study.

In interpreting its charge, the committee sought to (1) consider all of the major national population-based child health/health care reporting systems sponsored by the federal government; (2) examine strengths and deficiencies of current federal data collection efforts and reporting systems; and (3) make recommendations for improving and strengthening the timeliness, quality, public transparency, and accessibility of information on child health and health care quality.

CONCLUSIONS

The committee reviewed multiple federal sources of data on the health and health care quality of children and adolescents, 24 core measures of health care quality recommended by the Secretary of HHS in 2010 for voluntary reporting by Medicaid and CHIP programs, and a number of private-sector efforts aimed at developing valid and reliable measures of health and health care quality for children and adolescents, as well as the salient research literature. As a result of this review, the committee formulated conclusions in three key areas.

The Nature, Scope, and Quality of Existing Data Sources

- Multiple and independent federal and state data sources exist that include measures of the health and health care quality of children and adolescents.
- The fragmentation of existing data sources impedes access to and timely use of the information they collectively provide.
- Existing data sources have their individual strengths and limitations, but no single data set derived from these sources provides robust information about the health status or health care quality of the general population of children and adolescents.
- Lack of standardization in the measurement of disparities in health and health care quality limits the ability to identify, monitor, and address persistent health disparities among children and adolescents.
- The absence of common definitions and consistent data collection methods impedes the standardization of common data elements (such as insurance coverage) across multiple settings, such as health care, education, and human services, in federal and state data sets.

Gaps in Measurement Areas

The conclusions in this area focus on the social and behavioral determinants of health and health care quality. Multiple longitudinal studies document the impact of physical and social environments (e.g., toxic exposures, safe neighborhoods, or crowded housing), behaviors (e.g., diet or the use of alcohol or drugs), and relationships (e.g., parent—child attachment) on the health status of children and adolescents and their use of health care services. Earlier IOM/NRC reports have documented the extent to which such information is lacking in existing federal health and health care data sets, and stressed that these contextual factors are key influences on the short- and long-term health outcomes of children and adolescents.

- Existing goal-setting efforts in the public and private sectors offer a foundation from which to develop national goals for children and adolescents in priority areas of health and health care quality.
- Quality measures for preventive services deserve particular attention for children and adolescents because most individuals in these age groups are generally healthy and because early interventions may prevent the onset of serious health disorders as the child or adolescent becomes an adult.
- Standardized measures of child health and the quality of relevant health care are important for all child health problems, but especially for preventable, ongoing, or serious health conditions.

- Variations persist in data elements pertaining to race, ethnicity, income, wealth, and education. Core data elements for socioeconomic status need to be identified that can feasibly be collected in a standardized manner, while introducing a life-course approach that can be applied across multiple data sets.
- The health of other family members, especially parents and other caregivers, may directly affect the health of children and adolescents, as well as their access to and use of health care services. Family-focused measures are a new frontier for research in the development of measures.
- With respect to social determinants of health, data are needed to determine those elements that offer timely potential for prediction of disparities.
- Race/ethnicity, socioeconomic status, primary language spoken at home, and parental English proficiency all affect disparities in health and health care and therefore are relevant topics for data collection for all children and adolescents.
- Measures of health literacy are important for adults' ability to understand information that is relevant for children's healthy development and in ensuring adolescents' understanding of their own health status, and deserve greater recognition in the identification of future research priorities and the testing of new measures in national surveys.
- Biological influences on the health of children and adolescents are an important focus for measures of health and health care quality; also important are measures of behaviors and levels of functioning. Measures focused on the needs of the "whole child," as opposed to individual clinical concerns, can address the distinct needs of children and adolescents, including their unique epidemiology, their dependent status, and their developmental stages.
- Measures of care transitions are important, especially for children with special health care needs.
- New areas of focus entail place-based measurement, targeting selected geographic regions and population groups at the state, county, and even neighborhood levels.

Methodological Areas That Deserve Attention

- Many data sources cannot be used to assess the status of specific groups of children and youth, particularly vulnerable populations who are at risk of poor health outcomes because of their health conditions or social circumstances.

- Implementing an integrated approach involves choosing specific criteria for selecting reference groups. The selection of reference group criteria would benefit from interactions with state and local health officials, as well as those concerned with the health and health care quality of children and adolescents in their region, particularly underserved populations. The selection of criteria could also be guided by the perspectives of families, consumers, and users, as well as those involved in data collection.
- Greater transparency is necessary to expose the strengths and limitations of different surveys in tracking the status of key child and adolescent populations of interest; in identifying appropriate reference groups over time; and in implementing innovative measurement practices that can adapt to changing conditions, changing populations, and opportunities for health improvement.
- Linking or aggregating databases offers opportunities to reduce variations among multiple data sources and to decrease the burden of data collection on individual states, providers, health plans, and households.
- While it is often difficult to connect data from the clinical records of children and adolescents enrolled in public health insurance plans to population health surveys and administrative data sets, such efforts will increase understanding of the social context and life-course influences that may affect children's health status and their access to and use and quality of health care services.
- Longitudinal data (with multiple observations for the same children/families over time) would enrich the quality of measures used in population health surveys and health care quality studies.
- Electronic data capture and linkage would greatly enhance future measurement activity. Expanding data collection beyond geographic and claims information to capture state-level policy and community-level characteristics would enable analysis of the variability and impact of coverage, eligibility, and payment policies. Special attention will be needed to ensure that advances in electronic data capture adhere to existing privacy and confidentiality guidelines and laws. Ongoing attention will also be needed to resolve emerging issues related to privacy and confidentiality in future measurement efforts.
- While electronic health records have potential for significant retrieval of selected variables across multiple records, they do not necessarily offer conceptual or metric precision. The data are locked in a multitude of disparate systems designed for purposes other than analyses of health and health care quality.

A STEPWISE APPROACH

The above conclusions provide the foundation for a stepwise approach to improving data sources and measures of health and health care quality for children and adolescents that in turn serves as a frame for the committee's recommendations. This approach is designed to stimulate and support collaborative efforts among federal and state agencies and key stakeholder groups in five key areas:

1. Set shared health and health care quality goals for children and adolescents in the United States;
2. Develop annual reports and standardized measures based on existing data sets of health and health care quality that can be collected and used to assess progress toward those goals;
3. Create new measures and data sources in priority areas;
4. Improve methods for data collection, reporting, and analysis; and
5. Improve public and private capacities to use and report data.

Each area requires attention to specific strategies, which are detailed below in the committee's recommendations. Some of these strategies represent actions that can be taken now; others require a longer-term effort. They are aimed at aligning the areas of measurement of the health of children and adolescents that are emerging in population health surveys and longitudinal studies—areas that go beyond health conditions to assess health functioning, health potential, and health influences—with existing efforts to measure health care quality for children and adolescents.

RECOMMENDATIONS

Step 1: Set Goals

Setting national and state-level goals for the health of children and adolescents would prioritize the next generation of health care quality measures and clarify the relative roles of health care services and improvements in health care quality in achieving those goals. These goals could be derived as a set of critical objectives for children and adolescents from such sources as Healthy People 2010 and Healthy People 2020. They could also be reported as part of the annual national quality strategy and national prevention strategy reports prepared by the Secretary of HHS.

In determining priority areas for these goals, the committee built on earlier work that goes beyond the traditional focus on such indicators as morbidity, mortality, and chronic and acute conditions and identified seven priority areas to inform the setting of goals for health and health care quality for children and adolescents:

- childhood morbidity and mortality,
- chronic disease conditions,
- preventable common health conditions (especially mental and behavioral health and oral health),
- functional status,
- end-of-life conditions,
- health disparities, and
- social determinants of health.

In addition, the committee recommends an overarching emphasis on a *life-course perspective* that is integral to all seven priority areas listed above. Because a life-course perspective provides a framework for understanding how health and disease patterns emerge within an individual's social and physical environments as the result of the accumulation of the effects of risk factors and determinants across the life span and across generations, it necessitates focusing on measures in each of the seven priority areas at various life stages within childhood and adolescence, as well as the transition to adulthood.

None of the seven priority areas is fully distinct; however, each presents unique measurement challenges and opportunities that merit separate consideration. Most existing measures focus primarily on the first two areas and draw extensively on administrative data sets. Yet important initiatives have emerged within population health surveys, longitudinal studies, and other research studies that provide data sources and opportunities to develop new measures in the remaining five areas. These initiatives warrant increased support because of their capacity to inform the next generation of health care quality measures, especially in areas that involve disparities, social determinants of health, and the life course, as well as the emerging health information technology (HIT) infrastructure. The use of such resources will require extensive collaboration among multiple agencies and the public and private sectors, as well as study participants and key consumers of the data.

It should be noted that the committee directed its recommendations to the Secretary of HHS to allow for flexibility and discretion at the highest levels. However, specific actions are also necessary within designated agencies to foster accountability for implementation. An initial action agenda for the implementation of each recommendation is therefore proposed in the full report.

Recommendation 1: The Secretary of Health and Human Services (HHS) should convene an interagency group to establish national health and health care quality goals for children and adolescents within a life-course framework.

Step 2: Develop Annual Reports and Standardized Measures Based on Existing Data Sets

Efforts to monitor and improve the health of children and adolescents are hampered by both the lack of annual reports that focus on child and adolescent health and health care quality and the absence of standardized measures and variation in salient data sources. Of particular concern are the lack of consistent measurement of disparities in health and health care quality to support the development of targeted interventions at the national and state levels and the retention of unnecessary or obsolete measures resulting from the adoption of nonstandardized core measure sets.

Existing Opportunities to Include Children and Adolescents in Annual HHS Reports

The Secretary of HHS is already required to make annual reports on health care quality and disparities, as well as on national prevention initiatives. These reports provide valuable opportunities to include specific consideration of children and adolescents and to draw attention to the ways in which their needs may differ from those of older populations.

Standardized Measurement of Disparities in Heath and Health Care Quality

Pervasive and persistent disparities exist in health and health care by race/ethnicity, socioeconomic status, special health care needs, primary language spoken at home, and parental English proficiency for all children and adolescents. Traditionally, such disparities have been measured through racial, ethnic, and geographic data. Assessment of children's and adolescents' health will benefit from efforts to (1) standardize definitions and measures of these characteristics, (2) routinely include socioeconomic data (minimally household income as an increment of the federal poverty level and educational attainment of parents), and (3) introduce data on language proficiency. All of these actions will be increasingly important in response to the growing poverty rate of younger populations. The percentage of U.S. children and adolescents (under age 18) who lived in poverty increased from 18 percent in 2007 to an estimated 20.7 percent in 2009.

The percentage is even higher among younger children (under age 6) and among children in selected geographic areas, such as rural communities or central city regions.

The increasing racial and ethnic heterogeneity of younger populations also deserves consideration. Compared with U.S. adults, U.S. children and adolescents are disproportionately of nonwhite race/ethnicity—a fact of particular significance because poor and minority children have disproportionately high special health care needs compared with their nonpoor and white counterparts. Children and adolescents in these groups also are more frequently insured through public health plans. For example, more than 40 percent of African American and one-third of Latino children have public insurance such as Medicaid or CHIP. Thus the development of health indicators that can provide a basis for considering the health status of these groups in relation to the general population of children and adolescents is a particularly urgent need.

> Recommendation 2a: The Secretary of HHS should include specific measures of the health and health care quality of children and adolescents in annual reports to Congress as part of the Secretary's national quality and prevention strategy initiatives.
>
> Recommendation 2b: These measures should include standardized definitions of race/ethnicity, socioeconomic status, and special health care needs, with the goal of identifying and eliminating disparities in health and health care quality within a life-course framework. Identifying and reducing disparities in health and health care will require collecting data on race/ethnicity, socioeconomic status, special health care needs, primary language spoken at home, and parental English proficiency for all children and adolescents.

A Periodic Review Process

The purpose of a periodic review of health and health care quality measures is to ensure that the system for child and adolescent health and health care quality measurement is achieving its information goals (public transparency, timeliness, accessibility, and quality); to identify obsolete, unnecessary, or redundant measures; to highlight emerging candidates for new measures; and to identify areas that deserve consideration in the development of valid and reliable measures in keeping with new health goals for children and adolescents. The review process provides an opportunity to address the need for effective and valid data collection approaches to ensure that respondents (especially parents and adolescents) are clear about the meaning and intent of questions being asked.

Recommendation 3: The Secretary of HHS should develop a strategy for continuous improvement of the system for collecting, analyzing, and reporting health and health care quality measures for children and adolescents. This strategy should include periodic review of those measures that are used, recommended, or required by the federal government.

Step 3: Create New Measures and Data Sources in Priority Areas

Ideally, child and adolescent health and health care quality measures and data sources should support analyses that can demonstrate how changes in funding levels for public insurance programs (such as Medicaid or CHIP) or in eligibility requirements, enrollment levels, or service procedures affect health outcomes, health care costs, and school achievement. They should make it possible to examine specific conditions and issues that are of particular importance to vulnerable and underserved children and adolescents, especially those served by Medicaid and CHIP. Such measures and data sources should also support analyses of whether and how the organization and delivery of health care achieve public goals of effectiveness, efficiency, safety, timeliness, equity, and patient-centeredness. Finally, they should be flexible enough to include possible emerging threats to child and adolescent health.

Collectively, the seven priority areas identified earlier can serve as a framework for assessing the comprehensiveness of any set of measures for child and adolescent health and health care quality. For example, in early 2010 the Secretary of HHS recommended a set of core measures of health care quality for children and adolescents that includes a strong emphasis on preventive services. These measures address, only minimally, oral health, mental and behavioral disorders, and substance use. Yet dental caries are the most prevalent childhood infectious disease, and some costly adult health outcomes (such as tobacco addiction and obesity) have their origins in youth. Early interventions to address these health issues in children and adolescents can help prevent such problems as coronary heart disease and diabetes. Thus, the life-course perspective advocated by the committee can pay dividends in savings to the health care system by addressing problems before they appear later in life.

The new National Prevention Strategy mandated in the Affordable Care Act of 2010 offers an opportunity to improve the quality of data sources for the measurement of preventive services for these and other conditions for children and adolescents. This effort will require collaboration among multiple agencies within HHS, as well as among multiple public- and private-sector stakeholders. Such will also be the case for measures targeting end-of-life conditions, health disparities, and social determinants of health.

Recommendation 4: The Secretary of HHS should develop new measures of health and health care quality focused on preventive services with a life-course perspective. These measures should focus on common health conditions for children and adolescents, especially in the areas of oral health and mental and behavioral health, including substance abuse.

Recommendation 5: The Secretary of HHS should support interagency collaboration within HHS to develop measures, data sources, and reporting focused on relationships between the social determinants of health and the health and health care quality of children and adolescents.

Recommendation 6: The Secretary of HHS should encourage interagency collaboration within HHS to introduce a life-course perspective that strengthens the capacity of existing data sources to measure health conditions, levels of functioning, and health influences (including access to and quality of care) for children and adolescents.

Recommendation 7: The Secretary of HHS should place priority on interactions between HHS agencies and other federal agencies to strengthen the capacity to link data sources in areas related to behavioral health and the social determinants of health and health care quality.

Step 4: Improve Data Collection, Reporting, and Analysis

Several strategies can be used to improve data sources and methods for data collection, reporting, and analysis: (1) data aggregation strategies, including the use of registries and data linkage opportunities; (2) the development of mechanisms to foster greater transparency of performance indicators; (3) the use of unique identifiers that allow analysts to link data on the same child from different administrative data sets to obtain a more robust profile of the family and neighborhood characteristics and his or her health and educational outcomes; and (4) greater use of longitudinal studies, which follow the same cohort of children over time to monitor their health conditions and the health care services they receive.

Creating opportunities to link data across multiple health care settings, as well as connecting health and health care data to education and human service data systems, would improve timeliness and facilitate analysis of the multiple factors that affect the well-being of children and adolescents. The success of such efforts will depend on both methodological and technical advances and the resolution of privacy and data sharing issues, as well as specific guidance from federal data collection agencies to create constructive remedies.

Likewise, longitudinal measurement fosters child-centered analysis, breaking down the divisions among data created by the different silos of the health care system and other service settings that engage the child and his or her family. Longitudinal measures are especially useful in monitoring care transitions, assessing whether the child's or adolescent's needs were identified and met within an appropriate care setting and developmentally tailored, and determining both the short- and long-term outcomes of care. While it may not be feasible to introduce longitudinal approaches into health care quality measures, longitudinal studies can identify specific data elements that merit consideration in the creation of new quality measures.

Finally, timely and transparent data systems can help engage parents in data collection efforts through explanation of the purpose of the effort and how the data will be used to assist their own and other children and adolescents throughout the country. This engagement and broad awareness are critical for ensuring that all segments of the population, including marginalized populations, will be fully represented in survey and administrative data sources.

> Recommendation 8: The Secretary of HHS should identify significant opportunities to link data across health care, education, and human service settings, with the goal of improving timeliness and fostering greater transparency as to the multiple factors that affect the health of children and adolescents and the quality of services (including health care, educational, and social services) aimed at addressing those factors.

> Recommendation 9: The Secretary of HHS should promote policy, research, and convening efforts that can facilitate linkages among digital data sets while also resolving legal and ethical concerns about privacy and data sharing.

Step 5: Improve Public and Private Capacities to Use and Report Data

The ultimate goal of improving data collection and reporting efforts is to develop national and state-based data collection systems, measures, and reports that are compatible and that provide a basis for comparing the health and health care quality of children and adolescents across different health plans and different states and other regions of the United States. It is therefore important to create conditions that will allow states to develop measures that are useful for their own purposes while moving toward a core set of national, standardized measures in key areas. It will also be important to develop an integrated approach that can blend measures of the health status of children and adolescents (drawn from population health surveys) with measures of health care quality for those services that are actually used by children, adolescents, and their families (drawn from administrative data sources or private health records). Measures are needed with which to compare the quality and utilization of services with the types and severity of children's health needs due to chronic health disorders or risk factors that make them vulnerable to adverse health outcomes. Measures are also needed to provide more precise information about the short- and long-term effects of preventive services within a life-course framework.

Efforts to build federal and state capacity for place-based measures (e.g., through geographic positioning data) can resolve some of the current difficulties in integrating health measures, social and physical environment measures, and other measures of influence that occur in health care settings. Such efforts will require innovative approaches to compiling and extracting data from existing surveys and databases. They will also require a conceptual framework with the ability to prioritize and operationalize key measures of social context, health influences, and preventive services. Necessary as well are criteria that can be used to designate the appropriate reference groups of common interest. At the same time, collaboration needs to be strengthened between those who collect the data and those who are expected to use the data to shape current and future interventions. Fostering this collaboration involves investing in the capacity of communities, states, providers, consumers, and others to use the data effectively to drive decision making in light of limited resources; to monitor changes given the introduction of new policies or investments over time; and to understand the importance of tailoring interventions to the needs of different racial/ethnic, geographic, and other segments of the population and tracking longitudinally how disparities respond to changes in health care resources, processes, and policies. Some states are prepared to serve as laboratories for the creation of new measures for difficult-to-measure indicators or difficult-to-reach populations, and they would benefit from the development of incentives that encourage voluntary compliance in these areas. The emerging HIT infrastructure offers an opportunity to emphasize the distinct needs of children and adolescents and to link those needs to family data in health information exchanges, as well as to supplement traditional electronic heath information with data from other sources (including parents). These linked data sets will need to track children across public and private data sources, as well as link with public health information systems through birth certificates and newborn screening data sets.

Recommendation 10: The Secretary of HHS should establish a timetable for all states to report on a core set of standardized measures that can be used in the health information technology infrastructure to assess health and health care quality for children and adolescents. Congress and HHS should formulate alternative strategies (through incentive awards, demonstration grants, and technical assistance, for example) that would enable states to develop the necessary data sources and analyses to meet such requirements.

FINAL OBSERVATIONS

The direction of policy and resources toward improving the health and health care quality of children and adolescents in recent years is an encouraging sign that the distinct needs and health priorities of these populations are being recognized. Opportunities are available now to incorporate these needs and priorities into emerging population wide health care quality initiatives while also enhancing separate data collection and analysis and research initiatives that address the unique characteristics and developmental requirements of these younger populations. Exploiting these opportunities will require strong national and state-based leadership. Much can be done with existing efforts, supplemented by modest additional resources, to go beyond traditional boundaries to incorporate data elements that can deepen our understanding of the complex interactions among health, health care quality, and the social determinants of health. Innovations in technology and data gathering methods enhance the potential to develop new measures that can inform our understanding of important health disparities, preventable health conditions, and the social determinants of health and enable a life-course approach to the assessment of health and health care quality for our nation's youth.

1

Introduction

The true measure of a nation's standing is how well it attends to its children—their health and safety, their material security, their education and socialization, and their sense of being loved, valued, and included in the families and societies into which they are born.

—Child Poverty in Perspective:
An Overview of Child Well-Being in Rich Countries
(UNICEF, 2007)

America's children are its greatest resource, and measures of child health are important indicators of the overall health and future prospects of the nation as a whole (CDC, 1991; Klein and Hawk, 1992; Nersesian, 1988; Reidpath and Allotey, 2003). Ensuring the health, safety, and well-being of children—at each critical stage of development—is a responsibility shared among individuals and families and across institutions and governmental jurisdictions. The vast number of public health initiatives, individual actions, community activities, advocacy campaigns, child- and adolescent-targeted programs and research, and policies and legislation focused on children would suggest the nation's desire to distinguish children's health as one of the highest national priorities.

STUDY CONTEXT

Monitoring the status of the health of children and adolescents is important because health matters both in and of itself—as a measure of a society's values and capabilities—and as a direct determinant of subsequent productivity and later longevity. Assessing the impact of policies, programs, and services that may influence child and adolescent health requires timely, high-quality, readily accessible and transparent indicators. Such information can be used to determine the relative health of the nation's children and adolescents; to support analyses of the health and access to high-quality health care services of selected population groups defined by geography, race/ethnicity, socioeconomic status, or other characteristics; and to drive

15

improvements in the quality of health care and other services so they can contribute to better health outcomes for children and adolescents.

Progress has been made in selected areas to improve measures of health and health care quality for younger populations, and interest is growing in developing standardized measures that could yield the information needed in these areas. The time is ripe, therefore, for a comprehensive strategy that can make better use of existing data, offer a basis for integrating or linking different data sources, develop new data sources and data collection methods for difficult-to-measure indicators and difficult-to-reach populations, and put a system in place for continuously improving the measures and the measurement system.

Several factors make this a particularly opportune time to mount an effort to strengthen existing measures and improve areas that require increased attention. First, Congress has emphasized improving health care quality as a strategy for obtaining greater value from public investments in health care services. Second, the health and health care of children and adolescents have become a particular focus as younger populations enrolled in public health plans such as Medicaid and the Children's Health Insurance Program (CHIP) have grown significantly. Third, the percentage of U.S. children and adolescents (under age 18) who live in poverty increased from 18 percent in 2007 to an estimated 20.7 percent (or 15.5 million children) in 2009 (DeNavas-Walt et al., 2010). The percentage is even higher among younger children (under age 6) and among children in selected geographic areas, such as rural communities or central city regions (Mattingly and Stransky, 2010).

Taking additional steps to improve health status and ensure quality health care for all U.S. children and adolescents is essential to achieving both optimal individual health and a healthy future for the nation. The health status of children and adolescents not only is an important determinant of their well-being, but also contributes to their school performance and their ability to become successful, productive, and healthy adults. Moreover, because children are dependent upon their adult caregivers, their families also bear the burden of inadequacies in access to and quality of health care services. Yet there are many indications that health and health care quality for the nation's youth fail to measure up to child and adolescent health outcomes and standards of care in many other developed countries (OECD, 2010a). Despite a broad array of efforts and significant investments in children's health, U.S. children and adolescents lag well behind their counterparts in other industrialized nations. According to UNICEF's report, *Child Poverty in Perspective: An Overview of Child Well-Being in Rich Countries*, the United States was in the bottom third of the rankings for material well-being, health and safety, educational well-being, family and peer relationships, and behaviors and risks (UNICEF, 2007). One possible explanation for the health lag is the severe disparities in socioeconomic status found in the United States (IOM and NRC, 2004). The United States also ranks at or near the bottom among industrialized countries on infant mortality and life expectancy (OECD, 2010b; Peterson and Burton, 2007). In 2004, the latest year for which comparable data are available, the United States had a higher infant mortality rate than 28 countries—including Singapore, Japan, Cuba, and Hungary—compared with 1960, when the U.S. infant mortality rate was higher than that of only 11 countries (NCHS, 2004). Evidence derived from meaningful data collection provides a platform for engaging a variety of stakeholders, including families and providers, in prioritizing and mobilizing for collective actions aimed at improving the health of the nation's youth.

STUDY CHARGE, APPROACH, AND SCOPE

These observations come at a time of great emphasis on the health of America's children as the U.S. Congress has passed, and President Obama has signed, the Children's Health Insurance Program Reauthorization Act (CHIPRA) of 2009. An important part of this reauthorization was a provision that the U.S. Department of Health and Human Services fund a study by the National Academies "on the extent and quality of efforts to measure child health status and the quality of health care for children across the age span and in relation to preventive care, treatments for acute conditions, and treatments aimed at ameliorating or correcting physical, mental, and developmental conditions in children."

The reauthorization of CHIP occurred just a few months before the enactment of the Patient Protection and Affordable Care Act and the Health Care and Education Reconciliation Act of 2010, signed by the President on March 30, 2010. The latter two pieces of legislation include provisions (both direct appropriations and authorizations) related to all three components of what most would consider the three principal elements of health care reform—access, quality, and cost. Taken together, these three pieces of legislation have major implications for the health of America's children and adolescents, although the latter two are broadly relevant to the health of and health care available to all Americans.

After the enactment of CHIPRA and in anticipation of the enactment of broader health care reform legislation some months later, the Congress directed attention in CHIPRA to two key questions: "How can we know that our programmatic efforts are having their intended impact on the health of the nation's children and adolescents?" and "Do we have data collection and analysis systems in place that would enable the accurate and timely assessment of the effectiveness and impact of those programs and services now made available to children and adolescents?" These questions reflect not only expectations that we can ascertain the short- and longer-term impacts of health care services and programs, but also expectations that we can effectively monitor the developmental aspects of child and adolescent health needs, health status, access to care, and important functional health outcomes to enable meaningful adjustments to these services and programs as they unfold over time.

Study Charge

The National Academies, specifically the Institute of Medicine (IOM) and the National Research Council (NRC), was contracted (by the Centers for Medicare and Medicaid Services [CMS] and the Agency for Healthcare Research and Quality [AHRQ]) to carry out a year-long study "to identify key advances in the development of pediatric health and health care quality measures, examine the capacity of existing federal data sets to support these measures, and consider related research activities focused on the development of new measures to address current gaps." This study, documented in this report, is part of an expanded effort within CMS and AHRQ to improve health outcomes and the quality of health care services for children and adolescents served by Medicaid and CHIP. The study was intended to complement these efforts by highlighting not only indicators of child health status and quality health care, but also the infrastructure that can support data coordination and integration strategies for measures of these indicators (see Chapter 2 for definitions of indicators and measures).

To conduct this study, the IOM and the NRC formed the Committee on Pediatric Health and Health Care Quality Measures. The committee was charged to

1. *consider all of the major national population-based child health/ health care reporting systems sponsored by the federal government* that are currently in place, including reporting requirements under federal grant programs and national population surveys conducted directly by the federal government;

2. *identify the information* regarding child health and health care quality that each system is designed to capture and generate, the study and reporting periods covered by each system, and the extent to which the information so generated is made widely available through publication;

3. *identify gaps in knowledge* related to children's health status, health disparities among subgroups of children, the effects of social conditions on children's health status and use and effectiveness of health care, and the relationship between child health status and family

income, family stability and preservation, and children's school readiness and educational achievement and attainment; and

4. *make recommendations* regarding improving and strengthening the timeliness, quality, public transparency, and accessibility of information about child health and health care quality.

Study Approach

The study committee included 16 members with expertise in pediatrics and clinical services, quality measures research, health policy, developmental and behavioral sciences, prenatal care and neonatal and infant health, adolescent health, nursing, public health statistics and systems-level metrics, health disparities, population health metrics, health finance, health information technology, decision making, and research on measurement. (See Appendix E for biographical sketches of the committee members.)

A variety of sources informed the committee's work. In conjunction with one of the committee's four formal meetings, a day-long public workshop was held on March 23, 2010 (see Appendix B for the workshop agenda), to obtain vital input from a broad range of relevant stakeholders, including parents; health care providers; public and private insurers; local, state, and federal agencies; and research experts. These stakeholders shared with the committee the experiences of federal, state, and local policy and decision makers and child health programs and advocates in using existing sources and methods for describing and measuring the health status of children and adolescents, determining access to and quality of health care for these populations, and performing outcome and impact assessments associated with these services. The committee also conducted an expansive review of the literature to identify key advances in the development of child and adolescent health and health care quality measures, examine the capacity of existing federal data sets to support these measures, and consider related research activities focused on the development of new measures to address current gaps.

Committee members brought to these deliberations their own perspectives on the nature of the problems in this area, as well as views on how the data collection and analysis systems relevant to child and adolescent health and health care can be made more timely, relevant, and useful. Workgroups of committee members pertinent to each of the chapters of this report were convened and met periodically throughout the course of the study.

In its deliberations and in the formulation of its findings, conclusions, and recommendations, the committee sought to balance ideas reflecting its hopes and aspirations for national data systems addressing child and adolescent health and health care with its understanding of the administrative, jurisdictional, financial, and even political exigencies that could delay or hinder the accomplishment of the goals and directions outlined in this report. The work described herein as essential to the nation's eventual ability to describe more fully health status and the health care experience and its impacts for children and adolescents is presented as a "journey," but one whose final destination may lay several iterations ahead. There will be many interim steps to achieve and many likely course corrections as well, but the journey itself will require a heightened level of consensus on why it is important to make this journey, what direction it should take, and what benefits it will have for each of the major stakeholders who will help make it possible. It is the committee's hope that this report addresses these issues in sufficient detail to make the enterprise important and worthwhile and to contribute to its ultimate success.

Study Scope

The committee was charged broadly with providing guidance on the state of efforts to measure child and adolescent health and the quality of their health care services. In approaching this task, the committee sought to gain an understanding of the full spectrum of influences, challenges, and opportunities facing current measurement efforts. The chapters that follow describe why such efforts are necessary and provide an overview of the key issues that must be addressed in the course of these efforts.

ORGANIZATION OF THE REPORT

This report reviews the array of current efforts to measure child and adolescent health, as well as the state of quality measurement of child and adolescent health and health care services. It presents the committee's findings; describes a new framework for assessing the health and health care quality of children and adolescents; and offers recommendations to state and federal agencies for enhancing the timeliness, quality, and public transparency and accessibility of information about child and adolescent health and health care services, with the ultimate goal of improving health outcomes.

The report has six chapters. Chapter 2 sets the stage for the remainder of the report by providing definitions of key terms, essential contextual information, the committee's argument for the need for a comprehensive approach to child and adolescent health, and initial observations.

Chapter 3 focuses on current data collection methods and sources used for measuring child and adolescent health and health care quality. It reviews the current inventory of federally supported population health data systems and provides illustrative examples of the challenges to data collection.

Chapter 4 reviews existing child and adolescent health indicators and key data sources for monitoring the health status and health outcomes of children and adolescents. This review is organized according to seven priority areas for measurement identified by the committee. The chapter describes the strengths and limitations of measurement within each priority area; the timeliness, quality, and public transparency and accessibility of the available data; and the extent to which national and state-based data sources are available within each priority area. It proposes using an integrated framework of health indicators to guide future quality measurement efforts and highlights opportunities to develop health measures that are responsive to local needs and health conditions while providing national and state profiles of the health status and health care quality of children and adolescents.

Chapter 5 focuses on measures of quality in child and adolescent health care. The chapter reviews prior measurement efforts, both public and private, in this area, as well as the current status of such efforts, highlighting strengths and limitations, including significant gaps. The chapter also addresses why quality measurement is important to a variety of audiences and actors—including health care providers, families, health plans, and policy makers—and how quality measures can be used to improve child and adolescent health care and, ultimately, health outcomes. Finally, the chapter highlights opportunities rooted in the emphasis on quality and accountability in recent legislation and resulting from emerging technologies.

Finally, Chapter 6 provides the committee's conclusions and recommendations for advancing the measurement of child and adolescent health and health care quality by addressing the gaps and inconsistencies detailed in the preceding chapters. It presents a stepwise approach to the development, collection, maintenance, and use of appropriate quality measures; the committee's recommendations for specific actions, including additional strategies that will be necessary to identify priorities, invest resources, integrate diverse activities over time, and evaluate progress; and immediate next steps that are feasible within the context of CHIPRA and health care reform initiatives.

The report includes several appendixes. Appendix A is a list of the acronyms used in the report. Appendix B contains the agenda for the March 2010 workshop. Appendix C reviews private-sector initiatives to advance health care quality and the development of quality measures. Appendix D provides an overview of data sources for measures of health care quality for children and adolescents. Appendix E provides biographical sketches of the committee members. Finally, Appendix F presents a detailed listing and description of existing population-based data sets for measuring child and adolescent health and salient influences, while Appendix G provides a detailed listing and description of sources of administrative data relevant to the quality of child and adolescent health and health care.

2

Setting the Stage

This chapter begins by providing definitions of key terms and essential contextual information. It then presents the committee's argument for the need for a comprehensive approach to child and adolescent health if measures of child and adolescent health and health care quality are to be improved. The final section offers initial observations that serve as the foundation for the rest of the report. The chapter provides the conceptual basis for addressing the strengths and limitations of current data sets that are used to measure health and health care quality for children and adolescents. It also summarizes the committee's perspectives regarding the ways in which these measures are derived from the structures, processes, and outcomes of health care services, as well as the social and behavioral determinants of health.

DEFINITIONS

Definitions for several key terms are foundational for this report. These terms include *child and adolescent health*, *functioning*, and *well-being*, defined below. They also include a number of terms related to data collection, defined in Box 2-1.

Children and Adolescents

In this report the terms *children* and *adolescents* are used to differentiate critical stages of development rather than precise age ranges. The terms include related terms such as childhood, teenagers, and youth. Adolescents

BOX 2-1
Terms Related to Data Collection

In addition to understanding what is measured, it is important to understand how data on these measures are collected. The terms defined below are used throughout this report; the specific methods of data collection are examined in greater detail in the following chapter.

Measures are specific data collection items within a survey/interview or administrative record system, including scales, numerators, and denominators, that serve to score survey results, medical records data, administrative data, and similar data sources. They involve such questions as: "Would you rate your child's overall health as excellent, very good, good, fair, or poor?," "What is the birth weight of U.S. infants?," "What is the average age, weight, or height of children served?," "Have you [an adolescent] ever used marijuana?," "Do you smoke cigarettes?," "Have you ever engaged in sexual intercourse?," and "How often do you take aspirin or medications like Tylenol for headache or other physical pain?"

Indicators are a collection of individual quality measures, consisting of a denominator and a numerator, that suggest a trend or pattern of health conditions, behaviors, or influences. Indicators of mental health status, for example, may consist of several individual measures of selected disorders, such as depression, attention-deficit disorder, and mental retardation.

Indexes are composites of indicators that are weighted to reflect assumptions about the relative value of selected indicators. One such example is body mass index (BMI), an index calculated on the basis of an individual's weight and height (and for children, gender and age) and used in the clinical assessment of obesity and overweight. Another example is the Consumer Price Index (CPI), which represents the total cost of a market basket of goods and services purchased by households at a point in time. Inflation is defined as a change in the CPI and is used by government, business, labor, and private citizens for many purposes. Some scholars have attempted to develop a Child Well-being Index (CWI) as a similar standard for assessing the general status (including health) of children over selected years. The CWI concept is based on a composite of indicators of well-being, including "economic well-being, safe/risky behavior, social relationships, emotional/spiritual well-being, community engagement, educational attainment . . . and health" (Land and FCD, 2010, p. 3).

Data systems are the collection of measures (e.g., surveys, indicators, and other reporting tools) that are used to examine the quality of child and adolescent health and health services. A data system may consist of several federally sponsored surveys, such as the National Immunization Survey (NCHS, 2011c), the National Health Interview Survey (NCHS, 2011b), and the Survey of Children with Special Health Care Needs (NCHS, 2009b). Data systems may require the linkage of several indicators or data sets to examine specific questions about the impact of children's health care quality on selected areas of functioning, such as: "What do we know about the impact of the quality of asthma care on the educational outcomes of school-aged children with asthma?"

are specified in the report because the scope of the task includes health conditions and behaviors that are unique to this age group. The age break in defining adolescent up to age 18 in this report is influenced by the age breaks currently associated with Medicaid data systems. Yet such definitions are frequently arbitrary. An earlier National Research Council (NRC) and Institute of Medicine (IOM) report *Adolescent Health Services: Missing Opportunities* (IOM and NRC, 2009a) described adolescence as a time of major transitions in which youth develop relational and behavioral skills and patterns that continue into adulthood and that critically impact future life experiences and outcomes. In earlier decades, adolescence was thought to begin with biological processes, namely the onset of puberty (generally around ages 12 or 13) and to end with the assumption of the social roles of an adult, such as the completion of education, the beginning of full-time employment, and the formation of relationships such as marriage and parenthood. In practice, multiple age breaks are used to define adolescence, such as the variations associated with the legal age of driving, underage drinking, military recruitment, voting, and so forth. Most of these eligibility criteria are determined by local customs or federal and state regulations that are not informed by the science of adolescent development.

The 2009 NRC and IOM report observed that adolescence is a theoretical construct that continues to evolve in response to historical events, cultural context, and biological changes. Disagreement persists among health care researchers, experts in adolescent health and development, practitioners, and policy makers on the specific age ranges associated with the terms *children* and *adolescents*. The lower range of adolescence has shifted in response to the earlier onset of puberty among boys and girls, calling into question the term that should be used to describe pre-teen children who exhibit signs of adolescent development. The widening delay in time between physical maturity and securing professional employment and independent living has also caused some researchers to designate the late teenage years and early 20s as a period of "emerging adulthood" (Arnett, 2000, 2004).

Before reviewing the current inventory of federally supported population health data systems in the chapters that follow, it is critical to understand what is meant by *child and adolescent health*. The World Health Organization (WHO) defines health as "not only the absence of infirmity and disease but also a state of physical, mental, and social well-being" (WHO, 1948). However, health involves more than physical wellness—it is affected by mental and emotional states as well. Moreover, those who are concerned with children's health status want to know about more than the presence or absence of specific health problems in the general child population at a given point in time. They also want to know whether children's health improved or diminished as compared with other periods. They often want to know as well how children with certain types of characteristics are faring. And increasingly, they want to know whether children are on track to grow into healthy adults. These multiple interests require an examination of the relationship between certain health conditions or behaviors and other child characteristics (such as age, race or ethnicity, gender, geography, and household income).

A growing literature documents the complex interaction among the genetics, environment, and developmental stages of children and the powerful impact of these factors on children's overall health. Transition points are also being recognized as key in children's health and well-being trajectory, including, for example, the transitions between childhood and adolescence and between adolescence and young adulthood (Ben-Shlomo and Kuh, 2002). Two other major factors are being recognized as influential—social determinants of health and life-course impacts.

An earlier IOM and NRC report, *Children's Health, the Nation's Wealth* (IOM and NRC, 2004), endorses an expanded definition of child health:

> Children's health should be defined as the extent to which individual children or groups of children are able or enabled to (a) develop and realize their potential, (b) satisfy their needs, and (c) develop the capacities that allow them to interact successfully with their biological, physical, and social environments. . . . (p. 4)

The report refers to three domains that are associated with the measurement of children's health: *health conditions, functioning,* and *health potential* (pp. 34–37):

- *Health conditions* denote disorders or illnesses of body systems.
- *Functioning* focuses on the manifestations of individual health in daily life.
- *Health potential* captures the development of health assets that indicate positive aspects—competence, capacity, and developmental potential.

In addition to these domains, that earlier report examines the relationships among a variety of physical, social, and policy influences and health status and outcomes. The IOM committee that developed the report formulated a conceptual model emphasizing the dynamic and developmental nature of children's health, focusing on the role of biology, the physical environment, and social and behavioral determinants in shaping the health and behaviors of children and youth (see Figure 2-1). While policy and health care services were also seen as key influences, they did not have a central role in that earlier study. The model of health used for Healthy People 2010 offers another approach to describing the interactions among

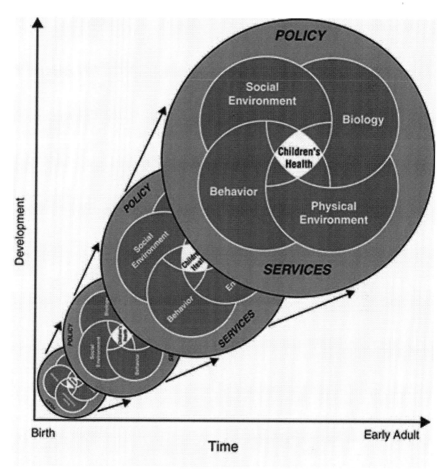

FIGURE 2-1 A model of children's health and its influences.
SOURCE: IOM and NRC, 2004, p. 42.

environmental factors and the biology and behavior of children and youth (HHS, 2000a).

While this committee endorses an expanded definition of child health, multiple definitions are in use. A number of challenges to current measurement efforts are a consequence of this lack of consensus on the definition of child health.

Different definitions of child health reflect different goals and yield distinct statistics. One systematic review found that the prevalence of chronic conditions among children in the United States ranges from less than 1 percent to as high as 44 percent across different studies, depending on the definition, sample, and methods used (Van der Lee et al., 2007). Assessment of the scope of selected health conditions through general population surveys is challenging, but it is equally difficult to estimate the prevalence of health disorders based on data from clinical service-based population surveys, such as hospital discharge or medical expense data studies.

In recent years, child and adolescent health indicators have expanded to include measures of overall levels of functioning and well-being—"a state broader than health that incorporates social, psychological, educational, behavioral, and economic dimensions" (IOM and NRC, 2004, p. 20)—especially in comparing the status of children and youth in the United States and in other developed nations. This approach led to a broadening of the concept of child health to include "the ability to realize aspirations, satisfy needs, and change or cope with the environment" (Starfield, 2004, p. 166). One result of this broader perspective is greater recognition of the different developmental stages of children and ways to enhance their successful transitions and navigation between childhood and adulthood, as well as greater appreciation of the importance of childhood antecedents of adult disease (such as the major role childhood obesity can play in cardiovascular disease and cancer, as well as in adult mortality). In addition, a focus on functioning and well-being encompasses interventions to minimize the impact of the experience of illness.

This distinction between the presence of a health problem and factors that lead to dysfunction resulting from that problem is articulated in the IOM report *Disability in America: Toward a National Agenda for Prevention* (1991). More recently, WHO extended this concept to say that every human being can experience a decrement in health and thereby experience some degree of disability. Disability is not something that only happens to a minority of humanity (WHO, 2010). According to WHO, this disability can reflect both biological and environmental factors. This formulation also emphasizes the dynamism of health as individuals experience and recuperate from health conditions (WHO, 2008). The fundamental shift in the types of morbidities facing children, from infectious to chronic conditions, as well as the impact of injuries on health, further requires a broadening of the definition of where health interventions need to focus, with increasing attention being paid to communities (e.g., neighborhood and housing characteristics), families (e.g., family structure and social support), and schools (e.g., school nutrition and physical education/activities). Considering child and adolescent morbidities within a community context, for example, allows for a more comprehensive examination of the clustering and interaction of risk factors (e.g., substandard housing conditions, poor air and water quality, poor social environment) and/or protective resources (e.g., access to affordable, healthy foods; affordable housing and transportation;

and essential services such as medical care and education) (Fielding et al., 2010; NRC, 2000).

The growing focus on children's levels of functioning or well-being has drawn attention to the complexity of assessing the nature and direction of interactions among children's health status, their access to and use of health services, and the impact of their physical and social environments on their health. In recent years, the quality of health care services provided to children in different settings, by different providers, and under different conditions also has been the subject of study.

For example, growing interest has focused on the use of a medical home, which the American Academy of Pediatrics defines as primary care that is "accessible, continuous, comprehensive, family centered, coordinated, compassionate, and culturally effective" (AAP, 2002, p. 184). The medical home concept may be especially useful for children with complex health care needs that require care coordination. Its utility as a measure of quality may be limited, however, in such areas as primary care and preventive services, where the identification of evidence-based and effective practices is still evolving, or in areas where the social or behavioral determinants of health may have greater impact than the use of health care services on health outcomes (such as in the areas of intentional or unintentional injury). The extent to which the medical home concept, by itself, can serve as a measure of the quality of the health care system also is questionable in the absence of more information about the extent to which other care arrangements, or other population health interventions, can effectively improve the health outcomes of children and adolescents.

The overall result of these shifts in focus is increased interest in identifying quality indicators of child and adolescent health and health care that are associated not only with traditional measures of child and adolescent health outcomes but also with broader indicators of well-being, such as school performance, risk behaviors, and childhood antecedents of adult disease. Greater attention also is being paid to the far-reaching costs and implications of childhood disease with respect to the productivity of caregivers, as well as the future productivity of children in whom the precursors of adult disease, such as obesity and smoking, are not addressed. For example, nearly a quarter of parents (23.8 percent) of children with special health care needs reported having to stop work or cut back hours at work because of their children's needs (HHS, 2008). These changes in employment had direct and significant consequences for family income, especially among lower-income families (HHS, 2008).

In focusing on data systems, the committee endeavored to examine the contributions of existing child health data collection efforts and to assess their relative strengths and limitations (see Chapter 4). The findings resulting from these efforts serve as the basis for changes recommended by the committee to improve the measurement of the health of children and adolescents and the quality of their health care services, especially in those areas of greatest concern to federal agencies and legislative policy makers. These findings also informed the committee's assessment of the potential for aggregating, synthesizing, and linking measures of specific health characteristics to reflect the general health status of children and adolescents (see Chapter 4).

BACKGROUND

As context for the remainder of the report, this section provides a current snapshot of children and youth in the United States, their health status and trends, and their access to and use of health services. It also presents the committee's argument for a comprehensive approach to child and adolescent health, the importance of measuring health and quality of health care for children and adolescents, and the need for a high-quality data system to collect these measures. Finally, it outlines challenges to creating such a data system.

Current Snapshot of Children and Youth in the United States

Children represent a substantial and growing segment of the U.S. population. In 2009, there were more than 74.2 million children and youth under age 18 in the United States, 1.9 million more than in 2000 (DeNavas-Walt et al., 2010). This number is projected to increase to 82 million in the next decade (FIFCFS, 2009).

Although children make up 25 percent of the total U.S. population, they represent 35 percent of those living in poverty (DeNavas-Walt et al., 2010). Compared with U.S. adults, U.S. children also are disproportionately of nonwhite race/ethnicity. According to the 2009 American Community Survey (ACS):

- In 2009, 55 percent of U.S. children were white, non-Latino; 22 percent were Latino; 15 percent were African American; 4 percent were Asian/Pacific Islander; 1 percent were American Indian/Alaska Native; 5 percent were multiracial; and 7 percent were identified as other race/ethnicity.
- The percentage of Latino children in the U.S. population continues to grow, and it is projected that one in every four children in the United States will be of Latino race/ethnicity by 2021 (FIFCFS, 2009).

Recent studies have focused on measuring disparities in terms of racial or ethnic differences, but disparities can also be measured along other dimensions, such as gender, household income, educational status of the child or parent, insurance type, and medical practice setting (Alessandrini et al., 2001; Merrick et al., 2001; Van Berkestijn et al., 1999; Wood et al., 1992). Some studies probe the importance of knowing more about the primary language spoken by parents and their children, since having English as a primary language frequently influences the success of efforts to navigate access to and use of health care services (Flores et al., 2000). For example, inequities and poor outcomes may be unobserved or understated with health care quality measures that are reported for those of Latino ethnicity without further subdivision by the child's or family's primary language.

Research has demonstrated that children in lower-income families have more severe health problems and worse health prognoses than children in higher-income families (IOM and NRC, 2004, p. 112). Yet few opportunities exist to collect data that provide a systematic understanding of differences in the health of children and adolescents based on their socioeconomic status. Several large population health surveys (such as the National Survey of Children's Health [NSCH] and the National Survey of Children with Special Health Care Needs [NS-CSHCN]) provide opportunities to collect this type of information, but their results cannot be integrated with the administrative data on health care services and expenditures that are routinely collected for Medicaid and Children's Health Insurance Program (CHIP) populations. Adding more data elements on race/ethnicity, socioeconomic status, special health care needs, primary language spoken at home, and parental English proficiency to administrative data sets for Medicaid and CHIP populations would provide a basis for comparing their health status and the quality of health care services they receive with the health and health care of other populations of children and adolescents.

Poor and minority children have disproportionately high special health care needs compared with their nonpoor and white counterparts, and they are more frequently insured through public health programs such as Medicaid and CHIP (Horn and Beal, 2004) (see Box 2-2 for a description of these programs). Recent estimates suggest that more than 40 percent of African American and one-third of Latino children are estimated to have public insurance (Horn and Beal, 2004). According to the census report on income, poverty, and health insurance coverage in the United States for 2009 (DeNavas-Walt et al., 2010):

- 20.7 percent of all children, or 15.5 million, lived in poverty in 2009 (p. 16);

BOX 2-2
Brief Description of the Medicaid and CHIP Programs

In the past 50 years, the U.S. Congress established two major health plans that extend health services to large groups of disadvantaged children and youth: Medicaid, established in 1965, and the Children's Health Insurance Program (CHIP) (formerly known as the State Children's Health Insurance Program, or SCHIP), established in 1997. Both programs were enacted by the Social Security Act (Titles XIX and XXI), which also established the Maternal and Child Health Bureau (MCHB) (Title V). Each of these programs involves substantial public investments by both federal and state governments, in contrast to Medicare and MCHB, which are administered and funded solely by a federal agency.

Medicaid

Medicaid is a joint federal–state program that provides access to affordable and comprehensive health care for targeted low-income people—primarily children, pregnant women, parents, the disabled, and the elderly (Villegas, 2011). Roughly 60 million people receive Medicaid benefits at "some point" during a given year, about half of whom—29 million—are children (Urban Institute and Kaiser Commission, 2010). Medicaid is administered by the states, although the federal government sets minimum eligibility standards and provides at least half of the funding (Villegas, 2011). Medicaid accounts for roughly one-sixth of the nation's total health care spending (Urban Institute and Kaiser Commission, 2010).

Children represent nearly half of all Medicaid enrollees but account for only 17 percent of total Medicaid expenditures. On the other hand, seniors and people with disabilities represent one-quarter of Medicaid enrollees but account for 70 percent of total Medicaid spending (in part because of the more intensive use of acute and long-term care services by these groups).

CHIP

SCHIP (now CHIP) was established in 1997 to provide a capped amount of federal matching funds to states for coverage of children whose family incomes were too high to qualify for Medicaid but for whom private health insurance was either unavailable or unaffordable. CHIP covers roughly 7 million children in a given year (KFF, 2008).

The Children's Health Insurance Program Reauthorization Act of 2009 (CHIPRA) was signed into law in February 2009 (see Box 2-3). CHIPRA extends and expands the original SCHIP program, adding $33 billion in federal funds for children's coverage over the next 4.5 years. The Congressional Budget Office (CBO) estimates that CHIPRA will provide coverage to an additional 6.5 million children under CHIP and Medicaid in 2013 (CBO, 2003).

In addition to providing significantly higher federal funding for children's health coverage, CHIPRA restructured the formula that determines how much CHIP funding states receive each year; the new formula bases allotments on actual expenditures and includes an "inflation factor," which is designed to take into account both the growth in per capita health care expenditures and the growth in the number of children in each state. The enactment of national health care reform in March 2010 extended CHIP funding through 2015 and continues the program through 2019.

- 9.3 percent of all children, or 6.9 million, lived in extreme poverty in 2009 (defined as income below 50 percent of the federal poverty level) (p. 19); and
- from 2000 to 2009, the poverty rate for children younger than 18 increased from 16.2 to 20.7 percent (p. 17).

Moreover, children in low-income families (typically operationalized as families with incomes less than 200 percent of the federal poverty level) share many of the adverse health characteristics and access problems of children in impoverished families. According to the Census Bureau's Current Population Survey from 1980–2008, 40 percent of children ages 0–17 lived in low-income families and 44 percent of children less than 6 years lived in low-income families (FIFCFS, 2010).

Equity is a feature of the initial health care quality framework set forth in *Crossing the Quality Chasm* (IOM, 2001a) and is also stressed in recent legislative guidance, as well as the CHIPRA domains for measurement. Previous IOM reports have identified the equitable distribution of health care services as an overarching concern in assessing health care in the United States (IOM, 2006b, 2006c, 2006d). One recent review found that all of the available data sets surveyed included items that could serve as the basis for analysis of patients at risk for poor outcomes in various categories of disparity (Beal et al., 2004). However, the authors noted that studies of equity in children's health care have relied on only a third of these data sets (Beal et al., 2004). And even these data sets have limitations that could affect their validity and reliability: only four of the survey instruments are available in languages other than English, and only one has undergone cross-cultural validation.

Child and Adolescent Health Status and Trends

Most children and adolescents in the United States are healthy (OECD, 2010b). Advances in medicine and more robust prevention efforts in the last half century have led to declines in infant and child mortality and improvements in overall child health. Dramatic improvements have occurred in survival rates for childhood conditions that previously had high fatality rates. Even in the short interval between 1985 and 1999, for example, mortality from cystic fibrosis fell by 61 percent for children aged 2–5, 70 percent for those aged 6–10, and 45 percent for those aged 11–15 (Kulich et al., 2003). Childhood cancer mortality has also seen substantial improvements. For the years 1975–1995, the reduction in mortality was greater than 50 percent for childhood leukemia (Linet et al., 1999). Overall, children experience lower rates of mortality, chronic illness, and disability compared with adults (Starfield, 2004).

BOX 2-3
Public Law 111-3, Title IV: Strengthening
Quality of Care and Health Outcomes

On February 4, 2009, the Congress enacted the Children's Health Insurance Program Reauthorization Act (CHIPRA) of 2009 (Public Law 111-3). Sections 401–403 call for a number of child health improvement activities for children enrolled in Medicaid and the Children's Health Insurance Program (CHIP), including the following:

- **Development of an initial core set of health care quality measures for children enrolled in Medicaid or CHIP**—The Centers for Medicare and Medicaid Services (CMS) and the Agency for Healthcare Research and Quality (AHRQ) will collaborate to make recommendations for an initial core set of children's health care quality measures (completed January 1, 2010). The initial core set will be used voluntarily by Medicaid and CHIP.
- **Quality Demonstration Grants**—CMS will implement a CHIPRA Quality Grant Program to establish and evaluate a national quality system for children's health care, which encompasses care provided through Medicaid and CHIP. This will be accomplished by awarding 10 demonstration grants to states, funded by CHIPRA. This funding opportunity will result in the establishment and evaluation of a national quality system for children's health care.
- **MACPAC**—CHIPRA establishes the Medicaid and CHIP Payment and Access Commission (MACPAC) to review Medicaid and CHIP access and payment policies, and submit reports and recommendations to Congress (KFF, 2008). MACPAC's purview was expanded in the Affordable Care Act.

The picture is not entirely or uniformly positive, however. For example, several studies document that African American children have the highest prevalence of asthma of any racial/ethnic group, and substantially higher than that of whites. Compared with whites, African Americans also experience substantially higher rates of asthma-related mortality, hospitalization, and emergency department and office visits, and these disparities have widened over time (Flores, 2010).

While children generally experience far less disease and disability than adults, new health indicators pertinent to the health experiences of early childhood, school-aged children, and adolescents are especially concerning:

- The United States has achieved significant improvements in infant mortality—declining from 20.0 to 6.7 deaths per 1,000 live births

- **Federal Quality Workgroup of the CHIPRA Steering Committee—** The Secretary of Health and Human Services (HHS) created a Federal Quality Workgroup of the CHIPRA Steering Committee to ensure that the expertise of key HHS entities would be brought to bear in efforts to improve quality measurement and quality health care for all children. This workgroup includes members from AHRQ, CMS, HHS's Office of the Assistant Secretary for Planning and Evaluation, the Centers for Disease Control and Prevention, the Health Resources and Services Administration, the Indian Health Service, the Substance Abuse and Mental Health Services Administration, and the Office of the National Coordinator for Health Information Technology.
- **Census activities—**CHIPRA includes $20 million for the Census Bureau to improve state-specific estimates of children's insurance status and requires a federal evaluation of this program.
- **Health information technology—**AHRQ and CMS will collaborate to develop an electronic health record format for children.
- **Development, validation, and improvement of pediatric quality measures—**AHRQ will create a program that uses grants and contracts to develop, validate, and improve pediatric quality measures. That program is to be in place by January 1, 2011, and completed by January 1, 2013, in time to produce a final core quality measurement set.
- **Technical support—**AHRQ will provide technical consultation to CMS as it reports on quality measures and recommendations for legislative changes, provides content for best practices related to the implementation of core measures, and prepares an evaluation of outcomes of demonstration projects aimed at improving the quality of health care for children.

from 1970 to 2007; however, the United States still ranks thirty-second in infant mortality worldwide (OECD, 2010a).

- The rising tide of childhood obesity has emerged as a major public health epidemic throughout the nation (IOM, 2005). At least 18 percent of U.S. children and adolescents are obese—an increase from approximately 5 percent in the 1980s (Ogden et al., 2010). Over the past three decades, the proportion of obese children has more than doubled for preschool children aged 2–5 and adolescents aged 12–19, and it has more than tripled for children aged 6–11 (IOM, 2005).
- An estimated 9 percent of children and adolescents have asthma—nearly twice as many as in the 1980s (Akinbami, 2006).
- The number of children and youth in the United States identified as having chronic health conditions has increased considerably in the

past four decades (Perrin, 2007). This trend may be the result of environmental changes, better survival rates for certain conditions, increased access to health care through Medicaid expansions and CHIP, or a combination of these factors (Van Cleave et al., 2010).

- More than 12 million U.S. children meet the definition of children with special health care needs—"those who have a chronic physical, development, behavioral, or emotional condition and who also require health and related services of a type or amount beyond that required by children generally" (McPherson et al., 1998, p. 138). This group accounts for roughly 15–18 percent of the child population and uses 80 percent of the health care dollars spent annually for all children (Newacheck et al., 1998a).

- While the number is difficult to estimate, as many as one in five U.S. children may have a mental disorder (Costello et al., 1996). It appears, however, that only about one-fifth of those with a need for mental health services receive a mental health evaluation, leaving as many as 7.5 million children with an unmet need for these services (Kataoka et al., 2002). A recent collaboration between the National Institute of Mental Health (NIMH) and the National Center for Health Statistics (NCHS) has led to the collection of population-based data on selected mental disorders in the National Health and Nutrition Examination Survey (NHANES), an important first step toward a national database on mental health in children and adolescents (Merikangas et al., 2010a).

- Unintentional injuries are the leading cause of morbidity and mortality among children in the United States. Between 2000 and 2006, more than 12,000 children (aged 0–19) died each year in the United States from an unintentional injury. During that same period, an estimated 9.2 million children annually made an initial emergency department visit for an unintentional injury (Borse et al., 2008). Approximately 20 million children and adolescents experience injuries that require medical attention or result in restricted activity each year; medical costs for these injuries exceed $17 billion annually (Danseco et al., 2000).

- Early exposure to smoking can greatly impact disparities in health outcomes (IOM, 2011a). An analysis of the National Health Interview Survey (NHIS) indicated that 30 percent of American children are exposed to secondhand smoke on a regular basis (at least 1 day a week) (Schuster et al., 2002). The amount of environmental tobacco smoke varies according to socioeconomic status, with children in households of lower socioeconomic status being twice as likely to be exposed as those in households of higher socioeconomic status (Mannino et al., 1996). According to the Surgeon

General's report on unintended health consequences of smoking, moreover, higher levels of cotinine (a biological marker of second-hand smoke exposure) were correlated with increased risk of sudden infant death syndrome (SIDS), lower birth weight, respiratory infections, decreased lung function, and other health problems (HHS, 2006).

The above evidence underscores the need to focus attention on measuring and improving child and adolescent health and the quality of their health care.

Access to and Use of Health Services

Children's health depends in part on their access to and utilization of health services, including routine physical examinations, preventive care, health education, screening, immunizations, and care for illness or injuries. Children with a usual source of health care—a regular provider to consult for treatment and preventive care—are more likely to receive timely and appropriate care (Hoilette et al., 2009; Newacheck et al., 1996). Chronic conditions are more likely to be identified and treated at early stages of development among children with a usual source of care, thereby preventing the serious consequences associated with hospitalization and emergency room use. Over time as children age, they and their parents also need to learn skills in navigating the health care system, as well as accessing confidential care for sensitive services. Increasingly, achieving access to care means that the usual source of care must be able to provide continuity and coordination of care as captured in the concept of the medical home.

Having health insurance, whether public or private is strongly associated with access to health care and use of health services among children (GAO, 1997; Newacheck et al., 1998a; Olson et al., 2005). According to an earlier IOM report, *America's Uninsured Crisis: Consequences for Health and Health Care* (IOM, 2009a, p. 5):

- Children with health insurance coverage are more likely to have access to a usual source of care, immunizations, and well-child care to prevent future illness and monitor developmental milestones; prescription medications; appropriate care for asthma; and basic dental services.
- Serious childhood health problems are identified earlier in children with health insurance.
- Insured children with special health care needs are more likely to have access to specialists.

- Children with health insurance receive more timely diagnoses of serious health conditions, experience fewer avoidable hospitalizations, have improved asthma outcomes, and miss fewer days of school.

The majority of children and adolescents have some form of health insurance coverage. In 2009, the percentage of children nationwide under 18 who lacked health insurance was 10 percent, or 7.5 million children. This figure was down from 11 percent, or 8.1 million, in 2007 and up, by just one-tenth of a percent (from 9.9 percent, or 7.3 million), since 2008, which saw the lowest uninsured rate and number of uninsured children recorded in more than 30 years (since 1987, the first year in which comparable health insurance data were collected) (DeNavas-Walt et al., 2010). Some children receive health insurance through a parent's employer or through a privately purchased plan; others are enrolled in public programs, such as Medicaid or CHIP. With the passage of the Affordable Care Act of 2010, the number of children and adolescents with health insurance coverage increased as a result of the inclusion of private-sector coverage through age 26, thereby accentuating the need to maintain access, utilization, and quality throughout this early adulthood transition period.

Children who lack health insurance of any kind or have intermittent health care coverage are more likely to be poor or near-poor and of minority race/ethnicity (DeNavas-Walt et al., 2010). Multiple interruptions in health care coverage are correlated with fewer or no well-child visits and increased likelihood of having unmet medical or prescription drug needs (Cassedy et al., 2008).

At the same time, having health care coverage is no guarantee that children will receive medical or dental care or that the care that they receive will adequately meet their needs or be of high quality. For example, the National Survey of Children's Health (NSCH) assesses the adequacy of children's health insurance coverage by asking parents about services and costs associated with their children's health insurance—whether it covers services and access to health care providers that meet their children's needs and whether the parents consider their out-of-pocket expenses for health care to be reasonable. In 2007, the NSCH found that nearly a quarter—23.5 percent—of currently insured children lacked adequate insurance (HHS et al., 2009).

These facts take on special significance given the strong evidence alluded to above that health status in childhood lays the foundation for health status throughout the life course. For example, if a baby born is too small or too early, then it is more likely to experience cognitive, behavioral, and physical challenges as a child, as well as develop chronic health conditions, including high blood pressure, heart disease, and diabetes as an adult (IOM, 2006c).

Despite the previous trend in increasing birth weight, the percentage of infants born preterm (birth at less than 37 completed weeks of gestation) and the percentage born with low birth weight (less than 2,500 grams, or 5 pounds, 8 ounces) declined slightly in 2007. The percentage of infants born preterm in 2007 was 12.7 percent (down from 12.8 percent in 2006), while the percentage of infants born with low birth weight in 2007 was 8.2 percent (down from 8.3 percent in 2006, the sixth consecutive year of increase and the highest rate recorded in 40 years) (FIFCFS, 2009; HHS et al., 2009). However, there has been no change in the proportion of infants born at greatest risk for adverse outcomes—those born at less than 32 weeks of gestation or of very low birth weight (less than 1,500 grams). Despite the recent declines, moreover, disparities in preterm birth and low birth weight have persisted by race/ethnicity, as well as by the age of the mother and health insurance status.

Another example of a factor influencing health status throughout the life course is childhood obesity. Over the past three decades, obesity has more than doubled among children aged 2–5 and more than tripled among those aged 6–11 and adolescents aged 12–19. The prevalence of obesity among children aged 2–5 increased from 5 percent in 1980 to 10.4 percent in 2008. Among children aged 6–12, obesity increased from 6.5 percent in 1980 to 19.6 percent in 2008. During that same period, obesity increased from 5.0 to 18.1 percent among adolescents aged 12–19 (NCHS, 2004; Ogden et al., 2010). Obese children are more likely to be obese as adults, placing them at risk for serious chronic diseases, including diabetes, heart disease, and stroke (Serdula et al., 1993). An overweight 10-year-old child has a 40–80 percent probability of being overweight at age 35 (Parsons et al., 1999). Moreover, overweight in adolescence is associated with a broad range of adverse health effects in adulthood that are independent of adult weight. Among men, for example, being overweight during adolescence is associated with approximately double the relative risk of mortality both from all causes and from heart disease (Guo and Chumlea, 1999).

Poor health in childhood may set the stage for a broad array of long-term outcomes that include not only future health, but also lower educational attainment, socioeconomic status, and productivity (McCormick et al., 2011). For example, beyond increasing the risk of significant morbidity in the newborn period, premature birth may also increase the probability of health problems such as asthma, or cognitive and behavioral problems that lead to lower school achievement. In recent Scandinavian studies, premature birth was associated with increased rates of hospitalization, work limitations due to disability, and lower rates of family formation (Moster

BOX 2-4
The Role of Health Care, Public Health Interventions, and Clinical Preventive Services in Child Health and Well-Being

The Role of Health Care

Health care comprises services provided by health professionals, including screening and prevention, treatment and disease management, and the maintenance of physical and emotional well-being. Children's health has improved markedly over the last century in part as a result of advances in health care, as well as in public health (see below).

A critical component of children's health care is the preventive services encompassed by regular well-child care, particularly as a lack of adequate well-child care visits often correlates with incomplete immunizations (Freed et al., 1999; Kogan et al., 1998). *Child Health USA*, the Health Resources and Services Administration's (HRSA's) annual report on the health status and service needs of America's children, tracks health care utilization. Highlights from the 2007 report underscore the differential rates of well-child care among children of different ages, household income, and racial and ethnic backgrounds:

- Nearly 26 percent of children under age 18 were reported by their parents not to have had a preventive, or well-child, medical visit in the past year, although this number ranges from 17.3 percent of those aged 4 or younger to 36 percent of those aged 15–17.
- During the past year, 20.2 percent of non-Hispanic black children and 25.9 percent of non-Hispanic white children failed to have a well-child visit. Hispanic children were least likely to have had a well-child visit (31.5 percent).
- In the past year, 25.7 percent of children with family incomes above the poverty threshold ($21,203 for a family of four in 2007) did not have a well-child visit, compared with 29.3 percent of children with family incomes below the poverty threshold (HHS et al., 2009).

The Role of Public Health Interventions

Numerous improvements in the health of the U.S. population have been accomplished through public health measures. The Institute of Medicine report *The Future of Public Health* established three core functions of public health: as-

et al., 2008; Selling et al., 2008; Swamy et al., 2008). Children with birth weights lower than expected for their gestational age may also be at risk for adult-onset cardiovascular disease and diabetes (Doyle and Anderson, 2010; Evensen et al., 2009; Hack, 2009). Moreover, the vulnerabilities incurred by premature birth reduce the ability to deal with adversity, particularly socioeconomic disadvantage. Absent appropriate intervention, then, the adverse outcomes of premature birth reflect an ongoing interplay sessment (e.g., conducting surveillance of disease/injuries, monitoring trends, and identifying needs); policy development (e.g., promoting evidence-based decision making and developing comprehensive public health policies); and assurance (e.g., requiring and providing needed services) (IOM, 1988).

Examples of public health achievements that have reduced morbidity and mortality and significantly improved quality of life among children include the control of communicable diseases; improvements in hygiene, sanitation, and food safety; and maternal and child health services. Clean water, for example, is credited with a significant reduction in infant and child mortality in major cities in the 19th and early 20th centuries—a three-quarters reduction in infant mortality and a nearly two-thirds reduction in child mortality (Cutler and Miller, 2004). Fluoridation of drinking water is another public health intervention that improves child health by effectively preventing tooth decay, regardless of socioeconomic status or access to care.

The Role of Clinical Preventive Services

Clinical preventive services also play a significant role in child health and well-being. For example, universal childhood vaccination programs helped control—and in the case of smallpox, eradicate—previously life-threatening illnesses. Dramatic declines in morbidity occurred for the nine vaccine-preventable diseases (smallpox, pertussis, tetanus, poliomyelitis [paralytic], measles, mumps, rubella, congenital rubella, and *Haemophilus influenzae* type b) (CDC, 1999).

Developmental screenings and mental/behavioral health screenings (e.g., screening for major depressive disorder among adolescents), which may increase the likelihood of early detection and timely intervention (if appropriate treatment is available), provide another critical pathway to improved child health and well-being (Sandler et al., 2001; U.S. Preventive Services Task Force, 2009). Among U.S. children, for example, an estimated 17 percent have a developmental or behavioral disability, such as intellectual disability or attention-deficit/hyperactivity disorder (ADHD). However, fewer than 50 percent of children with such a disability are identified as having the problem before starting school, by which time significant delays may already have occurred and opportunities for treatment missed (CDC, 1999). As a group, adolescents receive limited clinical preventive screening services, although many of their behaviors place them at particular risk, including tobacco and alcohol use and sexual activity (IOM, 2009c). However, receipt of service is not an end unto itself; access to a system that provides poor-quality care will not improve health outcomes (Mangione-Smith et al., 2007).

of a combination of biological and social factors with a cumulative impact on adult functioning.

Chapter 4 addresses in detail the relationship between childhood events and outcomes observed in adulthood, as well as the intergenerational transmission of health and well-being. Box 2-4 summarizes the role of health care, public health interventions, and clinical preventive services in child health and well-being.

NEED FOR A COMPREHENSIVE APPROACH TO CHILD AND ADOLESCENT HEALTH

Taking a life-course perspective and considering the social context in which health develops helps to provide a comprehensive picture of child and adolescent health. In considering how measures of child and adolescent health and health care quality might be improved, the committee concluded that taking such a comprehensive approach is an essential step to that end.

The Life-Course Approach to Health

As noted above, many adult health conditions originate in childhood, and several conditions that occur in childhood impact adult health. A recent IOM report, *Leading Health Indicators for Healthy People 2020 ("Leading Health Indicators")* (2011b), offered the following concise description of the life-course approach:

> The life-course approach is based on two concepts: first, the impact of specific risk factors and determinants of health varies during the life course; and second, health and disease result from the accumulation of the effects of risk factors and determinants over the life course. The combination of these two components produces a life-course health "trajectory" that represents the cumulative effect of risk factors and determinants at each point in the life course. Typically, the health trajectory "rises" during childhood, adolescence, and early adulthood, plateaus during middle age, and then declines with advancing age. This trajectory can be improved through the reduction of risk factors and the promotion of health through individual and population level (i.e., societal) actions, applied at specific points or during specific stages of the life course, especially during the early years of life (Ben-Shlomo and Kuh, 2002; Halfon and Hochstein, 2002; Halfon et al., 2002; IOM, 1999; Wise, 2009). There is also evidence to suggest that the impact of factors during early life and at other points in the life course is not immutable but can be influenced by other factors later in the life course (Ben-Shlomo and Kuh, 2002; Wise, 2009).

As described above, the life-course approach considers how an individual's current and future health (or "health trajectory") may be affected by the dynamic interaction among social, biological, and environmental influences over time. It underscores the importance of multiple risk and protective influences, and considers how the presence or absence of these influences during critical and sensitive stages of development (e.g., the prenatal period, early childhood, and adolescence) may affect the health of individuals or selected populations.

The life-course approach encompasses consideration of interactions among multiple determinants of health over time, including factors operating at the individual, family, community, and societal levels. It provides a basis for interpreting how distal influences, such as the context of individuals, affect current or future health outcomes and contribute to health disparities over time. It also provides a bridge between individual and population health measures, highlighting opportunities for preventive or treatment interventions to have significant effects on the well-being of selected groups. The committee's use of the life-course perspective provides an appropriate lens through which to view measures of child and adolescent health and health care quality.

While life-course research, particularly in the United States, is in its infancy, the rationale for the life-course approach is well supported in the literature (Ben-Shlomo and Kuh, 2002; Braveman and Barclay, 2009; Guyer et al., 2009; Halfon and Hochstein, 2002; Kuh and Ben-Shlomo, 1997; Shonkoff et al., 2009), and this approach is emerging as an important framework for national health policy goals. For example, the Healthy People 2020 agenda includes an overarching goal to "promote quality of life, healthy development and healthy behaviors across all life stages," which inherently demands using the life-course approach. Likewise, the MCHB within the HHS has developed a strategic plan that incorporates the life-course perspective as the foundation for MCHB, its grantees, and its partners over the next 5 years.

The life-course approach shaped the seven priority areas recommended by the committee in Chapter 4 as the focus for efforts to measure the health and health care quality of children and adolescents. These cross-cutting priority areas represent selected life stages within childhood and adolescence, as well as the transition to adulthood. Chapters 4 and 5, respectively, describe the limited number of existing measures and data collection efforts related to measuring health and monitoring health care services across the life course.

A recent report, *The Foundations of Lifelong Health Are Built in Early Childhood*, describes how "personal experiences, environmental conditions and developmental biology work together in early childhood to influence the roots of lifelong physical and mental well-being" (CDCHU, 2010, p. 5). The report notes that "a considerable body of research suggests that adult disease and risk factors for poor health can be biologically embedded in the brain and other organ systems during these sensitive periods, with resulting health impairments appearing years, or even decades, later" (p. 6).

Illustrative Examples

This section presents two illustrative examples of the life-course approach: childhood obesity and adolescent health care. These examples demonstrate how assessing maternal, child, and adolescent health across the life course provides valuable insights into the multiple points of intervention (e.g., environmental, behavioral, socioeconomic), multiple stages of the life course, and various levels of intervention (e.g., individual, family, community, state, federal) that are salient to improving child and adolescent health trajectories.

The Life-Course Perspective and Childhood Obesity

Childhood obesity, with its associated increased risk for adult obesity and type 2 diabetes, illustrates the value of using the life-course approach. Consider, for example, the biological influences on obesity. The life-course approach to measurement in this area would include assessing relevant exposures (e.g., maternal malnutrition before or during pregnancy, or childhood experiences of food insecurity) across critical or sensitive periods of development from preconception through adolescence. The specificity and sensitivity of selected biological processes that occur during these periods may result in greater risk for obesity from adverse exposures than would be the case at other times. Prior to conception, for example, maternal weight and diet can influence a child's risk of obesity later in life (Gillman, 2005; IOM and NRC, 2009b; Kitsantas et al., 2010; Ludwig and Currie, 2010). Similarly, gestational weight gain during the prenatal period is associated with childhood obesity and overweight (IOM and NRC, 2009b).

Environmental and behavioral influences offer another example. The life-course approach to measurement would include assessing relevant exposures (e.g., stress, poverty, environmental toxins, or access to appropriate nutrition) across the same critical or sensitive periods of development. Again, the specific biological processes that occur during these periods influence the ways in which adverse environmental and behavioral exposures may produce a significant risk for obesity. For example, certain feeding practices in early childhood are associated with risk for overweight and obesity later in life (Dietz, 1994; Gaillard et al., 2008; Owen et al., 2005a, 2005b). Likewise, increased and cumulative levels of individual, maternal, and family stress in early and middle childhood are associated with increased risk of adolescent overweight and obesity (Garasky et al., 2009; Gundersen et al., 2008; Lohman et al., 2009). Moreover, these effects are amplified among children in low-income households who experience food insecurity (Lohman et al., 2009).

The Life-Course Perspective and Adolescent Health Care

Adolescence is a critical period of transition that includes numerous biological changes (e.g., those associated with puberty and brain development) and the development of important cognitive functions (e.g., formal operational thought and maturation of higher executive function) that lay the foundation for future health (Arnett, 2006; IOM and NRC, 2009a). As noted in an earlier IOM and NRC report, "the health care system plays an important role in promoting healthful behavior, managing health conditions, and preventing disease in adolescence" (IOM and NRC, 2009a). Behaviors established during adolescence can have a profound influence (either protective or detrimental) not only on current health status but also on the risk of developing chronic diseases in adulthood (Mulye et al., 2009); the quality of adolescent health care therefore may have significant life-course implications.

The health care system can identify and address certain health conditions and risk factors that have particular importance during adolescence and implications for adult health, including sexually transmitted infections, chronic mental health conditions, substance abuse/use, disordered eating, unprotected sexual intercourse, and overweight/obesity, among others. Consider, for example, adolescent pregnancy, which has serious adverse consequences for the mother, including curtailing her educational attainment, which constrains her life chances and predicts worse health in adulthood (AHRQ, 2003). Early childbearing also has been linked to significant negative social, educational, economic, and other outcomes for the child, with ripple effects that impact health care access, educational opportunities, and risk behaviors (Baydar, 1995; IOM, 1995). Although social factors are crucial determinants of adolescent pregnancy (IOM, 1995), health promotion services, access to counseling, or access to affordable and confidential family planning services can help prevent unintended pregnancies (Kirby, 2007). The quality of hospital and postpartum care (e.g., breastfeeding education and support) strongly influences breastfeeding and the subsequent interpregnancy interval (Hack, 2009; Hack et al., 2002; Joyce et al., 2000). All of these services have a multigenerational impact on maternal and child health trajectories (Sable and Herman, 1997).

Policy Implications of the Life-Course Approach

The life-course approach has emerged in the national agenda for improving the health of all Americans, as reflected by the Healthy People 2020 goals and objectives. Similarly, MCHB is engaging states and local health agencies in exploring the applications and implications of the life-course approach for overall efforts to improve the health and well-being of current and future generations of women, children, adolescents, and families. A recent concept paper prepared for MCHB provides an "organizing framework" for using the life-course approach to guide the work of the Bureau and its grantees (Fine and Kotelchuck, 2010). The life-course approach also reflects growing international consensus on the importance of the behavioral and social determinants of health and their critical influence at different stages of development, including their influence on health disparities (Frieden, 2010; Marmot et al., 2008; Miller et al., 2009; WHO, 2008).

Behavioral choices influence health throughout the life course. Engagement in high-risk or illegal activities, early sexual activity, use of substances (e.g., tobacco, alcohol, illicit drugs), and participation in violent crime contribute to negative health consequences (FIFCFS, 2010a). Early sexual activity can expose children and adolescents to sexually transmitted infections, pregnancy risk, and diminished physical and emotional health (Meier, 2007). According to the National Statistics for Family Growth (NSFG), teen pregnancies were experienced by 70.6 per 1,000 women in 2005; although this was a historic low, pregnancy in this age group is associated with morbidity, mortality, and health care costs (Ventura et al., 2009). Furthermore, one in five births to adolescent mothers are repeat pregnancies (Abma et al., 2004), a statistic that suggests the urgent need for access to and utilization of reproductive services among at-risk individuals.

The *social determinants* of health, or "the conditions in which people are born, grow, live, work and age, including the health system," also are critical to understanding child and adolescent health and development (WHO, 2010). A significant and growing body of evidence demonstrates the links and interactions among social structures, environments, economic systems, and health (Braveman et al., 2011; Kawachi and Berkman, 2003; Marmot and Wilkinson, 1999; WHO, 2008). For example, researchers have found that family income and educational attainment are associated with adults' health status, as well as the health of their children. Specifically, higher educational attainment and higher income are associated with longer life expectancy in adults and lower rates of infant and child mortality (Blumenshine et al., 2010; Braveman et al., 2010), and children of parents with higher educational attainment experience better health (Braveman et al., 2010).

Like income and education, neighborhood conditions are linked to health outcomes. For example, poor neighborhood conditions (e.g., substandard housing and excess community violence) are associated with inferior health status (Diez Roux and Mair, 2010; Miller et al., 2011). Conversely, adequate neighborhood resources (e.g., access to healthy foods and safe, walkable neighborhoods) are associated with positive health behaviors, including healthier diets and increased physical activity (Diez Roux and Mair, 2010; Laraia et al., 2004; Larson et al., 2009; Morland et al., 2002).

Finally, the social environment (the social context and/or social interaction) is associated with health. For example, a poor social environment (e.g., neighborhoods and communities with low levels of social interaction) may have a negative impact on residents' health; this effect has been observed with asthma (Cagney et al., 2007; Williams et al., 2009) and health risk behaviors, including smoking (Chuang et al., 2005; Pickett and Pearl, 2001) and sexual and reproductive health behaviors (Averett et al., 2002; Lindberg and Orr, 2011). By contrast, a positive social environment (e.g., neighborhoods and communities with high levels of cohesiveness and social order) is associated with better health outcomes (Anderson et al., 2003; Giles-Corti and Donovan, 2002; Story et al., 2008).

Reflecting the above-noted international consensus on the importance of social determinants of health, those determinants are emerging as a central focus in the national agenda for improving the health of all Americans. For example, "social determinants of health" is a new topic area in Healthy People 2020 for which specific objectives are currently under development. Recently, the Centers for Disease Control and Prevention's (CDC's) National Center for HIV/AIDS, Viral Hepatitis, STD (sexually transmitted disease), and TB Prevention (NCHHSTP) published a paper outlining its planned activities to reduce health disparities related to these diseases by addressing the social determinants of health (HHS, 2010a). Finally, in fiscal year 2010, HHS's Office of Minority Health announced more than $16 million in grants aimed at eliminating health disparities, with a special emphasis on the social determinants of health.

Figure 2-2 illustrates the behavioral and social determinants of health across the life course, tying together the important concepts described above.

Measuring Health for Children and Adolescents

Changing demographic trends among America's children and youth; new health problems in the general population; persistent health disparities; and dynamic interactions among health, health services, health influences, and child functioning all contribute to the need for timely and accurate data systems that can document the health of children and adolescents. Questions have been raised about the capacity of existing data collection efforts to uncover key problem areas and disparities, as well as trends over time and fundamental changes that may contribute to their severity or amelioration. Significant questions also arise regarding the scope, sources, and specificity of data that are available at the national, state, and regional levels to monitor the status of children and youth, especially those at high risk of poor health outcomes.

The measurement of health for children and adolescents requires attention to multiple data sets that collect health information about specific populations, often sorted by age ranges, gender, race, ethnicity, or geography. The information is frequently derived from responses to survey questions from parents or reviews of health records and claims-based data,

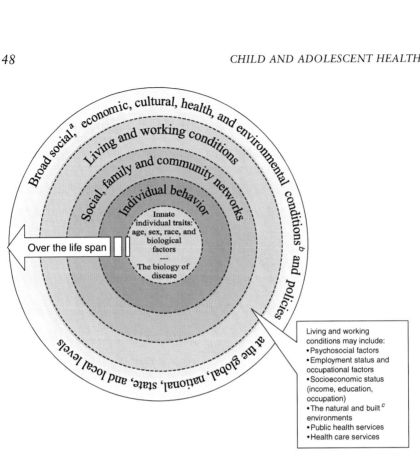

NOTES: Adapted from Dahlgren and Whitehead, 1991. The dotted lines between levels of the model denote interaction effects between and among the various levels of health determinants (Worthman, 1999).

[a] Social conditions include, but are not limited to: economic inequality, urbanization, mobility, cultural values, attitudes and policies related to discrimination and intolerance on the basis of race, gender, and other differences.

[b] Other conditions at the national level might include major sociopolitical shifts, such as recession, war, and governmental collapse.

[c] The built environment includes transportation, water and sanitation, housing, and other dimensions of urban planning.

FIGURE 2-2 The determinants of health across the life course.
SOURCE: IOM, 2003a, 2011a.

as discussed in Chapter 3. Many existing health data sets offer useful snapshots of specific conditions and selected populations, such as the number and geographic or age distribution of children with diabetes or asthma, or the ages and gender of adolescents who engage in unhealthy behaviors such as underage drinking, risky driving, or substance abuse.

However, the nation lacks the capacity to identify and monitor significant trends in many areas that involve the health status or health outcomes of children and adolescents. This is especially so for underserved populations—such as poor children; racial/ethnic minority children; children in rural settings; children in immigrant families; and children subject to multiple risk factors, such as abuse or neglect, who experience special barriers to care. Many current health and health care data sets are responsive to past concerns instead of providing guidance for questions on current or future needs, such as

- What are the general health and educational outcomes of low-birth-weight or premature infants as they become older?
- How many children or adolescents experience symptoms of mental, emotional, or behavioral disorders?
- How many children with chronic health conditions are able to function effectively in school?
- Do exposures to risk factors in early, middle, and/or late childhood contribute to the onset of adolescent health disorders?

Measuring Health Care Quality for Children and Adolescents

Measuring health care quality involves information about the types of health care services offered to children and adolescents, the settings in which these services are based, and the outcomes associated with the utilization or absence of selected care processes. A classic paradigm for assessing quality is derived from the Donabedian model, which identifies three basic components of the health care system: structure, process, and outcomes (Donabedian, 1988). Measures of the quality of each of these three components are thought to yield measures of the quality of the health care system. While this model is particularly useful in assessing the performance of health care services in meeting the needs of children and adolescents with special health care needs, as well as assessing the value and effectiveness of preventive services offered to general populations of children and adolescents in clinical settings, it may have limited value in determining the level of unmet health or health care needs of selected populations.

Health care quality measures can address such questions as

- Are immunization programs effective in protecting children and adolescents from infectious disease?
- Under what conditions do early preventive intervention services for populations of at-risk children produce better health outcomes than the delivery of treatment services after a chronic condition has been diagnosed?

- Do asthma education programs reduce the number of children with asthma who require emergency care or hospitalization?
- Does the early identification of mental health conditions through routine primary care screening lead to better long-term outcomes?
- Can school dropout rates or juvenile crime rates be reduced through early preventive intervention services for young children or adolescents?
- What interventions can reduce or eliminate significant disparities in health and health care quality?

The measurement of health care quality requires rigorous attention to the settings in which services are provided (structure) and the specific types or sequence of selected services (process) in order to understand the ways in which they influence health outcomes. Health care quality data frequently are collected from administrative or claims records or abstracts from medical records. Such data can also be derived from population health surveys of providers, patients, or their families. While multiple measures of health care quality are currently available, measures that rely heavily on abstraction from medical records are costly and are not feasible for use in large-scale data sets.

Many policy makers and researchers may be particularly interested in selected health outcomes or health trends within the general population of children and adolescents, but it is equally important to have rigorous measures of structures and processes of care in order to acquire greater understanding of the relationship between the utilization and quality of health care and health outcomes. This rigor requires the creation and use of valid, reliable, and well-specified measures that are feasible to implement, generally focusing on specific activities that occur within a selected health care setting or on interactions among health care providers in addressing a specific health condition through treatment or prevention interventions.

Using Population Health Measures for Action and Accountability

A recent IOM report, *For the Public's Health: The Role of Measurement in Action and Accountability,* highlights the importance of developing an information enterprise to drive knowledge and to improve the health of the U.S. population. Citing research demonstrating that "clinical care alone is neither responsible for poor health outcomes nor the sole solution to the problem" (IOM, 2011a, p. 35; Lalonde, 1981), the study identifies information needs of the health system and the capacities and limitations of the nation's population health statistics and information system to address these needs. The basic components of the population health information system include data sources such as vital records systems; surveillance systems (e.g., for acute conditions such as HIV/AIDS); clinical care data sources, including administrative claims databases; electronic health records data; and federal surveys summarizing population health outcomes (NCVHS, 2010). Key reports and other products associated with these systems include *Healthy People 2010* and *Healthy People 2020* (HHS, 2010b; Koh, 2010); the annual NCHS report *Health, United States, 2009* (NCHS, 2009a); and Health Data Interactive, a web-based site that provides access to multiple population health data sets (NCHS, 2011a).

According to the IOM committee that produced *For the Public's Health*:

> One of the persistent challenges to measures of health outcomes, and one of the obstacles to any attempt to nurture a level of standardization in the field, is that there are many different phenomena that may be measured, but the field is much more advanced in the area of distal health outcomes (e.g., mortality, cancer incidence) and intermediate outcomes (or individual-level and behavioral determinants of health) such as smoking and overweight, than in developing a knowledge base and valid useful indicators of more upstream determinants of health (social cohesion, social support, the quality of housing, green spaces, stress). (IOM, 2011a, p. 59)

The population health emphasis on intermediate and distal determinants of health, such as those that are influenced by social and economic factors or individual behaviors, is now beginning to shape the types of data that are collected within health care quality data sets as well. But significant challenges exist in striving to integrate health or health care quality data sets that have been designed for different purposes.

Using Metrics to Drive Improvements in Health Outcomes

The U.S. health care system comprises a diverse set of programs, services, policies, and practices that draw on resources and personnel in both the public and private sectors. Within this complex system, there is a growing emphasis on measuring health processes and outcomes and their determinants at both the individual and community levels, drawing largely on population health data sets that can support community-based analyses at the local, state, national, and even international levels. There is also a substantial body of work associated with the development of metrics focused on processes of care that can provide the basis for comparing the health outcomes and quality of services associated with individual providers and care settings, such as hospitals or regional networks of providers. In addition, interest is growing in the development of metrics that can provide a basis for analyzing the health outcomes and quality of care associated with different health plans or levels of public or private investment in health care services. These analyses can help identify whether children and adolescents who receive care through Medicaid or CHIP plans, for example, achieve health outcomes comparable to those whose clinical services are reimbursed through private health plans.

Each of these initiatives is developing metrics and indicators for different purposes. They draw on different data sources and direct their analytic efforts toward different audiences. Those who are concerned with strengthening the capacity of public health agencies to improve population health outcomes, for example, will often focus on ways in which community-based resources and preventive strategies can contribute to lower rates of obesity or infant mortality (see, for example, IOM, 2011a). Those who want to improve the use of evidence-based care in clinical services and care settings will emphasize the need to identify specific processes and organizational practices that can improve the effectiveness, safety, and efficiency of health care services. And those who want to achieve better health outcomes for patients who depend on public health plans will emphasize the need to monitor the health status and quality of care for groups of patients with similar health conditions in ways that can support analyses and help identify opportunities for interventions at the regional and national levels.

Although each of these efforts draws on different data sources for different objectives, they all share a common interest in using data and indicators to drive improvements in the performance of the health care system. In the public health sector, for example, there is evidence of growing interest in developing common metrics and strategies that "align potentially divergent interests towards a shared goal at local (city and county), state, and national levels" (IOM, 2011a, p. 19). Similarly, the emphasis on improving measurement of the quality of health care in clinical services has stimulated the creation and use of metrics and indicators that can be used to assess the safety, timeliness, effectiveness, and efficiency of care across diverse public and private health care settings.

Despite these common interests, the nation has yet to develop a strategy or framework that can combine the metrics associated with population health efforts with those that are focused more directly on the quality of clinical care. The population health measures advanced in Healthy People 2010 and 2020, for example, are not used by the clinical care delivery system or health insurance plans as outcome sets. One reason for this may be concern about accountability for health outcomes, especially for underserved and vulnerable populations, whose health conditions may be affected by behavioral or social determinants of health as well as the quality of care they receive. The notion of shared or partial accountability of the clinical care setting for achieving community health outcomes is not yet well established, particularly in drawing on a life-course perspective.

In this report, the committee examines specific ways to improve the measurement of health and health care quality through the lens of the clinical services supported by Medicaid and CHIP. At appropriate times, opportunities to align this work with other measurement improvement efforts, such as those now emerging in population health, are identified.

Need for a High-Quality Data System

Addressing questions such as those listed earlier requires a coordinated and meaningful quality measurement system, one that can capture and monitor key indicators and support analyses of selected population groups on the basis of age, race/ethnicity, gender, education, household income, geographic location, and other characteristics. Given the high—and growing—rates of participation of children in public health insurance programs, it will become increasingly important to know whether and how these plans contribute to the health and well-being of the nation's children and youth. Furthermore, given the extent of variations in public and private health care plans in terms of benefit designs, eligibility criteria, health care practices, and different types of health care providers seeing and treating children, it is necessary to understand the consequences of differences in health services that result from these variations.

People concerned with the health and well-being of today's children and youth, as well as their parents, educators, community leaders, future employers, and many others, want to know more about the extent to which existing investments result in improved health and health care outcomes. They also want to know whether the presence or absence of services that are covered by public plans such as Medicaid and CHIP make significant differences in child and adult health outcomes. They are particularly interested in knowing more about the relationship of selected health care structures and processes to child and adolescent health outcomes, such as the relative value of treating children with selected conditions in primary care versus specialty settings, or the outcomes associated with early preventive interventions for large populations of at-risk children compared with treatment services for identified conditions. Within a life-course framework, it is also reasonable to ask whether early prevention services financed by Medicaid or CHIP can reduce long-term Medicare costs by preventing avoidable health conditions in the nation's aging population.

Certain criteria need to be defined in developing such a high-quality child health data system. For example:

- What are the basic characteristics of *healthy development?* Healthy children—especially in early childhood—experience rapid cognitive, emotional, social, and physical development. A data collection system needs to reflect the dynamic state of child health across different developmental periods, including transitions between childhood and adolescence and adolescence and young adulthood, in ways that can be used to examine health status over time. Furthermore, the system needs to have the capacity to identify and monitor important racial/ethnic and gender differences in health status and functioning.

- What are the *essential health services* that contribute to healthy development? Certain services that are associated with the prevention of infectious disease (such as immunizations) are much easier to monitor and classify than services that contribute to higher levels of functioning or enhance positive development. As traditional threats to child health, such as polio and measles, were successfully addressed, attention began to focus on new health problems that require greater emphasis on interventions in such areas as nutrition, mental health, social behavior, functioning, and self-regulation. As these areas present enormous challenges to standardized measurement and data collection, a broad, longitudinal approach may assist in addressing this question.

- How should *preventive services* be defined and measured? The dynamic nature of interactions between children and their families, as well as their physical and social environments, presents major challenges to the identification and measurement of risk and protective factors. Formulating quality indicators for preventive services may be especially important for certain periods of development, such as pregnancy, early childhood, and adolescence, when the timing or sequence of such services may interact with certain biological or psychological changes that influence the desired outcomes. It is also important to consider the challenges that may exist in reaching children at critical stages of development. As many early childhood interventions are not identified or initiated until a child enters elementary school, screening and other preventive services may help capture opportunities when such interventions are likely to be most effective (NRC, 2000).

Challenges to Creating a High-Quality Data System for Child and Adolescent Health and Health Care Quality

Evidence indicates that the health care system in the United States is underperforming for children and that, as discussed above, considerable variation exists in access to care, care quality, and health outcomes (Kavanagh et al., 2009; Mangione-Smith et al., 2007; Schuster et al., 2005). A previous study by the President's Advisory Commission on Consumer Protection and Quality in the Healthcare Industry noted inadequacies in the measurement and monitoring of quality measures for children's health care (PAC, 1998).

Further study indicated that a failure to properly document both the quantitative and qualitative characteristics of health and health care services for children and adolescents would mean that health care improvement efforts will not lead to anticipated results or may fail to occur at all (Dougherty and Simpson, 2004). Yet several persistent challenges must be met in creating a high-quality data system for child health and health care quality. Below are brief descriptions of the primary challenges, which are addressed in greater depth in the chapters that follow.

Gaps in the Development of Indicators and Measures

While recent efforts have shown progress, the development of key health and health care quality indicators for children and adolescents still falls far short of where it should be. The majority of current indicators are related to routine outpatient care, yet nearly 40 percent of U.S. health care spending for children in 2004 was for inpatient care. This dichotomy points to the importance of developing and using quality indicators for high-cost, low-incidence areas of care, such as neonatal intensive care and treatment of childhood cancers (Hartman et al., 2008), although focusing only on severe and rare conditions will not allow assessment of health care quality for a majority of children. In addition, quality measures ought to focus on high-prevalence issues, such as high-quality preventive services. Moreover, many measures currently in use focus on the *process* of providing health care, with varying degrees of evidence regarding the linkage to the true *health outcomes* or functional status of America's children.

To date, few health indicators exist for important subpopulations of children and youth. One important such subpopulation is children with special health care needs. As a group, children with special health care needs are difficult to define precisely, although a definition was developed by MCHB and adopted by the American Academy of Pediatrics (McPherson et al., 1998). National surveys have estimated that children under 18 with chronic physical, developmental, behavioral, or emotional conditions, the basis for the MCHB definition, make up 13.9 to 16.0 percent of the pediatric population and account for more than one-third of total health care costs (Dietrich et al., 2008; Newacheck and Kim, 2005). The use of the MCHB definition, however, cannot be universal, as defining those children who are at risk for developing a chronic condition is highly dependent upon which criteria are used in identifying at-risk children.

Similarly, there are few well-defined and measurable indicators for child and adolescent mental health. A national inventory of mental health quality measures includes no measures for children and adolescents supported by "good research evidence" and few (eight) supported by "fair research evidence," as defined by the Agency for Healthcare Research and Quality

(AHRQ) (CQAIMH, 2010). Because of the limitations posed by the availability of evidence, HHS's initial core set of children's health care quality measures includes only two measures directly related to mental/behavioral health (i.e., follow-up after hospitalization for mental illness and follow-up care for children prescribed attention-deficit/hyperactivity disorder [ADHD] medication) (CMS, 2010).

Quality indicators focused on educating parents and caregivers of very young children about safety and child development are also in short supply (Kavanagh et al., 2009). Providing this type of education may prevent inappropriate care and accidental injury, as well as allow early identification of potential learning or behavioral problems (Gardner, 2007).

Lack of Parental and Adolescent Perspectives in Identifying Priority Measures

The preferences of parents and especially adolescents are not reflected in the existing array of measures of health and health care quality for children and adolescents. Adolescents' reports of their own health status, as well as their experiences with health care providers and settings, have been shown to be valid and reliable in reflecting the care they have received (IOM and NRC, 2009a). Parents also have been shown to be reliable informants in describing the extent to which their child's needs were met—especially when seeking treatment for severe or chronic health problems (IOM and NRC, 2009a).

Lack of Integration/Coordination of Data Gathering Efforts

Although numerous agencies, states, insurers, organizations, and delivery systems are engaged in measuring the quality of health and health care services, they lack a common approach to measurement. Analyses of data also are limited by a lack of comparable data across states or benchmarks from national sources that might be used for performance improvement. Additionally, most systems and agencies lack the ability to access important data from multiple sources. And while integrating multiple administrative data sources is elemental to understanding the complex needs of children and families with multiple issues and those involved with more than one system of care simultaneously, few agencies or jurisdictions are able to accomplish such integration.

Limited Capacity to Monitor Significant Trends Over Time

Most data collection efforts lack the capacity to integrate sets of data or are limited by factors such as the ability to conduct medical record abstraction on a large scale. Hence, most current measures gauge only whether care is provided/offered and yield little information about the receipt of care, adherence to regimens prescribed or recommended, or the long-term impact of care.

Gaps in Monitoring of Disparities

Several different types of disparities deserve consideration in monitoring health and health care equity issues among children and adolescents. These include differences in socioeconomic factors, such as household income, accumulated wealth, education, and occupation; racial and ethnic disparities; and disparities in English proficiency. Each area requires consistent and precise definitions to make it possible to track trends within and between selected populations, as well as to follow trends across different time periods. Interactions may occur among each of these areas, and all may be affected as well by the powerful role—as mediators and/or moderators—of social conditions within a specific community (Braveman, 2006). Considerable evidence indicates that these conditions and social factors operate through diverse, often complex pathways, including biological mechanisms, pathways involving access to health-promoting or health-damaging resources, and pathways involving psychosocial phenomena.

Scores of studies published in the medical literature over the past several decades document that numerous racial/ethnic disparities in children's health and health care persist, even after adjusting for all relevant covariates, including socioeconomic status. The 2003 IOM report *Unequal Treatment: Confronting Racial and Ethnic Disparities in Health Care* (IOM, 2003a), for example, states that "racial and ethnic minorities tend to receive a lower quality of healthcare than non-minorities, even when access-related factors, such as patients' insurance status and income, are controlled" (p. 1). Likewise, the American Academy of Pediatrics Committee on Pediatric Research published a technical report in 2010 stating that "racial/ethnic disparities in children's health and health care are extensive, pervasive, and persistent, and occur across the spectrum of health and health care" (Flores, 2010, p. e1015). The report identifies numerous studies documenting stark racial/ethnic disparities for these populations, after adjusting for socioeconomic status and other relevant covariates.

A substantial body of research also documents a range of deleterious effects that language barriers can have on the health and health care quality of children and adolescents, including inferior medical and oral health status; greater odds of having no medical or dental insurance; a lower likelihood of having a usual source of medical care; and impaired patient understanding of diagnoses, medications, and follow-up (Baker et al., 1996; Burbano O'Leary et al., 2003; Crane, 1997; Flores and Tomany-Korman,

2008; Hu and Covell, 1986; Kirkman-Liff and Mondragon, 1991). For example, language barriers are associated as well with medical errors, injuries, and other patient safety events, including increased risk of serious medical events and physical harm (Cohen et al., 2005; Divi et al., 2007). Available evidence indicates that optimal communication, the highest patient satisfaction, the best outcomes, and the fewest errors of potential clinical consequence occur when patients and families with limited English proficiency have access to trained professional interpreters or bilingual health care providers (Flores, 2005).

An emerging literature points to the value of considering additional variables when assessing disparities in health care quality, access, and outcomes among children and adolescents. These include socioeconomic status, school density and status, parental education, literacy, family structure, and environmental quality at the neighborhood level with respect to safety and other social determinants that impact the health of children and adolescents. As CDC notes in a 2011 report on health disparities, "although the combined effects of changes in the age structure, racial/ethnic diversity, and income inequality on health disparities are difficult to assess, the nation is likely to continue experiencing substantial racial/ethnic and socioeconomic health disparities" (CDC, 2011, p. 3). A greater emphasis on improving precise measures of a broader range of variables may enable clearer causal inferences and intervention points than are possible with current measures of health disparities alone.

Several studies document the adverse effects that racial discrimination can have on the health and health care of racial/ethnic minorities (Williams and Sternthal, 2010). A recent review of the literature reveals that racism can result in racial/ethnic disparities in child health (Pachter and García Coll, 2009). Disparities exist in other areas that have received less attention—from special health care needs to sexual orientation—and share analogous issues of underreporting and insufficient and inconsistent data collection. For example, states collect data on health and health care disparities in a variety of nonstandard ways, which can make it challenging to identify, monitor, and address disparities at the national level.

Challenges in Translating Data into Practice and Action

The limited data that are available today are not well translated into practice and action. This translation requires unique skills and capacity, as well as quality improvement strategies. As the available data reflect a wide set of indicators, communities and providers often must prioritize the health conditions on which to focus, determine how to use the data to improve service delivery, and build the capacity for evidence-based practice. For asthma, for example, while an individual care plan may help ensure that a child is receiving the most effective treatment regimen, attention must also be focused on addressing factors known to be associated with preventable asthma hospitalizations, including avoidance of known disease triggers, inferior housing conditions, poor air quality, lack of adequate parental education, inadequate access to prescription refills, and lack of follow-up with health care providers (Flores et al., 2005a).

Challenges of Relying on the Appropriate Key Informant

Whereas parents/primary caregivers are clearly the most knowledgeable about their children's health status, they may encounter a variety of barriers to understanding crucial health care concepts for their children, including low health literacy due to medical jargon, language barriers, low literacy overall, and low educational attainment, as well as pressures related to social acceptability (e.g., respondents may provide answers that they feel are more "appropriate" or "acceptable"). These barriers may create issues of validity and/or reliability for many measures. (See Box 2-5 for a detailed description of low health literacy issues.)

A second issue is that when adolescents seek care for sensitive services, such as mental health issues, drug or alcohol dependency, and sexually transmitted infections and contraceptives, their parents may or may not be aware of these health-seeking behaviors or their children's health status. This lack of awareness may lead to inaccurate reporting or underreporting of risk behaviors and/or health conditions.

INITIAL OBSERVATIONS ON CURRENT DATA SYSTEMS ADDRESSING CHILD AND ADOLESCENT HEALTH AND HEALTH CARE

The committee recognized from the outset of this study that in efforts to address important issues related to child and adolescent health status, health care access and quality, and outcomes of care, attention must be paid to decades-old problems within the data collection and reporting systems. At present, there is no shortage of child health data, but it is exceedingly difficult to aggregate these data in a form that is optimally useful for either sound policy decisions or health care program management. To address these issues, the committee noted that several steps will need to be taken, some requiring new and increased funding and others requiring intergovernmental coordination that is often considered difficult to accomplish. These steps are captured in the initial observations detailed below.

Initial Observation 1: *A general conceptual map of the critical dimensions of child and adolescent health (including health status; health*

BOX 2-5
Challenges Posed by Low Health Literacy

Health literacy is integrally linked to social determinants of health and the contexts in which families live. People who lack basic functional health literacy, defined as those who possess insufficient reading and writing skills to function effectively in everyday situations, are more likely to have never attended or completed high school (Nutbeam, 2000), live in poverty, have limited English-language proficiency, and be non-Caucasian (Kutner et al., 2006). Low health literacy affects a large portion of the U.S. population. According to the most recent national assessment of health literacy among those aged 16 and older, 30 million (14 percent of the adult U.S. population) failed to meet standards for basic health literacy (Hawkins et al., 2010).

Low health literacy has important implications for parents who are charged with seeking preventive or treatment services for their children or adhering to prescribed treatments. Although one in five adults reads at the fifth-grade level, most health information is communicated in writing and at the tenth-grade level (Hawkins et al., 2010). Research has shown that low levels of functional health literacy are associated with increased hospitalizations, greater use of emergency services, lower likelihood of obtaining preventive vaccinations, diminished ability to read and comprehend prescription labels and health messages, poorer oral health status, and lower likelihood of enrolling in social welfare programs designed to improve child health and family well-being (AHRQ, 2011; Mejia et al., 2010; Miller et al., 2010; Pati et al., 2010). Consistent with these findings, the estimated excess health care cost associated with low health literacy in the United States is $50–73 billion (Weiss and Palmer, 2004). These findings suggest that even when parents have access to and receive information from pediatric providers, health care quality will likely be compromised by the parents' inability to use the information effectively, leading to poorer outcomes, greater health disparities, and increased health care costs.

The problem of low health literacy levels may be interpreted by providers as evidence that health education is an ineffective strategy for promoting health. As health information becomes more available to the public through the Internet and other media, however, parents' capacity to access and understand the information, to decipher its meaning and accuracy, and to feel confident in their ability to use the information effectively has never been more important. Unfortunately, identifying families with low levels of health literacy is a challenge since many individuals with low literacy skills feel ashamed and do not want others to know. Moreover, extant health literacy measures are flawed; a recent review cites numerous weaknesses related to their psychometric quality and problems with wide variations in how relevant aspects of health literacy are defined and measured (Jordan et al., 2010).

Given the challenge of identifying individuals in the health care system with limited health literacy skills and the likelihood that as more immigrant families enter the health care system, more children will be affected, it is imperative that innovative strategies for the delivery of health information be developed. These strategies may include greater use of audio and video recorded messages, pictures, maps, diagrams, and large print with simple words that are easy to understand (Hawkins et al., 2010).

care access, utilization, and quality; and health care outcomes) will need to be developed, widely adopted, and implemented by federal, state, and local health and health care agencies, as well as private-sector organizations.

There is considerable value to be derived from conceptual frameworks presented in a graphically understandable form. One such framework upon which the committee decided to build was developed by the IOM committee that produced *Children's Health, the Nation's Wealth* (IOM and NRC, 2004). This diagram, reproduced earlier as Figure 2-1, offers a perspective on how children's developmental stages over time have important (and different) health implications for four spheres of influence on child/adolescent health (biological factors; the child's social environment; the physical environment in which the child lives and matures; and health-relevant behaviors, some of which are health-promoting, while others pose threats to health status and the processes of healthy physical and emotional/mental development).

This committee did not attempt to reconceptualize these important facets of child health and development but used this earlier framework to begin addressing the questions posed by the Congress and the federal agency sponsoring this study (see Chapter 1). In embarking on its charge, however, the committee noted that, despite the focus of the earlier IOM report on child health status and the multidimensional factors that, together, influence health status, the diagram in Figure 2-1 does not illustrate the complexities associated with interactions between health care services and interventions and health outcomes. Thus it fails to address access to and availability of relevant services for children; understanding of the presumptive value of such services by parents or guardians; the actual provision of those services and their quality; and the impact of access to and use of those services on child health outcomes, such as functional health status. The committee determined that it was necessary to complement the conceptualization of children's health and its influences with an approach that would capture additional facets of health care services, including access, use and quality of services, and impact.

The committee began this discussion with the now axiomatic formulation of the late Avedis Donabedian of the University of Michigan (Donabedian, 1988), who identified structure, process, and outcomes as the key dimensions of health care quality. Using these Donabedian domains, the committee identified three key foci for the collection, analysis, and use of child and adolescent health and health care quality measures: (1) access to care/services; (2) levels of utilization and quality of care/services (including underlying processes); and (3) outcomes of service access, use, and quality (see Figure 2-3). This initial formulation led to an elaboration of the es-

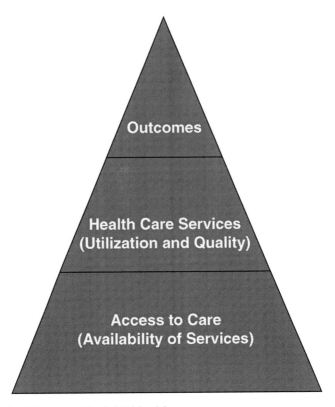

FIGURE 2-3 The pyramid of child health care.

sential content and meaning of each of these three interrelated dimensions (see Figure 2-4).

The committee quickly concluded that a comprehensive attempt to characterize the principal (and priority) components of a national data system to address the key components of child and adolescent health care—including access to and utilization of quality services and the outcomes of such access and use—would be an effort of considerable complexity, beyond the scope of this study. This effort would need to identify not only measures of evidence-based health care services but also the extent to which such services were available or provided in an effective manner to the appropriate populations of children and adolescents, including indicators of overuse and underuse of such services. Including these types of data system components would represent an extension of the four major categories of influence on child and adolescent health depicted in the diagram from the earlier IOM study, *Children's Health, the Nation's Wealth* (Figure 2-1),

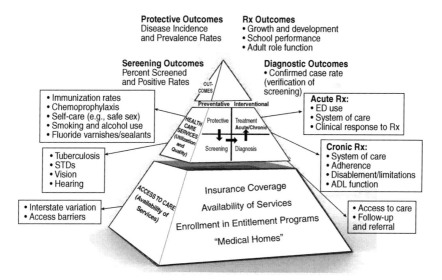

FIGURE 2-4 Changing the structure and emphasis in child and adolescent health care access and quality measures.

NOTE: ADL = activities of daily life; DX = diagnosis; ED = emergency department; STD = sexually transmitted disease.

and introduce even greater complexity, cost, and anticipated difficulties in implementation.

In its deliberations, the committee assumed that an important outcome of its efforts would be the promulgation of one or more conceptual models for a comprehensive data system for child and adolescent health and health care quality. To be successful, such conceptual models would need to be widely accepted and applicable at all levels (federal, state, and local) so as to promote efforts at each level to develop useful child and adolescent health data systems for the future.

Initial Observation 2: *The identification of critical dimensions of child and adolescent health and health care services will require consensus around specified goals for this population.*

Many of the objectives of such a system, however, are of high priority. A planning process will be necessary to prioritize needs for data on child and adolescent health status, health care needs, service availability and accessibility, utilization and quality of care processes, and outcomes of care that will make it possible to address urgent public policy issues surrounding new program initiatives and entitlement expansions for children and adolescents. In this report, therefore, the committee attempts to identify concrete steps that can be taken to meet these needs.

> **Initial Observation 3:** *Once consensus is reached on the best and most reliable indicators of key variables in this conceptual map, federal, state, and local health and health care agencies, as well as the private sector, will need guidance on the feasibility of incorporating these indicators and associated measures as requisite data items (i.e., minimum basic data items to be collected on child and adolescent health) in existing health and health care data sets.*

An important initial step in enabling immediate progress toward a national approach to child and adolescent health and health care quality data was undertaken by an expert advisory panel convened by AHRQ. This panel, known as the Subcommittee of the National Advisory Committee (SNAC), recommended an initial group of core measures for health and health care quality for children and adolescents. (A detailed review of the SNAC effort is provided in Chapter 5.) The SNAC identified 24 key indicators (referred to as "the initial core set") of health and health care service utilization that are currently available from federal agency sources and could serve as a useful starting point for a national approach to the development of a child and adolescent health data system.

> **Initial Observation 4:** *Standardized, annual (or more frequent) reporting of these standard measures (minimum basic data items) is necessary. In some cases, high-quality measures are already available and being collected in some but not all jurisdictions. In other cases, less than optimal data collection strategies may exist that can be improved through additional funding and collaboration among local, state, and federal agencies.*

As the committee began its work, it soon realized that the task before it would involve consideration of additional (and perhaps new) statistical measures of various indicators of child and adolescent health and health care quality that would fill gaps in current federal data sources. Thus it would be important to lay the groundwork for the definition of a minimum basic data set for child and adolescent health and health care quality that would be enabled by the standardized collection, analysis, and reporting of comparable data of high statistical quality from every state. Clearly, the implementation of a new national effort to collect, analyze, and report data on child and adolescent health and health care quality that involves federal, state, and local collaboration would require time, expertise, and financial support.

SUMMARY

A commitment to improving the health and health care of children and adolescents requires careful and thoughtful measurement to gauge progress, existing gaps, and future directions. The increasingly diverse population of the United States necessitates that data be collected routinely; consistently; and with special attention to identifying, monitoring, and addressing racial/ethnic, socioeconomic, linguistic, and special health care disparities. Changing definitions of health, the changing sociodemographic profile of the nation's next generation, and significant changes in health conditions call for improved measures in the nation's health care and population-based information systems. The improved measures will need to address the availability of and access to health care services, the utilization and quality of health and health care services and their underlying processes, and the outcomes associated with their use.

Initial observations about the current state of measurement of child and adolescent health and health care quality suggest that conceptual work is necessary to organize data on child and adolescent health and health care quality; to identify priority goals in these areas; to reach consensus on valid and feasible measures for these goals; and to standardize reporting of these measures in federal, state, and local reports. These observations provided the starting point for the committee's deliberations.

3

Current Data Collection
Methods and Sources

Summary of Key Findings

- There is a lack of comparable, standardized data (due in part to a lack of consistent definitions) in the measurement of health status and quality of health care for children and adolescents.
- Many health conditions and health care processes that are important to children appear in rates/numbers that are too small to be adequately represented in survey data sets.
- Improving linkages among administrative record systems and between those systems and population-based survey data sets would facilitate comprehensive assessment of child and adolescent health and health care quality.
- The use and interoperability of electronic health records are expected to increase dramatically over the next 5 years, creating a robust source of data that can be readily analyzed and acted upon.

Imagine that you are driving a complex piece of machinery. You want to know the direction in which you are headed, your rate of speed, how much fuel you have, the engine temperature (and possibly the external temperature as well), and whether the engine is performing as it should. If you are flying a plane, you want to know more details, such as your altitude and the wind speed. If you are under water, you want to know other things. The display that signals whether you are on track is derived from hundreds of intricate gauges, sensors, computer chips, and monitoring devices. Each mechanism is designed to collect certain types of performance data; these data are then compared against standard specifications, and the results are analyzed to determine whether the data are signaling a problem that requires the operator's attention. Some gauges are large and dominate the operator's routine field of vision; others are more peripheral and show alerts only when significant problems arise.

The above analogy is useful in considering the monitoring systems that are used in determining the quality of child and adolescent health and health care services. The clinician examines an individual child and collects data from numerous sources—temperature, heart rhythm, height, weight, sleeping and eating habits, and so forth—before concluding whether the child is "healthy" or requires attention for some specific reason. In much the same way, health professionals and policy makers examine data from a variety of population surveys and administrative data sets in making judgments about the health and health care of children and adolescents. Yet the data system used to measure the quality of child and adolescent health and health care services is not as finely developed as the instrumentation in the above analogy or the collection of clinical data. Indeed, it may be inappropriate even to refer to the existing data sets on child health and health care services as a "system," since these data sets consist of multiple, independent efforts that are largely uncoordinated and unrelated to each other. In many cases, data sets were designed for specific objectives without regard to how they fit within the larger landscape of child health measures. Furthermore, child and adolescent health data sets are not harmonized or coordinated with efforts that collect data about other aspects of development, education, or family and social contexts. The result is a tremendous wealth of data about many different specific dimensions of child and adolescent health and well-being, significant gaps with respect to important areas of health and selected populations, and the absence of an analytic framework that can provide routine guidance for general or even specific areas of concern.

The remainder of this chapter begins with a brief review of current methods used to collect data on health and health care. It then describes existing sources of these data for children and adolescents. Next, the chapter examines the limitations of these data sources. The final section argues for the need for a coordinated approach to integrate measures of child and adolescent health and health care quality.

DATA COLLECTION METHODS

Methods used to collect data on health and health care can be characterized by the following features:

- **Sample versus census**—Some data are collected for the entire population to which they apply; such data are sometimes referred to as *census* data. One example is the actual decennial census, which aims to obtain counts by geographic location and basic demographic characteristics for the entire resident population of the United States. However, the term *census* may be used to refer to any data collection aimed at collecting data for every unit in the population of interest (i.e., a subset of a larger population of emphasis). Conversely, many data cannot be collected for the entire population without excessive cost and/or a burden on respondents. Instead, the data are collected from a subset of the population, or a *sample*, that is selected (usually by randomization) in a way that makes it representative of the entire population; thus, estimates can be calculated from the sample that approximate those for the entire population.

- **Based on administrative records versus respondents**—Some data are extracted from records that already exist because they are necessary for the administration of a program or intervention. Examples are government records (tax files, social security and Medicaid enrollment, school enrollment, accident reports), commercial records (health plan enrollment files, medical claims), and medical records (from physicians' offices, hospitals, and other providers of health care). Other data are collected directly from respondents, for example, by interviewing individuals about their experiences. The line between the two may not be entirely distinct; for example, a physician might be asked to provide data derived from the medical records she uses in her practice; thus the data collection is respondent based, but the data are ultimately derived from administrative records. In the case of children, most respondent-based data are collected from proxy respondents (e.g., parents and caregivers). A third category to consider is that pertaining to clinical data, such as observational studies.

- **Population- versus service-based**—Some data collection efforts focus on a general *population* defined only by broad demographic characteristics, such as all children under age 6 or all adolescent girls. (Note that *population-based* in this sense could encompass data collection using sampling, and thus is unrelated to census data collection from an entire population.) Other data collection

TABLE 3-1 Data Collection Methods

	Source	Census	Sample
Population-based	Administrative records	Vital statistics	Some components of Medical Expenditure Panel Survey (MEPS) cost data; national samples of discharge abstracts, etc.
	Respondents	Decennial census	Most national surveys (e.g., Behavioral Risk Factor Surveillance System [BRFSS], MEPS, National Health Interview Survey [NHIS], National Immunization Survey [NIS], National Survey of Family Growth [NSFG], Pregnancy Risk Assessment Monitoring [PRAMS])
Service-based	Administrative records	Some Healthcare Effectiveness Data and Information Set (HEDIS) measures (those available in plan billing records)	Some HEDIS measures (those requiring medical record review)
	Respondents	Health plan collection of race/ethnicity data	Consumer Assessment of Healthcare Providers and Systems (CAHPS) measures

SOURCE: Committee on Pediatric Health and Health Care Quality Measures.

efforts in health and health care operate only through specific sites or administrators of services, such as health plans or clinics; such *service-based* data collection can cover only subpopulations defined by their attachment to the service providers.

While the above three features (summarized in Table 3-1) are not unrelated in practice, they are nonetheless conceptually and practically distinct. Two examples follow:

- **Census and administrative records**—Given the costs and burden of respondent-based data collection, census (100 percent) data collection for a specific population is almost always limited to administrative records that can be accessed inexpensively and efficiently. However, not every data collection from administrative records is a census; cost, access, or confidentially issues may necessitate use of a sample of records.
- **Respondent-based and population-based**—For some data needs, the relevant administrative records are service based. To obtain general population coverage, either records must be consolidated across providers or a respondent-based collection must be conducted. However, many respondent-based data collections are aimed only at coverage of a set of service providers, not a general population.

It should also be noted that none of these distinctions bears a perfect relationship to the distinction between health and health care data. Compared with health care data, health data tend more often to be population based (at least in objective) and respondent based; however, many examples of health care data are population or respondent based, while many examples of health data are based on administrative records or service based. Furthermore, the same data on health might be regarded as a population measure or as a measure of quality (through sentinel care processes) for a health care provider, depending on how they are collected and reported. For example, immunization rates are both a population measure and a measure of system performance.

Assessment of child and adolescent health and health care quality relies on data collected through a variety of the methods discussed above and from a variety of sources. Sources may include primary or secondary sources, surveys or registries, and voluntary or required reports. They may include parents or health care providers, as well as older children and adolescents who self-report their own data. Surveys may be conducted by telephone or through interviews with children and their families in health care or other service settings. Some surveys may involve a review of health records in providers' offices or claims records submitted to public or private health plans. Surveys may be conducted at one point in time, or they may recur annually or over other time periods. The reporting source may change over different time periods, or the same population may be surveyed or interviewed on multiple occasions. Data may be retrospective, based on respondents' recall of certain events or conditions, or prospective, which involves collecting data at multiple intervals over time to monitor changes in health characteristics. Surveys may be administered to a universal or randomized sample of children on a national, state, or local basis; or they may focus on selected populations, such as underserved children, children with special health care needs, or children with specific demographic characteristics. Registries are another common source for data on health and health care, especially when a specific procedure (such as immunization) can be recorded electronically in a central data collection site.

The consistency and rigor of the measurement method are directly associated with the quality of the data collected. In examining child and adolescent health and health care, therefore, it is important to know details about the sampling strategy, data collection method, and reporting source associated with surveys or reports.

EXISTING DATA SOURCES

The federal government supports numerous surveys and information systems that collect data about selected aspects of child and adolescent health and health services. Prior studies have reviewed many of these data sets, often with detailed analyses of their sampling strategy, periodicity, and specific data components (IOM and NRC, 2004; NRC, 1998, 2010; NRC and IOM, 1995).

Federal Population Health Data Sets

The committee developed Appendix F, a table briefly describing the major population health data sets that include information about child and adolescent health and health care services. In developing this table, the committee examined the following sources:

- *Children's Health, the Nation's Wealth: Assessing and Improving Child Health* (IOM and NRC, 2004), which identifies 30 federal data sets used for measuring children's health and relevant influences and includes a gap analysis of specific measures for 12 of these data sets;
- data sets reviewed by the Federal Interagency Forum on Child and Family Statistics, which produces the annual *America's Children* reports (FIFCFS, 2010a);
- the *Directory of Health and Human Services Data Resources*, prepared by the Department of Health and Human Services' (HHS') Data Council (HHS, 2003);
- a list of federal data sets and repositories available on the research portal of the National Information Center on Health Services Research and Health Care Technology (NICHSR) at the National Institutes of Health (NIH, 2010a);

- three research papers examining selected federal data sets for children, youth, and families (Hogan and Msall, 2008; NRC and IOM, 1995; Stagner and Zweigl, 2007);
- a review of longitudinal data sets compiled during the planning for the National Children's Study (The Lewin Group, 2000); and
- a list compiled by the Agency for Healthcare Research and Quality's (AHRQ's) Data and Surveys web site (AHRQ, 2010a).

This inventory includes surveys of health and health care services administered for children and adolescents (aged 0–18) within the past 20 years (beginning in 1990). Data sources for these surveys include information provided by children, adolescents, parents, caregivers, and health care providers. Some surveys involve reviewing health records. Only surveys administered within the United States to sample sizes greater than 1,000 are included in the above list.

The largest number of population health surveys, registries, and studies are administered by HHS. Other federal agencies collect child health data as part of their administration of information systems for other purposes, such as environmental quality (Environmental Protection Agency), education (U.S. Department of Education), or occupational injuries (U.S. Department of Labor). In addition, some federal agencies collect data on health influences, such as poverty (Census Bureau), housing and homelessness (U.S. Department of Housing and Urban Development), and motor vehicle safety (U.S. Department of Transportation).

Longitudinal Studies of Children and Youth

In addition to data systems administered directly by federal agencies (or their contractors), federal funds have supported hundreds of longitudinal studies examining selected aspects of child health, frequently focusing on small populations that are followed intensely over several years or even decades. No central source exists that can catalogue the information gleaned from these longitudinal studies, although many of these studies have been described in earlier reports (NRC, 1998).

One example of a longitudinal study is the National Children's Study (NCS), launched in January 2009. The NCS is the largest long-term study of environmental and genetic effects on children's health conducted in the United States. A nationally representative probability sample of 100,000 births will be followed from before birth to age 21. Data will be collected on multiple exposures and multiple outcomes using repeated measures over time (NIH, 2010c).

Other longitudinal studies include the National Longitudinal Study of Adolescent Health (Add Health) and the Great Smoky Mountains Study

(GSMS). Add Health, which began in 1994, examines how social contexts (such as families, friends, peers, schools, neighborhoods, and communities) influence adolescents' health and risk behaviors (NICHD, 2007). The GSMS, a population-based community survey of children and adolescents in North Carolina, estimates the number of youth with emotional and behavioral disorders, the persistence of those disorders over time, the need for and use of services for those disorders, and the possible risk factors for developing them (Costello et al., 1996) (see Appendix F for additional information on selected longitudinal studies of children and adolescents).

Administrative Data Sources

In addition to the population health and longitudinal studies described above, data on child health and health care services can be derived from service-based records. These data sets include those prepared for administrative purposes, such as vital statistics (birth and death records), medical records, health plan payments, and quality measures. They also include surveys of populations from selected service settings, such as children or youth who are enrolled in specific health plans (e.g., Medicaid or CHIP), children who are hospitalized, or children who are identified in cases of abuse and neglect.

The committee identified and catalogued these service-based data sets by reviewing the sources on population health described above and drawing on a commissioned background paper (MacTaggart, 2010). Appendix F provides a listing of the individual data sets derived from service-based studies, which include, for example, Healthcare Effectiveness Data and Information Set (HEDIS) measures, National Committee for Quality Assurance (NCQA) measures, and hospital administrative data.

LIMITATIONS OF EXISTING DATA SOURCES

Estimates of the scope and severity of certain health conditions are sometimes derived from service-based information sources rather than general population surveys. Existing data sources have a number of limitations related to standardization, data collection, the ability to capture disparities, case mix adjustment, and data aggregation methods.

Standardization

There is no lack of standards; rather, there are multiple standards that are competing and conflicting in nature. The same is true of existing quality performance measures. A range of such measures exist for children and adolescents, and the administrative requirements for their collection vary with respect to which measures are collected, the sources of the data (based on administrative records or respondents or a mix of the two), validation of the data sources, and the reporting period. The lack of comparable, standardized data has limited the ability to develop benchmarks from national or state sources.

Interstate issues are significant as a result of variations in state reporting requirements, state information technology (IT) infrastructure capacity and specifications, state collection methods, cross-state access to data, and the way various parameters are defined. For instance, the definition of "fully" immunized and the components of a newborn screening can vary by state; therefore, the data elements that are collected and tracked may vary and not be comparable (Ferris et al., 2001). Data are more likely to be equivalent if claims data are used as the source and the services are provided in the same setting; however, the conversion from the ninth to the tenth edition of the *International Classification of Diseases* (ICD-9 to ICD-10) in the coming years will require additional scrutiny to ensure continued comparability.

One of the greatest challenges is standardizing the definition of children. For Medicaid early and periodic screening, diagnosis, and treatment (EPSDT), a child is defined as up to age 21. For the Children's Health Insurance Program (CHIP), a child is defined as up to age 19. For the Consumer Assessment of Healthcare Providers and Systems (CAHPS) (Berdahl et al., 2010), a child is defined as age 17 or younger. And the Federal Interagency Forum on Child and Family Statistics (FIFCFS) of the National Center for Health Statistics defines teens as those aged 12–17 (FIFCFS, 2010a). Family structure likewise is not standardized across funding mechanisms and time.

Other problems occur in attempting to compare similar health issues across data sets. These problems illustrate both the advantages and difficulties of attempting to standardize definitions and data collection methods. For example, Bethell and colleagues' (2002) characterization of good health raises concern about how the information is obtained. Many national surveys have converged on using a single question on how the individual rates his/her own health or parents rate their child's health along a spectrum of excellent, very good, good, fair, or poor (Anderson et al., 2001; Andresen et al., 2003; Hennessey et al., 1994; NCHS, 1973; Roghmann and Pless, 1993). Such convergence allows for comparison over time and across age groups. However, little variation in the responses is seen, and the measure is insensitive to fairly major differences in health. A more nuanced measure that captures more dimensions of perceived health status would be useful, but its use might sacrifice the value of comparability. Addressing such issues would require ongoing methodological work on assessing and refining measures and establishing comparability over time, as is done with changes in the ICD (Anderson et al., 2001).

Likewise, the Maternal and Child Health Bureau has developed a short screener to identify children with special health care needs (Bethell et al., 2002). While ensuring comparable ascertainment across populations, the use of this instrument hinders comparisons with data sets that rely on diagnoses. Standardized measures of child health and the quality of relevant health care are also important for all child health problems, but especially for those children with preventable, ongoing, or serious health conditions (Kuhlthau et al., 2002). Child health problems include a large number of relatively rare conditions (see Chapter 4). Moreover, the implications of the existence of a health condition may vary with child development (IOM and NRC, 2004). Thus, an early sign of a health problem may be slower rates of physical growth, but later implications may include poorer school achievement, perhaps due to repeated absences (Byrd and Weitzman, 1994; Weitzman et al., 1982), and may be associated with behavioral issues that may further impede school success (Gortmaker et al., 1990). In addition, conditions may vary in severity across different children and over time and have implications for adult health.

Criteria for the design of health measures are identified in *Children's Health, the Nation's Wealth* (IOM and NRC, 2004, p. 43):

- importance to current and future health,
- reliability and validity,
- meaning in terms of the special aspects of child health and development,
- cultural appropriateness,
- sensitivity to change, and
- feasibility of collection.

Inherent in these criteria is the challenge of a measurement system that speaks to the various parties engaged in improving the health of children. Diagnoses (ICD codes), for example, may be meaningful to health care providers but less so to parents, who, in turn, may be concerned about functional implications, including management strategies. Both types of information may be critical to the development of an education plan for special education students.

Data Collection

The use of administrative data to assess child health and health care quality is limited to some extent to certain dimensions of quality, such as access and some process measures. The combining of medical records and claims data through the development and operation of electronic health record (EHR) systems and electronic health information exchange (e-HIE) will appreciably reduce this limitation. The evolution to ICD-10 coding will also expand the value of claims data. Data linkages resulting from Medicaid Transformation Grant initiatives, Children's Health Insurance Program Reauthorization Act (CHIPRA) provisions, and American Recovery and Reinvestment Act (ARRA) funding are providing critical data elements. For example, the opportunity to collect some measures more efficiently is enhanced through the linkage of Medicaid with vital statistics, state laboratories, and registries. In addition, the availability of web-based interfaces expands options for the collection and transmission of data.

Given that the cost of quality oversight and performance measurement reporting is a cost to public and private purchasers and providers, the fiscal impact as well as efficiency of using standardized, formatted data through an ongoing infrastructure is considerable. However, the realization of these benefits assumes that the data are collected and documented at the site of care, which is not always the case. Also assumed is that the individual is identifiable. A current issue is that Medicaid requires coverage of newborns under their mother's identification until their own eligibility can be established, which may take up to a year. Data coded to a mother's identification may or may not be tracked back to the newborn when the child becomes individually enrolled.

Another factor that can potentially affect the data collected is a change in payment methods. For example, while there is significant interest in episode-of-care payment methods, there is a risk that some of the previous detailed claims data may be lost. A lesson learned from the transition from individual to bundled payments for prenatal visits and delivery was that the requirement to collect and track the number of prenatal visits through administrative data no longer existed.

Identification and Monitoring of Disparities

As discussed in Chapter 2, it is crucial to identify and monitor health and health care equity issues among children and adolescents. Racial/ethnic and linguistic disparities in children's health and health care cannot be identified, tracked, addressed, or eliminated without consistent collection of race/ethnicity and language data on all patients (Flores, 2009). Yet, one-third of all health plan enrollees (28.7 million individuals) are covered by plans that collect no race/ethnicity data (AHIP and RWJF, 2006). A national survey of 272 hospitals found that only 39 percent collected data on patients' primary language (Hasnain-Wynia et al., 2004), and no information is available on what proportions of hospitals or health plans collect data on English proficiency. Parental limited English proficiency (defined by the U.S. Census Bureau [Shin and Kominski, 2010] as the self-rated ability to speak English less than "very well") has been shown to be superior to primary language spoken at home as a measure of the impact of language barriers on children's health and health care (Flores et al., 2005a).

Although the Office of Management and Budget (OMB) requires highly discrete breakdowns of race and ethnicity, many current Medicaid eligibility systems are old legacy systems that fail to collect or retain this information, even if it is collected at the time of application. A particular difficulty is addressing American Indians/Alaska Natives and the lack of integration of their health care delivery systems and health care coverage data with other systems and data. Because much of their health care is delivered through the Indian Health Service or tribal-sponsored facilities, it may or may not be included in the Medicaid/CHIP data sets, although where it is included in claims data, it is easily identifiable as it is reimbursed and tracked for 100 percent federal financial participation (Hasnain-Wynia et al., 2004).

Despite the large body of evidence indicating the importance of socio-economic factors in health, very limited resources have been directed to obtaining adequate socioeconomic information in the ongoing sources of surveillance data or one-time studies. Wealth could have important health effects not captured by income, which is temporary, and yet very few data sources include information on both health and wealth (Pollack et al., 2007). Similarly, socioeconomic conditions in early childhood, which are likely to play a major role in chronic disease in adulthood (see Chapter 2), are rarely described (Braveman and Barclay, 2009). And neighborhood socioeconomic conditions may influence health behaviors and health status, yet generally are not included in most health studies.

Even just using income as a measure of socioeconomic status presents methodological challenges. For example, children in low-income families, typically operationalized as families with incomes below 200 percent of the federal poverty level (FPL), share many of the health characteristics and access problems of children in impoverished families. The 2010 Annual Social and Economic Supplement (formerly called the March Supplement) to the Current Population Survey (CPS) includes online estimates for the number of children living in families with incomes below 200 percent of the FPL (DeNavas-Walt et al., 2010): fully 40 percent of children aged 0–17 and 44 percent of children under age 6 live in low-income families (FIFCFS, 2010a). Using this income break helps underscore the prevalence of economic disadvantage among American children. The federal poverty standard is widely acknowledged as inadequate in representing household resource sufficiency, yet many states vary in the extent to which their Medicaid or CHIP plans will cover children and adolescents up to 200 percent of the FPL (or higher).

Wealth, early childhood, and neighborhood conditions all vary markedly by race/ethnicity. The absence of information on all of these factors can lead to erroneous assumptions about the relationship between an independent variable such as race/ethnicity and health outcomes. Federal investment in the development of feasible and valid measures of a range of key socioeconomic, racial/ethnic, and English proficiency factors is needed to achieve progress in understanding and addressing health disparities (Braveman et al., 2005). Particular attention is needed to determine for what and for whom racial and ethnic characteristics are a proxy in terms of health care quality, access, and outcomes, although many studies over decades of research document that race and ethnicity are independently associated with multiple disparities in health and health care. The confusion created when inadequate and inconsistent definitions of race, ethnicity, and language proficiency are used can lead to erroneous conclusions.

Case Mix Adjustment

Nearly all outcome measures are affected by some characteristics of the population to which they are applied, including age, gender, race, ethnicity, income, education level, and geographic jurisdiction. Thus, for example, developmental measures such as cognitive ability are associated with age; the prevalence of a condition or functional limitation is likely to be associated with age and in some cases with gender; and the probability of receiving a clinical or remedial service is related to having a condition or functional limitation that makes that service appropriate. In a comparison of two populations with different distributions of characteristics, if one (for example) has more older children or more children with functional limitations, measures of cognitive ability or service receipt may reflect these differences in population characteristics as well as differences in the outcome of interest for otherwise similar children. For purely descriptive purposes (e.g., how many hours of services are used in each school), such effects might be ignored. However, when the focus shifts to policy inferences (e.g., did service provision increase over time? Was it more intensive in school A than school B?), some effects may become extraneous to the questions of interest because of changing or differential population characteristics. Thus, it may be desirable to use analysis methods that prevent these characteristics from confounding comparisons. Such methods go by a number of different names depending on the setting, types of predictor and outcome variables, and specific methodological approaches. Here the general term "case mix adjustment" is used to encompass a wide variety of such methods, which include the following:

- **Adjustment implicit in measures**—Some measures are constructed in a manner that inherently adjusts for certain demographic characteristics. For example, IQ is normed in relation to abilities of children of the same age; if this norming is done correctly, comparisons can be made across groups with differing age distributions. The same can be said of a measure such as "reads at or above grade level."

- **Restriction to homogeneous populations**—Some measures can be made comparable by restriction to a homogeneous population. For example, childhood immunizations typically run on strict age-based schedules and are appropriate for essentially all children in the age window; hence the measure can be calculated from a specific age group, and no age adjustment is needed. One can then compare immunization rates in different states at that single age.

- **Stratified reporting**—There might be several groups of interest for a measure, each of which is homogeneous. For example, one might be interested in immunization rates across a range of ages, but recognize that younger children are more likely than older ones to have immunizations complete. A simple comparison of childhood immunization rates across states could be confounded if one state has a higher proportion of young children. Instead, one might stratify reporting by age, that is, prepare a separate measure for each of several nearly homogeneous age groups. Unconfounded comparisons could then be made for each stratum.

- **Direct standardization**—Stratified reporting might be impractical for any of at least three reasons: (1) there might be insufficient data with which to calculate measures for each of the relevant strata with adequate precision for stratified reporting; (2) stratified reports might provide more detail than is desired (for example, comparing 51 states in 10 age strata involves cognitively processing 510 measures, obscuring overall state differences); and (3) when a control variable has many levels or several control variables must be considered at once, the number of strata can become very large, exacerbating both of the previous problems. A set of stratified measures can be consolidated into a simpler single measure by combining measures across strata with fixed weights corresponding to some reference population. To develop a single immunization measure for comparison of states, for example, one might combine immunization rates by year of age with weights based on the national age distribution. Then no state would receive a higher score simply because it had a larger proportion of young children.

- **Model-based standardization**—Direct standardization may fail when the number of observations per cell is small or zero. Model-based (regression) standardization is a generalization that can be more robust against such problems (Little, 1982). Regression standardization can accommodate simultaneous adjustment for multiple variables. A variety of models are appropriate for use with different kinds of data.

Given the existence of technical methods for implementing case mix adjustment in a variety of settings, the key scientific or policy question is which variables to adjust for in reporting any particular comparison. Since case mix adjustment is a method of removing extraneous compositional effects from a comparison, the key is to figure out which effects are extraneous for a given purpose and which are of interest. For example, it is common to adjust for severity of illness and comorbidities when using outcome measures to evaluate the quality of care provided by hospitals. Without such adjustment, hospitals that treat more severely ill patients might be rated as worse than those of similar quality that treat mildly ill patients. Similarly, when evaluation is based on a measure of process, it is appropriate to adjust for patient variables associated with either the degree of appropriateness of the process or the difficulty of applying it.

To consider a slightly more complex example, one might be interested in unadjusted rates of severe emotional distress (SED) if one simply wanted to determine how to distribute funds for mental health services across schools. If one wanted to compare schools on their psychological climates, one might want to adjust for age distributions (if age is a predictor of a determination of SED). If one wanted to evaluate schools on how well they (and their associated support systems) help children cope with stressors that tend to engender SED, one might further adjust for known stressors such as family poverty or instability.

While adjusting for age is rarely controversial, adjusting for socioeconomic or race/ethnicity variables raises more subtle issues. Suppose, for example, that low-income patients with a certain condition at each hospital are less likely than upper-income patients at the same hospital to obtain a service equally needed by both. Without adjustment of two hospitals that perform identically on a measure of this service, the one with a greater proportion of low-income patients would receive a worse quality score. By the logic of the previous examples, adjustment for patient composition by income group might be considered. It has been argued that such adjustment obscures and excuses inferior performance for disadvantaged (low-income, in this case) patients (Romano, 2000). On the other hand, by hypothesis in this example and perhaps empirically in many cases, inferior performance for low-income patients is a systemwide failure, not just a failure of the hospitals that see many such patients. Such a systemwide failure might arise, for example, from a lack of insurance coverage for needed medications, a lack of resources required to enable less educated patients to master complex treatment regimens, or unconscious discrimination against such patients. Indeed, such a pattern of inferior treatment within each hospital is not discernible in unadjusted hospital-level reports, which combine income groups. (If some hospitals serving many low-income patients have generally inferior performance—that is, for each income group—this could be observed in either adjusted or unadjusted reports.) Reports stratified by income for each hospital would reveal the pattern, albeit only after further analysis, and become subject to the disadvantages discussed above. In fact, the pattern would be revealed most explicitly in the coefficients of the case mix regression model, which summarize the within-hospital differences in a single number (Zaslavsky, 2001). The point here is that hospital (or other unit-specific) reports are good for some purposes but are best examined in conjunction with analysis of more general patterns.

Another controversy concerns the applicability of case mix adjustment in assessment of racial/ethnic health and health care disparities. It is logical to age- and sex-adjust intergroup comparisons of health, and similarly to adjust comparisons of health care for clinical characteristics affecting need and outcome. However, the IOM report *Unequal Treatment: Confronting Racial and Ethnic Disparities in Health Care* (2003a) argues that it is not appropriate to adjust for socioeconomic measures (that is, remove their effects) in such comparisons since worse socioeconomic status is one of the aspects of disadvantage imposed on disadvantaged racial/ethnic groups and a mediator of effects on health, treatment, and outcomes. Others have argued for adjustment for socioeconomic variables, thus more or less explicitly taking a much narrower view of what counts as a disparity that excludes effects mediated through socioeconomic differences between groups at variance with the IOM-endorsed definitions (Satel and Klick, 2006). This controversy illustrates how important scientific and normative principles may arise in case mix adjustment.

Data Aggregation Methods

Any analysis of data used to measure health or health care quality requires aggregation of the data. These data may be collected with the primary goal of measurement, using any combination of tools and design approaches as described previously; in this case, the time-consuming and expensive process of data collection for measurement must be balanced against the rigor with which these data can be collected. In many cases, secondary data, such as those collected for clinical, billing, research, or other purposes, may be used secondarily to assess health or health care quality. These data are often less well validated and may contain errors or formats that compromise data analysis; for some data types in some populations, however, secondary data are the only accessible source of the needed information. In either case, IT often plays an important role. Databases, medical data registries, and clinical health information technology (HIT) are three common approaches to data aggregation and reuse.

Databases, defined as a structured collection of organized, retrievable, and (typically) machine-readable information (Frawley et al., 1992), are a common tool for assembling data before conducting analyses. Database software is specifically designed to support the storage, manipulation, and retrieval of data, and is a critical tool for the biostatistician dealing with large data sets. One of the key features of databases is the ability to define relationships among data elements. For example, databases allow billing system data that include provider identifiers and sites of care to be combined with survey data that may include a provider name. These two collections of data can be combined because the provider name and date of visit may match the provider name and date of completion in the survey. This relationship allows the site of care to be linked to the survey, thereby supporting a variety of analyses that compare some measure across sites of care.

Medical data registries are a specialized type of database designed to contain data collected in the course of caring for a specific patient population (Drolet and Johnson, 2008). Because the goal of medical data registries is often to support secondary data analysis, they feature well-characterized data collection methods and carefully constructed data fields that rely on controlled terminologies to support the aggregation of data in ways not always defined *a priori*. Medical data registries also characteristically support longitudinal data collection (i.e., the collection of data on a particular patient over time), as well as cross-sectional data collection (e.g., survey results on functional status after hip replacement in clinics across the country). Finally, the use of a medical data registry implies attention not only to the quality of the data, but also to the rigorous policies of human subjects assurance, the Health Insurance Portability and Accountability Act (HIPAA), and internationally sanctioned approaches to privacy and security.

Clinical HIT has received significant attention because of its potential impact on quality and safety (IOM, 1999). EHR and, more recently, personal health record (PHR) systems are primary data sources that provide a rich source of information about health and health care quality. These systems promote the collection of comprehensive, patient-specific data on active medications, allergies, medical diagnoses, encounter summaries, referrals, and laboratory tests, as well as other longitudinal data. As utilization of EHRs and PHRs continues to grow, they will provide an important opportunity to integrate data across specialty care, such as care for mental health and substance use disorders.

In addition to the above three approaches, the adoption of controlled terminologies, such as the Systematized Nomenclature of Medicine (SNOMED) or the ICD, together with relatively structured formats for encounter summaries or document types, makes it possible to aggregate data across patients, sites of care, and even entire regions, as demonstrated by numerous health information exchange demonstration projects around the United States (Denny et al., 2009; Doan et al., 2010). These systems may catalyze the formulation of new health and health care quality measures and may radically lower the implementation cost of measurement. Moreover, through the use of algorithmic approaches to data analysis, researchers are beginning to demonstrate near-real-time feedback of quality measures to providers at the point of care (Roberts et al., 2009; Starmer and Giuse, 2008; Starmer and Waitman, 2006; Zaydfudim et al., 2009).

Unfortunately, as of 2008, fewer than 20 percent of providers were using a comprehensive EHR in their practice (DesRoches et al., 2008). Similarly, demonstration projects of e-HIE have achieved usage for under 20 percent of encounters (Johnson et al., 2008; Vest, 2009), although with recent federal incentives, the adoption of both EHRs and e-HIE is expected to increase dramatically over the next 5 years.

The promise of these technologies suggests that measurement researchers should modify validated measures to support them and investigate how best to integrate efforts to collect valid and reliable data with available populationwide data samples that may be of lower quality. Furthermore, issues surrounding privacy and access to state-based Medicaid data continue to underscore challenges in EHR and e-HIE implementation. While the issues of privacy and confidentiality are of critical concern, detailed discussion of these issues is beyond the scope of the report. (For a more comprehensive discussion of privacy and confidentiality issues, see *Engaging Privacy and Information Technology in a Digital Age* [NRC, 2007] and *Beyond the HIPAA Privacy Rule: Enhancing Privacy, Improving Health Through Research* [IOM, 2009b].) HIPAA and the regulations that followed protect personal health information held by third parties and give patients an array of rights. They also established a range of administrative, physical, and technical safeguards to ensure the confidentiality, integrity, and availability of electronic health information.

HIPAA was followed by the Patient Safety and Quality Improvement Act of 2005 (PSQIA), which established a voluntary reporting system to resolve patient safety and health care quality issues: "To encourage the reporting and analysis of medical errors, PSQIA provides Federal privilege and confidentiality protections for patient safety information called patient safety work product. Patient safety work product includes information collected and created during the reporting and analysis of patient safety events" (HHS, 2011a).

Both of these pieces of legislation represent the policy consensus and technical capabilities at the time they were enacted. It is unlikely that new legislation will be enacted in the near future to refine and update this policy consensus and incorporate technical advances. In the meantime, well-designed systems that produce robust data with strong privacy protection will be able to meet the needs and protections encompassed by these two pieces of legislation, but also self-adjust to adapt to the needs and challenges of the future.

At present, privacy protections can conflict with attempts at data aggregation. The adolescent population poses special data collection issues, particularly with regard to privacy and security concerns, as confidentiality is known to be a significant and necessary component when interviewing adolescents. Conflicts also exist at the state and local levels with respect to accessing Medicaid and vital statistics data; there is marked variation in the way states have interpreted recent guidance from the Centers for Medicare and Medicaid Services (CMS) regarding access to and the availability of Medicaid data. Successful future efforts to conduct cross-state quality measurement will require specific guidance from CMS to the states regarding the priority associated with these efforts. Although necessary safeguards for patient confidentiality are essential, they need not preclude the ability to develop and utilize analytic methods to conduct both cross-sectional and longitudinal comparisons among states. The failure of CMS to facilitate the comfort of states in providing limited yet essential access to Medicaid data would restrict the ability to perform quality measurement across the nation for this important patient population.

Illustrative Examples

This section presents two illustrative examples of the challenges discussed above: an assessment of a state-based demonstration program and measurement of health insurance coverage.

Hypothetical State-Based Demonstration Program

The first example is a hypothetical state-based demonstration program designed to examine the effect of changes in insurance coverage strategies aimed at reducing preventable hospitalizations and hospital costs among low-income children. To conduct such an assessment would require data on the details of insurance coverage; on the details of hospitalizations; and on personal characteristics of each child's family, notably income, by state. The Medical Expenditures Panel Study (MEPS) is carried out by interviewing parents of a nationally representative sample of children about their children's health and health care use (AHRQ, 2010b), the parents' employers about insurance benefits, and health care providers about the children's use of services and charges. Thus, this data set would appear to contain all the necessary data. In 2006, however, the sample included only 12,609 individuals younger than 24, slightly fewer than half of whom were from low-income families. Moreover, hospitalization is a relatively infrequent event for children: only 6.5 percent of children younger than 5 and 1.5 percent of those aged 5–17 have any hospital expenditures. With such small samples, further winnowing by specific diagnoses (e.g., those preventable), by subgroups of interest (e.g., by race/ethnicity or type of insurance coverage), and by state would preclude stable or meaningful estimates.

Two state-based data systems might prove more useful. The Kids' Inpatient Database (KID) contains data on all admissions for those younger than 20 from 38 states in the most recent compilation (HCUP, 2006). Data elements include primary and secondary diagnoses and procedures, admission and discharge status, demographic information such as age and gender, hospital characteristics, length of stay and charges, and expected source of payment on 2–3 million discharges per year. While providing a substantial window on hospital use by children, however, this data set has significant limitations. Among these is the characterization of socioeconomic status, as the income data reflect the median income of the zip code of the hospital, not the income of the child's family, and the insurance data (expected source of payment) may not be for the final payer. In addition, the data set does not permit linkage of multiple hospitalizations for the same child, nor does it provide much information on the events before and after hospitalization. Even with substantial numbers of events, quality indicators designed to parallel those used for adults may not occur in sufficient numbers to yield information on safety (Scanlon et al., 2008) or to support stratification by important covariates such as race/ethnicity, income, or insurance status (Berdahl et al., 2010).

Other state-based assessments of child health can be obtained from the series of surveys funded by the Maternal and Child Health Bureau on general child health (NCHS, 2009c) and the health experience of children with special health care needs (NCHS, 2009b) based on the State and Local Area Integrated Telephone Survey (NCHS, 2009a). These surveys are designed to provide robust samples for analysis at the state level and a wealth of data on health conditions and functional status, insurance coverage, use of medical care and other services, and individual family health behaviors for children generally and for the more vulnerable subgroup of those with special needs. As with the MEPS, however, the data come from parent reports and may be limited on any one issue because of the breadth of the topics covered. Unlike the MEPS, moreover, these surveys include no longitudinal component, so that assessing changes in health status or use of care is not possible. For the purposes of assessment of a hypothetical state-based demonstration program, virtually no data on costs of care are available except for out-of-pocket costs for families with children with special needs. Thus, each of these data sets might provide some insight, but none would be sufficient to support a comprehensive assessment.

Measurement of Health Insurance Coverage

Another example of the limitations imposed by the fragmentation of current data collection systems is measurement of health insurance coverage. Currently, there is no agreement on the number of children who are uninsured (CBO, 2003; Kenney et al., 2006; SHADAC and RWJF, 2009). Confusion as to the number of uninsured children arises in part because a range of different insurance concepts are relevant, in part because there is no proven method for collecting health insurance information, and in part because multiple surveys produce coverage estimates for children on an annual basis.

A number of different insurance coverage concepts exist—for example, the number of children who are uninsured at a particular point in time, the number of children who have been insured for a year or longer, the number of children who experienced short periods (less than 12 months) without coverage in a 12-month period, and the average number of children who are uninsured over a particular period in time. A priori, one would expect the number of uninsured children to depend on the particular concept: the number of children who are uninsured for a full year is expected to be smaller than the number of children who are uninsured at a particular point in time, which in turn is expected to be smaller than the number of children who experienced any period without coverage in a given year. Indeed, according to one source, which includes measures of two different insurance concepts, the number of children who are uninsured at a particular point in time is 1.6 times larger than the number of those who are uninsured for a full year (Davern et al., 2009; Klerman et al., 2009).

Each of the different insurance concepts provides valuable information about the nature of the coverage problem facing children. In particular, estimates of the number of children who are uninsured at a particular point in time are useful for budgeting purposes (Orszag, 2007). For example, when Medicaid and CHIP programs assess how eligibility expansions could affect program enrollment and spending, they rely on estimates of how many children are uninsured in the targeted income group. Similarly, knowing how many children are uninsured for a full year or longer provides important information on the extent to which uninsurance is a chronic problem for children, whereas knowing how many children experience short bouts of uninsurance could provide key insights about program operations related to churning (how individuals move back and forth between having and not having insurance) and retention (Tang et al., 2003).

Since there is no proven method for accurately measuring a given insurance concept, moreover, each survey's approach to measuring the uninsured differs along a number of dimensions that likely affects the estimated number of uninsured children. In particular, surveys differ in the wording

of the insurance questions they include, the names used to designate different Medicaid and CHIP programs, the order of the questions, whether
the insurance questions pertain to a specific child or to multiple individuals
in the family, who is providing information on the insurance coverage of
a particular child, what survey mode is used to collect the data (e.g., mail,
telephone, in person), whether the survey is cross-sectional or longitudinal
(which likely affects duration-dependent concepts such as the number of
children who have lacked insurance coverage for a full year), how missing
data on coverage are handled, how a response that requires some interpre-
tation is coded (e.g., when respondents reply that they have both private
coverage and Medicaid), and whether an explicit attempt is made to adjust
for what appears to be a systematic underreporting of Medicaid and CHIP
coverage in household surveys (Kenney et al., 2006; SHADAC and RWJF,
2009). The factors listed here shape the coverage estimates that emerge
from a particular survey.

Four federal surveys—the CPS, the American Community Survey
(ACS), the MEPS, and the National Health Interview Survey (NHIS)—
currently provide annual estimates of the number of children who are
uninsured. The ACS, MEPS, and NHIS all ask explicitly about coverage
at the time of the survey, which corresponds to the point-in-time concept.
The MEPS and NHIS also include measures of full-year uninsurance, with
the MEPS tracking coverage over the course of a year through multiple
interviews at 3- to 4-month intervals and the NHIS collecting information
on current and prior coverage from a single interview. In principle, the
CPS provides an estimate of the number of children who were uninsured
for a full year. However, the survey's long recall period (14–16 months)
may lead to inaccurate responses, especially among individuals who were
enrolled in Medicaid for a brief period in the previous calendar year or at
the beginning of the previous calendar year (DeNavas-Walt et al., 2009;
Klerman et al., 2009).

For 2008, the most recent year for which official estimates are available
from each of these surveys, the number of uninsured children aged 0–17
at a particular point in time ranges from 6.6 million on the NHIS to 10.7
million on the MEPS (the CPS [unadjusted] and ACS estimates are both
7.3 million). Not only is there disagreement about how many children lack
health insurance coverage at a particular point in time nationally, but state-
level estimates vary across surveys as well (Blewett and Davern, 2006; Call
et al., 2007).

THE NEED FOR A COORDINATED APPROACH TO INTEGRATE MEASURES OF CHILD AND ADOLESCENT HEALTH AND HEALTH CARE QUALITY

Much progress has been made in developing and expanding the scope of measures of child and adolescent health and health care quality. However, a comprehensive set of ideal measures does not yet exist for children and adolescents that can support the types of analyses needed in both of these areas. What is available instead is a patchwork of measures of health and health care quality drawn from different population surveys, administrative data sets, and longitudinal studies of children and adolescents, each of which was designed for different specific purposes, as reviewed above. In the absence of a framework that can prioritize selected measures of health outcomes, health services, or care processes, it is difficult to achieve an appropriate balance between population-based measures of health and service-based measures of health care quality. Separate efforts to strengthen both systems of measurement are currently under way at the federal, state, and local levels, as well as in private-sector initiatives (see, for example, How et al., 2011; IOM, 2011a; NQF, 2011). But the nation lacks a coherent strategy and process for coordinating these efforts and for establishing national priorities to guide emerging health informatics efforts at the federal, state, and local levels. One example of the latter activity is the new Health Indicators Warehouse, part of the Community Health Data Initiative (Bilheimer, 2010), which is aimed at improving data transparency and timeliness and access to federal health and health care data sets.

The committee believes a coordinated approach is needed to link these data sets and recommended measures to accomplish several objectives:

- prioritize the health domains that should inform the next generation of quality improvement efforts;
- suggest strategies by which child health indicators could be developed from existing child and adolescent data sources; and
- identify gaps that should be addressed through future research on health measures or enhanced data collection efforts.

Any effort to create such an integrated approach is challenged by multiple factors:

- a lack of consensus on the fundamental areas of health that are important to monitor both for the general population of children and adolescents and for vulnerable groups;
- the absence of high-quality state-level data that make it possible to monitor the health status of children and adolescents over time;

- a growing realization that children's and adolescents' health status and levels of functioning are frequently influenced by social and economic factors;
- methodological challenges in establishing relationships among children's and adolescents' health status, insurance status, use of health care services and their quality, care processes, and health outcomes;
- the recognition that access to and utilization of high-quality health care services may be insufficient to compensate for adverse social and economic conditions within families and communities; and
- the persistent inability within various data sets to link measures of children's and adolescents' health status with measures of social and economic status and family conditions.

A coordinated approach is a necessary step toward building consensus on the definition of health and the types of health indicators that are important to monitor in assessing the health status of children and adolescents, especially those from disadvantaged and underserved communities.

SUMMARY

This chapter has provided an overview of current methods used to collect data and demonstrated how the consistency and rigor of measurement methods are directly associated with the quality of the data collected. In examining the measurement of child and adolescent health and health care, the committee identified several key findings that highlight areas in which current measurement efforts fall short. In particular, the evidence reveals a need for greater consistency, standardization, and interoperability of data.

From its examination of the evidence, the committee determined that consistent standards for data elements, based on common definitions of key concepts, are necessary to facilitate the integration of data across health care systems and geographic areas. In particular, greater consistency is needed in measuring such characteristics as insurance coverage. Improving linkages among administrative record systems and between population-based survey data sets and administrative records would enhance the comprehensive assessment of child and adolescent health and the quality of their health care. Finally, the emergence of EHRs and personal health records (PHRs) has the potential to provide an important and novel source of primary data for assessing health and health care quality. The committee believes that the use and interoperability of EHRs and PHRs will create a robust source of data that can be readily analyzed and acted upon.

4

Existing Measures of Child and Adolescent Health

Health is not bought with a chemist's pills,
nor saved by the surgeon's knife.
Health is not only the absence of ills,
but the fight for the fullness of life.

—*P. Hein Prologue at the celebration of the 40th anniversary of the World Health Organization (1988), Copenhagen*
(Reprinted with permission by WHO)

Summary of Key Findings

- Multiple data systems capture information on specific health conditions, but there appears to be overlap in their populations and content. Moreover, measures are inconsistent across states, and no current mandate exists for comparability and standardization.
- Current data collection systems for monitoring health frequently fail to address important social and environmental factors that influence children's health outcomes. Likewise, data collection systems that monitor educational performance or children's well-being frequently omit health data.
- Multiple recommendations for improving health measures for children and adolescents have emerged in recent years. However, current federal surveys do not yet include a robust set of measures of positive health, functioning, development, and health potential within a life-course framework.
- Significant disparities in health status and health care quality currently exist for a variety of racial, ethnic, and sociodemographic populations of children.

91

- Social and economic conditions influence child health. Such conditions include not only household income and educational level, but also such factors as racial and ethnic identity, family structure, immigrant status, urban/rural location, and health literacy.
- Multiple environmental factors influence child health, many of which are outside the purview of the health care system.
- Data on community factors are frequently available in non-health surveys (e.g., environmental surveys, educational surveys, or child victimization surveys).
- A life-course approach provides a basis for understanding the relationships among early health conditions, health influences, and later health status.
- Child health is strongly influenced by family and especially maternal health (e.g., maternal depression).

The development of conceptually sound and reliable health measures for children and adolescents is of critical importance for policy makers, researchers, clinicians, and families, as well as community leaders and the general public. Child and adolescent health measures can be used to assess the effects of disease or injury on health; to identify vulnerable children in clinical practices and vulnerable population subgroups in health plans or geographic regions; to measure the effects of medical care, policy, and social programs; and to set targets for improving health care (Szilagyi and Schor, 1998). Health measures also can identify general health trends over time to highlight areas of progress as well as emerging areas of concern.

Until the middle of the 20th century, data on infant and child mortality provided a reasonable assessment of child health (Guyer et al., 2000). The neonatal segment of infant mortality (number of infant deaths at less than 28 days per 1,000 live births) provided a window on conditions related to fetal development, complications of pregnancy and delivery, and the newborn period; the postneonatal segment helped in understanding conditions influencing child health through the preschool years (Black et al., 2003; Heron et al., 2010).

The middle of the 20th century saw a decrease in the influence of infectious diseases on child health. A different pattern of morbidity emerged, termed the "new morbidity" (Haggerty et al., 1993; Palfrey, 2006). The conditions dominating child health today often reflect behavioral and developmental problems and chronic conditions, as well as associated social conditions, which are poorly captured in vital statistics systems.

This same period saw the emergence of a wealth of measurement tools in developmental psychology for assessing normal child development, including Ages and Stages Questionnaires (ASQ), Bayley Infant Neurodevelopmental Screens (BINS), Parents' Evaluations of Developmental Status (PEDS), and the Wechsler Preschool and Primary Scale of Intelligence (WPPSI), among others. The application of these measures, however, has been limited by both conceptual and practical issues. The conceptual issue is that theories of developmental psychology are still evolving and do not agree on the selection of appropriate domains for assessment. A comparison of several well-established child health measures, for example, reveals 14 separate dimensions of child health (Landraf et al., 1996). Moreover, many of the dimensions, such as learning disabilities, require sophisticated testing by trained examiners. Practical issues include provider time, reimbursement, and differential skill requirements for administering the instruments.

Early efforts focused specifically on measures of child health status that would capture issues related to functional abilities were patterned after more well-established adult measures (Eisen, 1980; Starfield et al., 1993). For example, many adult health function measures inquire about the impact of health issues on work and can be adapted to inquire about school for older children. For preschool children and infants, however, such adaptation is limited, as the activities of younger children are focused more on attaining developmental skills necessary to attend school and participate in other activities. Further, data on the validity and reliability of even established measures are relatively sparse for pediatric outcomes. Validity is established most commonly by the ability of the instrument to yield different scores when administered to healthy children and those with established diagnoses. Most instruments have not been used in a longitudinal fashion, moreover, so that information on predictive validity is lacking, and little has been done to validate responses against clinical observations. For example, if a mother reports that her child has difficulty in play activities, does this indicate a lack of stamina, a lack of coordination, or a lack of social skills? Alternatively, does it reflect the mother's lack of understanding of what developmentally appropriate play looks like at that age?

Since the adoption of quality improvement initiatives under the Children's Health Insurance Program Reauthorization Act (CHIPRA), as well as new quality efforts authorized under the Patient Protection and Affordable Care Act (ACA), the Congress and public and private health agencies have begun searching for valid, reliable, and accessible health and health care measures that can support the implementation and evaluation of these efforts. Ideally, such indicators would provide the capacity at the national, state, and local levels both to monitor the overall health of children and adolescents and to analyze the quality of health care services offered to both the general population and vulnerable groups of children and adolescents.

An ideal set of health measures would inform comparisons of the status of children and adolescents served by different health plans (both public and private) and the types of health issues associated with different providers (pediatricians versus nurse practitioners and primary versus specialty care) and health settings (such as hospitals or ambulatory care settings). These measures would provide opportunities for states or regions of the country to monitor the conditions of children and adolescents in areas relevant to their own circumstances.

Ideally, robust health indicators would reveal significant trends and changes in health status over time for the general population of children and adolescents, as well as special groups that are at particular risk for poor health outcomes and frequently are not identifiable in the major population-based data sources. Such groups of vulnerable children include those whose health may require special attention because of particular or multiple conditions of disadvantage, such as those in certain income categories; those in certain racial or ethnic groups (such as American Indians or Alaska Natives); those who live in homes in which English is not the primary language spoken; those in residential or institutional care (such as foster care); those who are uninsured or underinsured; and those who reside in certain geographic areas, such as selected census tracts, rural environments, or regions with low numbers of health care providers (underserved communities).

Finally, in an ideal world, child and adolescent health measures would support analyses of the ways in which economic and social circumstances influence health status. Such analyses might include the relationships among children's insurance status, their access to health providers, and their use of and the effectiveness of health care, as well as the relationship between child health status and family income, family stability and preservation, and children's school readiness and educational achievement and attainment. The measures would also make it possible to examine relationships between the health status of children and adolescents and their educational performance, their social behaviors, and their future health status and productivity as adults.

The remainder of this chapter examines the current status of child and adolescent health measures; measures of health care quality are discussed in Chapter 5. The first section takes a detailed look at existing measures, including their strengths and limitations. Issues of the timeliness, quality, public transparency, and accessibility of currently available data on child and adolescent health are then addressed. Next, the chapter turns to the challenges of aggregating, synthesizing, and linking multiple sources of these data. This is followed by a review of efforts to make the data more meaningful by linking population health indicators and public health interventions.

EXISTING MEASURES OF CHILD AND ADOLESCENT HEALTH

In preparing a review of existing measures of child and adolescent health, the committee identified seven priority areas for measurement, current related measures, and the existing sources that provide data on these measures. The priority areas are based on the committee's collective judgment and emerged through careful deliberations, a thorough review of the literature, workshop presentations from a variety of engaged stakeholders and experts, and an extensive review of existing data sets. The committee considered the strengths and limitations of measures within each priority area, as well as the extent to which national and state-based data sources are available within each area. The seven priority areas are

- childhood morbidity and mortality,
- chronic disease conditions,
- preventable common health conditions (especially mental and behavioral health and oral health),
- functional status,
- end-of-life conditions,
- health disparities, and
- social determinants of health.

In addition, the committee considered the life-course approach, discussed in detail in Chapter 2, to be an overarching priority area that is integral to all seven areas listed above. The committee therefore contends that measurement should be informed by a life-course perspective and includes in this section a review of the limited number of existing measures and data collection efforts related to the life course.

Using these priority areas as a starting point for examining the existing array of measures and data collection efforts differs from previous approaches. For example, the IOM-NRC report *Children's Health, the Nation's Wealth* (2004) focuses on the specific measures of child health included in selected national surveys (e.g., up-to-date immunizations or nutrition adequacy). Instead, the approach used in this report enables those who are interested in a particular aspect of child and adolescent health (e.g., preventable common health conditions) to readily identify the most relevant currently available data sources. The sections that follow review child and adolescent health measures and data sources according to the seven priority areas, as well as the life-course approach; a more comprehensive review of the relevant data sets is included in Appendix D.

Childhood Morbidity and Mortality

A considerable amount of data related to child and adolescent morbidity and mortality is routinely collected and analyzed. Surveillance of injuries and fatalities among young people, for example, provides insight into one aspect of how children are doing and underscores how their epidemiology differs from that of adults. While unintentional injuries are a leading cause of death among Americans of all ages, they are the leading cause of death among children and adolescents aged 1–19 (Bernard et al., 2007) (see Box 4-1). Young children (under age 4) are especially vulnerable to life-threatening injuries (e.g., suffocation, drowning, and injuries related to motor vehicle crashes) (CDC, 2006).

Three primary sources of data are used nationally to track morbidity and mortality: the National Vital Statistics System (NVSS), the Medical Expenditure Panel Survey (MEPS), and the Healthcare Cost and Utilization Project (HCUP).

BOX 4-1
Leading Causes of Death Among Children and Adolescents

Accidents* are by far the leading cause of death among children and adolescents. The top three causes of death by age group are listed below.

Ages 0–1:
- Developmental and genetic conditions present at birth
- Sudden infant death syndrome
- All conditions associated with prematurity and low birth weight

Ages 1–4:
- Accidents/injuries
- Developmental and genetic conditions present at birth
- Cancer

Ages 5–14:
- Accidents/injuries
- Cancer
- Homicide

Ages 15–24:
- Accidents/injuries
- Homicide
- Suicide

---

* The preferred term for "accidents" is "unintentional injuries."
SOURCE: NIH, 2010b.

The NVSS is maintained by the National Center for Health Statistics (NCHS) within the Centers for Disease Control and Prevention (CDC). Federal reports frequently use data from the NVSS to monitor trends in child and adolescent mortality on a regional, national, and international basis. NVSS data are collected through ongoing reports from vital statistics officers in 50 states and the District of Columbia and reflect the cause of death that is recorded on individual death certificates, providing the basis for analyses of the leading causes of childhood morbidity and mortality. The data are organized by age and gender, as well as selected racial and ethnic groups. The NVSS relies on *International Classification of Diseases* (ICD) codes to describe health conditions, disorders, diseases, and injuries. For the most part, the ICD codes are organized by disease or injury categories, such as different types of cancers or congenital conditions, infectious and parasitic diseases, endocrine conditions, mental disorders, disorders of pregnancy and childbirth, poisonings, drowning, and so forth.

Hospitalization data for children and adolescents are collected through such data sources as the MEPS, as well as such syntheses of public–private data collection efforts as the HCUP. MEPS data are collected through a nationally representative survey of U.S. civilian households. The data provide information on the utilization and cost of health services, as well as on the cost, scope, and breadth of private health insurance held by and available to the U.S. population. HCUP data include a census of hospital discharge billing records collected from 40 states. The data provide information on reasons for hospitalization, length of hospital stays, procedures during hospitalization, and treatments received for specific conditions while in the hospital.

As a part of HCUP, the Agency for Healthcare Quality and Research (AHRQ) developed a database specifically designed to allow in-depth studies of children's hospitalizations—the Kids' Inpatient Database (KID). The KID is a stratified probability sample of pediatric discharges from 2,500–4,000 community hospitals in the United States (defined as short-term, nonfederal general and specialty hospitals, excluding hospital units of other institutions). The purpose of KID data, which are drawn from an all-payer (Medicaid, private insurance, and uninsured) inpatient care database for children, is to identify, track, and analyze national trends in utilization, access, charges, quality, and outcomes for inpatient hospital services.

Large claims-based data sets available from insurers and vendors also are commonly used in research on health care utilization and on prevalence of disease. Examples include the Medstat Marketscan data set and the data sets of Blue Cross Blue Shield, Wellpoint/HealthCore, and Kaiser Permanente.

Data collected by the HCUP and the KID reveal the most common reasons for admission to the hospital among children aged 17 and younger.

The overwhelming majority—approximately 95 percent—of these admissions are for the birth of infants (Owens et al., 2003). Newborns, or children 30 days of age or less, account for approximately 4.8 million hospital stays or 73 percent of all childhood admissions (Elixhauser, 2008). Affective disorders, including depression and bipolar disorders, are the sixth most common reason for hospital admissions among children, accounting for 82,500 discharges. Adolescent pregnancy is one of the leading causes of hospitalization for females younger than 17. For adolescent boys, hospitalization occurs primarily as a result of unintentional injuries (Owens et al., 2003).

Strengths

NVSS data provide a rigorous classification scheme for deaths associated with an array of health conditions, including pregnancy, abortions, and various types of injuries that are common among children and adolescents. The data can be pooled and analyses conducted over multiple years by gender, race and ethnicity, and geographic location (state and county level) to highlight trends that may not be apparent within a single time period. The NVSS E-codes provide supplemental information about the cause of injury (such as motor vehicle crash or child maltreatment). The rigor of the data classification and the ongoing data collection support analyses of trends among racial and ethnic minority groups that are often difficult to detect in studies that rely on household surveys or other data sources. For example, one CDC study of fatal injuries among children by race and ethnicity (1999–2002) highlighted disproportionate rates of deaths due to motor vehicle injuries among American Indian/Alaska Native children, as well as higher rates of drowning deaths among black infants and American Indians/Alaska Natives aged 1–19 (Bernard et al., 2007). Linked death and birth records permit the examination of infant deaths by characteristics of the parents and can be used to compare the mortality experience of different subpopulations (IOM, 1993). Linked records also provide insight into access to prenatal and delivery care and some outcomes of pregnancy (Marquis and Long, 2002; Schoendorf and Branum, 2006).

Data collected through the MEPS and HCUP may be more accurate and reliable than survey data. For example, data obtained directly from providers, such as specific diagnoses and treatment, are less likely to be affected by recall bias than comparable data obtained from surveys based on self-reports (Cohen, 2004). Hospital discharge data can often be linked to other data sets, including data from the social services, criminal justice, education, housing, and other sectors (Schoenman et al., 2005).

The KID's large sample size enables analyses of both common and rare conditions. The database comprises more than 100 clinical and nonclinical variables for each hospital stay, including primary and secondary diagnoses and procedures, admission and discharge status, patient demographics (e.g., gender, age, race, median income for ZIP code), expected payment source, total charges, length of stay, and hospital characteristics (e.g., ownership, size, teaching status). The KID contains clinical and resource use data included in a typical discharge abstract, but excludes data elements that could identify individuals directly or indirectly. Analyses of HCUP and KID data on rates of hospital admissions for specific conditions per population or rates of specific events per procedure can provide the hospital and reimbursement perspective on health care quality in terms of effectiveness and patient safety (Berdahl et al., 2010). Children can be identified by age in the Household Component of the MEPS, allowing most MEPS analyses to be performed for children. In 2001, a Child Health and Preventive Care section was added to the survey. It contains questions previously included in the 2000 Parent Administered Questionnaire, selected questions related to children that had been asked in previous years, and additional questions related to child preventive care.

Limitations

Morbidity and mortality data provide information for only the most severe health consequences, which involve a relatively small number of children and adolescents. Those who are concerned with children's health status often want to know more than just the presence or absence of specific health problems in the general child population at a given point in time. They want to know the sequence of health conditions that may contribute to morbidity and mortality events, as well as the relationship between selected health conditions and certain social characteristics. They want to know whether children who have access to certain family resources, certain types of health care providers, or certain environmental and social conditions fare better than those who do not. And increasingly, they want to know whether children are on track to become healthy adults, especially those young people who display early signs of poor health conditions that are associated with adverse health outcomes and chronic disease in older populations.

While NCHS can link vital statistics data with other data sources (including census data, Supplemental Nutrition Program for Women, Infants, and Children [WIC] program data, and hospital discharge data), NVSS data alone are limited in the information they can provide. For example, NVSS data do not capture fetal mortality experience by special populations (e.g., populations that are relatively small in number). Furthermore, challenges to data collection, including frequent item nonresponse, variation in state reporting requirements, and racial misclassification, may limit the overall quality and utility of NVSS data (Hoyert and Martin, 2002). The NVSS also does not collect information about family or other household characteristics (e.g., socioeconomic status), nor does it collect data on the types of health plans associated with selected health conditions or injuries. Hospital discharge data, of course, are limited in that they capture only those events that occur in a hospital. Moreover, the HCUP does not include data from all states, and less populous states are underrepresented. Further, the HCUP is not designed specifically for pediatric issues and does not allow for longitudinal studies of individuals. It is unclear whether the KID has the capacity to capture a representative sample of uncommon and rare diagnoses.

Chronic Disease Conditions

The number of children and youth in the United States identified as having chronic health conditions has increased considerably in the past four decades. Data from the 2009 National Health Interview Survey (NHIS), for example, indicate that 14 percent (more than 10 million) of children in the United States aged 17 and under have ever been diagnosed with asthma and that 10 percent (7.1 million) of children still have asthma. The 2009 survey also found that 9 percent (5 million) of children aged 3–17 had attention-deficit/hyperactivity disorder (ADHD) (Bloom et al., 2010). More than 12 million U.S. children meet the definition of children and youth with special health care needs—those at "increased risk for chronic physical, developmental, behavioral, or emotional conditions that require health and related services of a type or amount beyond that required of children generally" (McCormick et al., 2011; McPherson et al., 1998, p. 138). This group accounts for roughly 15–20 percent of the childhood population and for 80 percent of annual health care expenditures for all children (Newacheck et al., 1998b). Whether the increase in the number of children and adolescents with chronic health conditions is the result of environmental changes, better survival rates for once-fatal conditions, or increased access to care through Medicaid expansions and the Children's Health Insurance Program (CHIP), it represents a significant trend (Van Cleave et al., 2010).

The NHIS is conducted annually and collects data on health indicators, health care utilization and access (including current health insurance coverage), and health-related behaviors for the U.S. civilian noninstitutionalized population. As a household survey, the NHIS collects data on all members of the household, including children, adolescents, and adults. Data collected through the NHIS are used to monitor trends in illness and disability and to track progress toward the achievement of national health objectives (Bloom et al., 2010).

The National Survey of Children's Health (NSCH), first introduced in 2003 and subsequently fielded in 2007, is one of the most comprehensive surveys of child and adolescent health that offers national as well as state-level data (NCHS, 2010b). Data collected through the NSCH support analyses of physical, emotional, and behavioral child health indicators, as well as contextual factors. The next NSCH survey, planned for 2011, will expand the measurement of insurance adequacy beyond "having coverage" to include items regarding the actual providers and services covered by the child's insurance policy, the costs of services not covered by the deductible, and the overall adequacy of benefits (Bethell and Newacheck, 2010).

The NSCH is complemented by two other national surveys—the National Survey of Children with Special Health Care Needs (NS-CSHCN) and the National Survey of Early Child Health (NSECH). The NS-CSHCN was first conducted in 2001 and again in 2005–2006 to monitor states' provision of services to children with special health care needs through federal programs, such as Title V and Supplemental Security Income (SSI) (Blumberg et al., 2003; van Dyck et al., 2002). The NS-CSHCN measures more than 100 indicators of children's health and well-being for children enrolled in these programs in six key areas: health status, health care, school and activities, family and neighborhood, young children (aged 0–5), and school-aged children (aged 6–17). The NS-CSHCN was developed to measure the prevalence among children of both chronic conditions (e.g., asthma; attention-deficit disorder [ADD]/ADHD; depression, anxiety, or other emotional problems; mental retardation; and seizure disorders) and functional difficulties (e.g., respiratory problems, behavioral problems, chronic pain, and self-care), as well as services received and satisfaction with care (Blumberg et al., 2003; CAHMI, 2006; van Dyck et al., 2002).

The NSECH is a nationally representative household survey of children aged 4–35 months that produces national and regional estimates. It was administered once, in 2000. Planning for a possible NSECH-II has been under way for several years, but no plan for its readministration has yet been developed. Survey questions include child developmental status, provision of recommended preventive services for which parents are valid reporters (e.g., anticipatory guidance, some screenings, and family-centered care), parenting behaviors and home safety, health insurance status, early childhood program enrollment, and utilization of services (Halfon et al., 2002).

The above three national surveys obtain national and state-based samples that are weighted to represent the general population of noninstitutionalized children and adolescents. They all rely on a household survey platform known as the State and Local Area Integrated Telephone Survey (SLAITS), which is conducted by NCHS to support the design and sampling frame for the ongoing National Immunization Survey. The SLAITS operates by calling household telephone numbers at random to identify households with one or more children under 18. In each household, one child is randomly selected to be the subject of the interview.

Strengths

Key strengths of the NHIS include its large and carefully constructed sample size, its well-tested questionnaire items, and the fact that it is conducted annually (IOM, 1993). Another strength of the NHIS is that it can be linked to other surveys and data sources, including the MEPS and death certificates in the National Death Index (NDI). These linkages to multiple years of data produce a rich database that includes medical care utilization data.

The NSCH, NS-CSHCN, and NSECH allow analysts to collect information from parents about the health and well-being of their children, as well as the social and economic conditions of the family, such as household income and type of insurance coverage (public or private), in a fairly short time period. By relying on the common sample pool developed by the SLAITS, these surveys can be conducted by telephone in English and Spanish at relatively low cost. The NSCH national data support analyses by gender, age group, race/ethnicity, household income, and insurance status, as well as type of insurance plan (public or private). Sample sizes in these surveys are sufficient for state-based analyses.

Limitations

The NHIS was redesigned in 1997, and the current survey differs somewhat from earlier versions in content, format, and data collection method. These changes can hinder comparisons between 1997–2009 NHIS estimates and those from earlier years (Bloom et al., 2010). Like other surveys, moreover, the NHIS relies on respondents' recall and self-reports of health status, which may be imprecise compared with health examination data or medical record abstracts (IOM, 1993).

While the NSCH sample is sufficient to represent the general U.S. population of children and adolescents, the survey does not adequately represent large numbers of disadvantaged children who may rely on Medicaid or CHIP health plans for their health services, nor does it include children or adolescents who reside in group homes or juvenile detention centers and who may be at greatest risk of poor health outcomes. For example, the sample is too small to document rates of chronic health conditions, such as sickle cell disease, that may be relatively rare in the general population but more common among certain racial and ethnic groups of children and adolescents. Moreover, the NSCH is a periodic survey, and its data are confined to the years in which the survey was conducted.[1] Also, because the NSCH

---

[1] Legislation to expand state-level indicators of child well-being has been introduced in the House (H.R. 2558) and Senate (S.1151). The legislation would expand the range of data collected in the existing NSCH and provide for collection of the data on an ongoing basis or annually (U.S. Congress 111th, 2009).

relies on the SLAITS platform, the data it collects are limited to residential telephone numbers (e.g., land lines), and parental participants are restricted to those who speak English or Spanish. In addition, cellular telephone technology may have a significant impact on the scope and quality of the survey data, especially in households that rely solely on cell phones and may not want to participate in national surveys because of time restrictions on cell phone use (Blumberg and Luke, 2007; Blumberg et al., 2006; Brick et al., 2007). In terms of specific measures, the NSCH does not collect data on neonatal or perinatal conditions or on child mortality. Nor does it collect data on the English proficiency of parents, so the impact of limited English proficiency cannot be assessed. As noted, the NSCH also is administered in English and Spanish only, which limits the conclusions that can be drawn regarding the primary language spoken at home. Finally, several limitations result from the fact that the survey is conducted with a parent or caregiver, which may contribute to under-, over-, or inaccurate reporting:

- Parental reports of child or adolescent health conditions, insurance status, or household income are not verified by a review of individual health or financial records.
- Parents may not be familiar with the type of insurance coverage in their health plan (e.g., managed care versus preferred provider networks).
- The survey relies on parental reports of diagnoses of their child's health conditions. Parents may not know the specifics of the health conditions affecting their child, may not be familiar with the types of screening instruments or early intervention services offered to their child, and may not recall specific aspects of their child's treatment and/or care.
- The parents of an adolescent may not be aware that their child has accessed confidential mental health, drug treatment, and/or reproductive health services.

Preventable Common Health Conditions (Especially Mental and Behavioral Health and Oral Health)

Apart from mortality and hospitalization data, as well as data on children with special needs and/or chronic health conditions, a number of population-based child health indicators are used as the basis for the early detection of health conditions that are likely to contribute to chronic conditions during either childhood or adulthood. Since 1980, CDC has established national health objectives for improving the health of all Americans (PHS, 1980). These objectives focus on a range of largely preventable health conditions that contribute to the leading causes of mortality and morbidity and are frequently associated with unnecessary hospitalizations among children, adolescents, and adults. Many of these health conditions are targets for specific health care interventions to prevent or delay the onset or reduce the severity of avoidable health problems.

A variety of national data sources suggest childhood trends that are particularly disturbing in some areas. For example:

- As discussed in Chapter 2, the growing epidemic of childhood obesity has emerged as a major public health problem throughout the nation (IOM, 2005).
- Another disturbing trend noted in Chapter 2 is the near doubling of the proportion of children and adolescents with asthma since the 1980s (Akinbami, 2006).
- While the oral health status of most Americans has improved over the last two decades, the prevalence of dental caries (or tooth decay) in primary teeth increased significantly among children aged 2–5 (from approximately 24 to 28 percent), and dental caries has remained the most prevalent chronic disease of childhood (Dye et al., 2007).
- A recent study providing "the first prevalence data on a broad range of mental disorders in a nationally representative sample of U.S. adolescents" estimated that one in five children and adolescents in the United States meets criteria for a mental disorder (see also Chapter 2). Among those surveyed, 31.9 percent met the criteria for anxiety disorders, 19.1 percent those for behavioral disorders, and 14.3 percent those for mood disorders (Merikangas et al., 2010a).

NCHS collects data from vital and medical records and interview surveys and through physical examinations and laboratory testing. These data provide important surveillance information that helps identify and address critical health problems. Major survey-based data collection efforts include the National Health and Nutrition Examination Survey (NHANES), the NHIS, the SLAITS, and the NSCH. These surveys measure children's health to varying degrees and occur at different intervals, annual and periodic. (See Appendix D for a comprehensive review of data sets that measure children's health and related influences.) The Pregnancy Risk Assessment and Monitoring System (PRAMS), another data collection effort conducted by CDC, provides state-specific, population-based information on women's health during pregnancy, birth outcomes, and the postpartum period. Thirty-seven states currently participate in the PRAMS (CDC, 2010d). The National Survey of Family Growth (NSFG) is a periodic survey of women and men aged 15–44 that collects data on factors related to birth and pregnancy rates (e.g., sexual activity, contraceptive use, and infertility) (Martinez et al., 2010); factors related to marriage, divorce, cohabitation, and adoption (Goodwin et al., 2010); and attitudes regarding sex, childbearing, and marriage (Martinez et al., 2006). In addition, the survey collects a range of social, demographic, and economic data (Lepkowski et al., 2010). The NSFG is considered a significant part of CDC's public health surveillance for women, infants, and children.

The NHANES is an annual survey that collects data on the health and nutritional status of U.S. adults and children. The survey is administered to a nationally representative probability sample of about 5,000 noninstitutionalized U.S. civilians each year. The NHANES is unique in that it combines interviews and physical examinations of sample respondents (NCHS, 2010a). The interview includes questions regarding diet and health, socioeconomic status, and demographics. The physical examination includes medical, dental, and physiological measurements, as well as laboratory tests. Data from the NHANES are used to determine the prevalence of major diseases and risk factors for diseases, including the prevalence and treatment of mental disorders (Merikangas et al., 2010b), trends in childhood obesity and the prevalence of high body mass index (BMI) (Ogden et al., 2010), and high asthma prevalence among subgroups of children and adolescents (Rodriguez et al., 2002).

The Youth Risk Behavior Surveillance System (YRBSS) monitors priority health risk behaviors among youth and young adults, such as those that contribute to unintentional injuries and violence, tobacco use, and alcohol and other drug use; sexual behaviors that contribute to unintended pregnancy and sexually transmitted diseases (STDs); behaviors that contribute to obesity (e.g., unhealthy dietary behaviors and physical inactivity); and those that contribute to asthma. Similar to the NHIS, the YRBSS monitors activities that constitute priority health risk behaviors because they "contribute to the leading causes of morbidity and mortality among youth and adults, often are established during childhood and adolescence, extend into adulthood, are interrelated, and are preventable" (CDC, 2008, p. 1). These behaviors are important to measure because they help in understanding the general quality of life for younger populations. They also provide insight into behavioral trends and health conditions that may evolve into significant health problems as these young people become adults.

In contrast to population health surveys based on diagnosed conditions that fit within the ICD-9 categories, surveys of risk behaviors are designed to identify the behaviors or settings that may contribute to future health disorders as children and youth become adults. In earlier decades, for example, smoking among adolescents was not a health behavior that elicited a medical response. But as the lifetime risks associated with the use of tobacco became well documented among adults, public health and clinical efforts emerged to encourage early intervention and preventive strategies that would reduce the onset and prevalence of smoking behaviors, especially in younger populations.

Strengths

The NHANES is one of the largest and longest-running national sources of health data from a nationally representative sample of U.S. adults. The survey's sample size is sufficient to detect differences among time periods. One of the survey's key strengths is its rigorous study protocol for data collection; physical examinations and the collection of biological and environmental specimens adhere to extensive quality control procedures, and technicians are trained and certified in all data collection procedures. To improve the statistical reliability of its estimates, the NHANES has relied on oversampling of certain subgroups, including Latinos, African Americans, adolescents (aged 12–19), adults aged 60 and older, and low-income whites (NCHS and CDC, 2006). As noted in the report *Children's Health, the Nation's Wealth*, both the NHANES and the YRBSS dedicate significant time to interviewing children regarding behaviors related to adverse outcomes (e.g., substance abuse) (IOM and NRC, 2004).

Multiple years of data are available for the NHANES, the PRAMS, the NSFG, and the YRBSS to support trend analysis. These trend data can help states, communities, and schools with program and policy decisions regarding child and adolescent health.

Both the PRAMS and the YRBSS generate state-specific data but also allow comparisons among states through the use of standardized data collection methods. For example, the CDC Model Surveillance Protocol establishes the data collection method for the PRAMS. Participating states follow the protocol but also can customize it to some extent to meet their needs (CDC, 2009). Similarly, the YRBSS questionnaire can be adapted from the CDC-developed core instrument. This flexibility allows states and localities to address their unique needs and goals. The NSFG is one of the few data sources that follow both men and women from adolescence through young adulthood and include service data as well as data on behaviors and outcomes.

Limitations

Surveys of risk behaviors involve more ambiguity and less precision than the collection of data on established conditions. Studies of sexual assault and intimate partner violence, for example, suggest that such experiences often are associated with emotional and mental disorders that are not detected until many years after the initial victimization experience. It is difficult, therefore, to establish clear thresholds for the criteria that should be used in deciding on the inclusion of such indicators in population health surveys.

Despite the need for timely and state-specific data on child health, current data collection efforts are limited in their ability to provide such data. The NHIS and the NSFG have samples that are too small to provide statistically reliable data for every state. It is therefore necessary to combine multiple years of data to obtain useful estimates for most states. The YRBSS and PRAMS are not conducted in every state. The YRBSS depends on local school authorities and state departments of education to conduct the survey, and the sample does not include children who have dropped out of high school or other adolescents who do not participate in high school surveys, a group whose health may be at greater risk relative to the general population. Further, the survey is anonymous, so it cannot be linked to other characteristics of the children sampled. Finally, the YRBSS lacks an established coding system with which to provide an overall "health score" for respondents.

The report *Children's Health, the Nation's Wealth* (IOM and NRC, 2004) provides a thorough explanation of the limitations of the NHIS and NHANES, including sample sizes that are too small to conduct analyses by racial and ethnic subgroups or by ages and stages of development. The report concludes that "neither of these surveys provides the information needed to develop a comprehensive picture of the health of young children, to better understand the role of various risk and protective factors during early childhood, to assess their access to personal or public health services, or to measure the impact of health care on health" (IOM and NRC, 2004, p. 113). Further, for small population groups and less prevalent conditions and diseases, data must be accumulated over several years to provide adequate estimates. The NHANES also lacks the ability to measure important behavioral and mental health conditions (IOM and NRC, 2004).

Some federal data sources monitor selected health behaviors, focusing on specific categories of risky practices, such as the use of alcohol or unsafe sexual behaviors. These federal data sources are scattered across multiple agencies, such as the National Institute on Drug Abuse, the National Institute on Alcoholism and Alcohol Abuse, and the Substance Abuse and Mental Health Services Administration. CDC strives to integrate data from these separate surveys as baseline measures for its Healthy People initiative. However, no single federal database currently monitors a comprehensive set of health behaviors that could incorporate trends involving all of the concerns discussed above.

Functional Status

The decline that has occurred in childhood mortality and the increase in the number of children and adolescents in the United States identified as having chronic health conditions have led to a greater need to measure functional status, or how well children are able to perform their daily activities and their ability to maintain health and well-being (Stein and Jessop, 1990). The report *Children's Health, the Nation's Wealth* defines functioning as "all aspects of physical, psychological, cognitive, and social functioning as they express themselves in children's daily activities and behavior" (IOM and NRC, 2004, p. 35). This increasingly important aspect of child and adolescent health can be used to estimate the extent of an injury and to gauge the impact of an acute and chronic health condition. Further, measures of functional status offer a fuller picture of how well children are doing compared with mortality and morbidity statistics, which are often single measures (e.g., infant mortality or incidence and prevalence of type 2 diabetes). Functional status measures offer a view into the impact of multiple conditions as well as the effects of their treatment, including side effects (IOM and NRC, 2004), and provide a common measure for assessing the health of children across conditions (Stein and Jessop, 1990; Stein et al., 1987).

There can be either mitigating or complicating factors in functional status, or both, depending on the condition and the affected individual. These may include factors intrinsic to the child (such as personality, genetic endowment, or the existence of comorbidities) or resources and/or conditions external to the child (such as his or her physical environment and support system or the availability of ameliorative medical equipment and medications).

Recent data regarding child and adolescent functional status underscore its significance:

- In 2007, approximately 8 percent of children aged 5–17 were reported by parents to have activity limitations due to chronic conditions (FIFCFS, 2009).
- More than 60 percent of children with special health care needs have health conditions that affect their daily activities (FIFCFS, 2009).
- According to one recent study, overweight and obese adolescents were more likely than adolescents with a normal BMI to report one or more functional limitations (e.g., limitations in attending school, limitations performing strenuous acts, and difficulty with personal care and hygiene) (Swallen et al., 2005).

- Approximately 1.4 million children with some kind of activity limitation were aged 14–17, a critical period for planning for the transition to adulthood (IOM, 2007).

Knowledge gained from measuring child and adolescent functional status is valuable both for individual- and population-based efforts. At the individual level, measures of functional status have great meaning because of their implications for caregiving, dependence, and the ability to participate in social roles. At the population level, measures of functional status provide insight into demands on systems of care and support, including early intervention and rehabilitation needs, distribution of resources, and housing and transportation issues (Altman et al., 2006). Understanding the functional status of children and adolescents is critical not only for providing support and services today, but also for planning to meet future demands, especially as adolescents' transition into adulthood (Lotstein et al., 2005).

Given the profound development that occurs over the life course of a child, accurate measurement of physical, psychological, social, emotional, and cognitive status presents significant challenges. Repeated measurement of a child's or adolescent's functional status is therefore necessary to determine the impact of a disease or condition over time (to gauge both improvements and deteriorations in health). One major challenge is to develop measures that are "well defined, quantitative, rapid, reliable, minimally dependent on subjective assessments, and applicable to as broad an age range as possible" (Pollack et al., 2009, p. e19).

Currently, health surveys assess functional status through single survey items or nested items (IOM and NRC, 2004). These questions are generally focused on limitations in functioning related to school or play, which are considered the main functional arenas of children. Ideally, functional status would include more complete descriptions of levels of functioning in a variety of settings and roles.

The primary sources of data on functional status are the NS-CSHCN, the NHIS, the NHANES, and the National Longitudinal Study of Adolescent Health (Add Health). Add Health is a longitudinal study of a nationally representative sample of adolescents. It was designed to examine the influence of individual attributes and the impact of social environments (e.g., families, friends, schools, communities, and neighborhoods) on health and risk behaviors. Add Health is currently the largest, most comprehensive survey of adolescents in the United States. The most recent phase of the study included the collection of biological data (e.g., biomarkers for metabolic, immune, and inflammatory processes). These data will provide additional insight into the interactions among social, behavioral, and biological influences on health over time; achievement outcomes in early adulthood; and childhood antecedents of adult disease (Udry et al., 2009).

Strengths

Generally, national health surveys include questions regarding some aspect of a child's physical health. In fact, measures of functional status are most often focused on measures of physical function (e.g., impairments or deficits in mobility; ability to perform usual activities; or deficits in hearing, vision, or speech). The NHIS, for example, includes questions on limitation of activity in its "child core" to determine limitations in movement and whether the causal impairment is expected to last a year or more. More recently, some surveys—including the NHIS, the NHANES, and to an even greater extent Add Health—have adopted a broader definition of child and adolescent health, and now evaluate aspects of cognitive, emotional, and even social functioning. The NS-CSHCN focuses exclusively on children with special health care needs, and some reports, such as *America's Children* (FIFCFS, 2009), which draws on data from a collection of national surveys, address this population. Overall, however, measures of functional status in these sources are relatively limited in nature. Measures that capture the broader perspective of what constitutes health, as defined by *Children's Health, the Nation's Wealth*, are more often included as the focus of issue-specific, one-time surveys rather than in ongoing surveys.

Limitations

One of the most significant gaps in the assessment of child and adolescent health is the evaluation of positive aspects of functional status (IOM and NRC, 2004). Many surveys include questions regarding impairments in functioning; relatively few include routine questions about positive functional trajectories. Overall, ongoing national surveys remain limited in their view of health, so that most of their questions focus on the absence of illness.

As noted earlier, surveys often ask about functioning in terms of limited activity (e.g., the amount of play for children under age 5), but seldom address *overall* health functioning. This is a significant gap because many children, even those with extreme impairments, are able to play and attend school. Therefore, these measures may be a poor estimate of their overall functioning.

Existing measures of child functional status are time-consuming (Bayley, 1993; Sparrow et al., 2006), apply to a limited age range (CFAR, 1993), or rely heavily on subjective clinician and caregiver assessments (Fiser et al., 2000a, 2000b). Moreover, current efforts to measure functional status do an inadequate job of reflecting the dynamic state of disease and recovery and fail to provide information needed to predict long-term health outcomes. Validation of measures has, for the most part, been restricted to cross-sectional examinations of how scores differ for children with different conditions, and few instruments are suitable for children younger than 5–7. With the exception of the disease-specific scales, little has been done to correlate reports of functional limitations with clinical observations; virtually no predictive validity work has been done that could demonstrate how a measure of functional status at a particular point in time has implications for planning for later services; and it is difficult to reconcile specialized assessments (e.g., developmental milestones, behavior problems, autism symptoms) with general health status. Thus, the lack of measures that assess health potential and provide a more comprehensive assessment of functioning is a significant gap (Pollack et al., 2009). To enhance current efforts to measure child and adolescent functional status, the report *Children's Health, the Nation's Wealth* suggests:

> The utility of existing data and a more complete range of data on physical, cognitive, emotional, and social functioning, as well as disability and restriction of activity, would be enhanced by adoption of the WHO International Classification of Functioning (ICF), as it becomes better known by practitioners and survey organizations. This system is designed to inventory different aspects of participation in a wide range of daily activities and to assess the structural and environmental barriers that impede or facilitate functioning. However, it has not yet been adapted to be rapidly used in clinical care or in surveys. (IOM and NRC, 2004, p. 103)

Because WHO's ICF considers contextual factors of disability—and not just medical or biological dysfunction—it can be used to develop public health goals, form functional status assessments, guide disability management in infectious disease programs, and improve disability statistics in a wide range of settings.

Another opportunity to enhance efforts to measure health functioning and quality of life is the National Institutes of Health's (NIH's) Patient-Reported Outcomes Measurement Information System (PROMIS). Although the activities of this network of NIH-funded primary research sites and coordinating centers focuses primarily on adults, its pediatric component is growing and suggests a likely direction for future measurement.

End-of-Life Conditions

Children may experience terminal conditions at various stages in their young lives. Some children start life with a reduced life expectancy, while others contract a life-threatening illness during childhood. The most recent final death counts from NCHS indicate that 53,287 children and adolescents (through age 19) died in 2007 (Xu et al., 2010). The most recent report with a breakdown of deaths among children and adolescents is from 2006. It suggests that end-of-life care likely was needed for the 14.8 percent of young patients (aged 5–14) who died of malignancies, 5.6 percent who died of congenital conditions, and 4.1 percent who died of heart disease (Heron, 2010).

Patients, their families, and physicians are likely to have a difficult time accepting a prediction of imminent death. This is particularly true for children and adolescents, whose families and medical providers do not want to give up on attempts at a cure (Stephenson, 2000). The situation is further complicated by the fact that it can be difficult for physicians to predict time of death with a great deal of accuracy, particularly for children. One study found that in only 20 percent of cases is the date of death reliably predictable within 6 months (Stephenson, 2000), while other authors have noted that this is particularly true for children (Feudtner et al., 2001, 2009). Part of the reason is that children and adolescents can go into and out of terminal illness phases, and in some cases, it may not be clear whether they will ultimately succumb to or recover from an illness (Stephenson, 2000).

According to a previous IOM report, *When Children Die*, "The National Center for Health Statistics, the National Institutes of Health, and other relevant public and private organizations, including philanthropic organizations, should collaborate to improve the collection of descriptive data—epidemiological, clinical, organizational, and financial—to guide the provision, funding, and evaluation of palliative, end-of-life, and bereavement care for children and families" (IOM, 2003b, p. 355). To date, no national data have been collected for these purposes. Without such data and related measures, it is impossible to monitor progress in helping dying children gain the best possible quality of life.

In 2004, the Nursing Home Survey added questions on advance directives and end-of-life care, and in 2009, the National Home and Hospice Care Survey added questions regarding end-of-life care. To date, no such questions have been included in national surveys of children and their families.

The committee considers it critically important to track end-of-life conditions for children and adolescents. The committee also recognizes that this is a frontier area for measurement in child and adolescent health. *When Children Die* outlines areas important to children and adolescents experiencing life-threatening and -limiting illnesses, and these areas could form the foundation for data collection and measurement (IOM, 2003b). Chapter 5 looks at end-of-life conditions as they relate to the quality of child and adolescent health care services.

Health Disparities

As for adults, disparities in health status and health care are pervasive in children, with important and often lifelong consequences (Pearlin et al., 2005; Shone et al., 2005). Such disparities exist based on race, ethnicity, primary language, special needs, socioeconomic status, and geography (Callahan and Cooper, 2004; Newacheck et al., 1996; Satcher, 2000; Shone et al., 2003). Each data source in the above five areas provides an opportunity to examine health disparities among selected populations, most frequently racial and ethnic minorities. In most cases, however, the pool of minority populations in the survey samples is not large enough for use in considering health issues that are of particular concern to certain groups or certain regions of the United States. The outcomes of the experience of illness among children and adolescents in poor households may be different from those among children and adolescents with access to greater social and economic resources, but these interactions are extremely difficult to examine. Similarly, health indicators for children and adolescents in urban and rural settings may differ significantly.

Another important characteristic of the major national health surveys is that they automatically exclude children and adolescents who reside in institutional or group care settings. In 2007, nearly half a million (492,818) children lived apart from their families in out-of-home care (CWLA, 2010). Following these children is particularly important as they are at increased risk for mental health disorders (Wasserman et al., 2004), poor developmental outcomes (Jones, 2004), and substance abuse (Shufelt and Cocozza, 2006) relative to children and adolescents in the general population (Otto et al., 1992). The underrepresentation and omission of key groups of vulnerable children and adolescents have prompted the development of targeted surveys that focus on the health status of specific populations, such as children and adolescents in poor households, those served by child welfare agencies, and those in juvenile detention settings.

As noted in Chapter 2, compared with U.S. adults, U.S. children are disproportionately of nonwhite race/ethnicity and more likely to live in poverty or low-income households, and the number of children in these economic circumstances is growing. Poor and minority children have disproportionately high special health care needs compared with their nonpoor and white counterparts, and they are more frequently insured through public health programs such as Medicaid and CHIP (Horn and Beal, 2004).

In 2010, the Committee on Pediatric Research of the American Academy of Pediatrics (AAP) reported that racial and ethnic disparities in children's health are "extensive, pervasive, and persistent and occur across the spectrum of health and health care" (Flores, 2010, p. 1). The AAP committee examined 111 original research papers published between 1950 and March 2007, focusing on health disparities involving four major U.S. racial/ethnic minority groups: African Americans, Asians/Pacific Islanders, Latinos, and American Indians/Alaska Natives. Health conditions of children and adolescents from each of these four groups were compared with health conditions of white children and adolescents. The AAP committee organized its findings into nine areas: mortality rates, health status, adolescent health, chronic diseases (particularly asthma and mental health), prevention and population health, special health care needs, access to care and use of services, quality of care, and organ transplantation. Highlights from the AAP report include the following:

African American children:

- African American children have the highest asthma prevalence of any racial/ethnic group. The prevalence rate in this population is substantially higher than that in white children, and the severity of the disease is worse as measured by rates of asthma mortality, hospitalization, and emergency department and office visits. The disparity in rates of asthma mortality and hospitalization has widened over time (Akinbami and Schoendorf, 2002).
- The mortality rates for young African American children (aged 1–4) are more than twice those for white children; disparities also occur for older children (aged 5–14) (Singh and Kogan, 2007). The mortality disparity ratio has increased in the past decade.

Latino children:

- Latino children exhibit a wide range of disparities in access to care and use of services in comparison with non-Latino white children, including greater adjusted odds of being uninsured (Flores et al., 2005b), having no usual source of care or health care provider, not having seen a physician in the past year, having gone a year or more since the last physician visit, making fewer physician visits in the past year (Shi and Stevens, 2005), not being referred to a specialist (Flores et al., 2005b), having a perforated appendix (Guagliardo et al., 2003), never or only sometimes receiving medical care without long waits, receiving timely routine care or phone help, and experiencing brief wait times for medical appointments (Brousseau et al., 2005).
- Relative to non-Latino whites, Latino children have a significantly higher unmet need for mental health care (Sturm et al., 2003) and lower odds of making any mental health visit (Kataoka et al., 2002), receiving an antidepressant prescription (Richardson et al.,

2003), and receiving treatment from a mental health specialist for any mental health condition or behavioral problem (Kataoka et al., 2002).

Asian/Pacific Islander children:

- Native Hawaiian children have a higher crude mortality rate than that of white children (Singh and Yu, 1996).
- Disparities have been reported for Asian/Pacific Islander children in the areas of injuries, lead intoxication, obesity, and nutrition (Lee et al., 2006; Neumark-Sztainer et al., 2002; Roesler and Ostercamp, 2000). These children have the highest proportion of elevated blood lead concentrations in the state of Rhode Island and were the only racial/ethnic group whose rate increased over time (Flores, 2010).

American Indian/Alaska Native children:

- American Indian/Alaska Native children have a firearm injury rate more than seven times higher than that of white children (Roesler and Ostercamp, 2000).
- These children have higher adjusted odds than white children of being in poor or fair health and the highest prevalence of these suboptimal health ratings of any racial/ethnic group (Grossman et al., 1994).

Oral health disparities parallel overall health disparities, with children of nonwhite race/ethnicity having higher levels of dental disease (HHS, 2000b). Further, oral health disparities by race/ethnicity among children and adolescents have been shown to exist independently of socioeconomic status and attitudes toward preventive care (Dietrich et al., 2008).

Health data from most national population surveys and administrative records include gender and racial/ethnic identifiers that support analyses of health disparities for these categories. However, many researchers have recognized that significant health disparities among children and adolescents result from social determinants associated with access to social or economic resources (Braveman et al., 2004).

One source of data on health disparities is the Survey of Income and Program Participation (SIPP), a continuous series of national longitudinal panels administered by the U.S. Census Bureau. The SIPP collects information on poverty, income, employment, and health insurance coverage from a representative sample of the U.S. civilian noninstitutionalized population. Each panel ranges in duration from 2 to 4 years and includes household interviews every 4 months. In addition to providing longitudinal data from the core survey, the SIPP includes topic modules that provide valuable cross-sectional data on a variety of subjects, including costs and characteristics of child care, adult and child well-being, child disability, general health status, and utilization of health care services (Weinburg, 2003).

The National Survey of Child and Adolescent Well-being (NSCAW) collects nationally representative longitudinal child- and family-level data from children in the child welfare system and their biological parents, caregivers, teachers, and caseworkers, as well as from administrative records. Data are collected through face-to-face interviews at baseline and subsequent annual intervals. The data set consists of two samples of children: those who were the subject of child abuse or neglect investigations conducted by child protective services agencies, and those who had been in out-of-home or foster care for approximately 1 year and whose placement had been preceded by an investigation of child abuse or neglect (NSCAW Research Group, 2002). The data collected address child and family risk factors, service needs and utilization, and agency- and system-level factors likely to be related to child and family outcomes. Child outcomes of interest include health and physical well-being, cognitive and school performance, mental health, behavioral problems, and social functioning and relationships. Multiple years of data are available for secondary analysis through the National Data Archive on Child Abuse and Neglect (NDACAN).

Most of the national surveys (e.g., NHIS, MEPS, and NHANES) also include measures of race/ethnicity and some measures of socioeconomic status that allow for robust analyses of disparities. When sample sizes are small, as is the case when the focus is on specific ethnic groups, these data sets have the advantage of being collected on an annual basis, thereby allowing for data aggregation across two to three years to achieve adequate sample sizes.

Strengths

One of the unique contributions of the SIPP is that, in addition to routinely collecting data on household earnings and employment, it collects data on household composition and medical expenses. Collectively, these data provide insights into disparities and social determinants of health. Further, the SIPP periodically collects data on such topics as shelter costs and assets that enhance understanding of the interplay between socioeconomic well-being and overall health and well-being. Both the SIPP and the NSCAW are longitudinal studies and therefore provide important information on participants over time. Like the SIPP, the NSCAW collects data on nonmedical determinants of health (e.g., community environment, family characteristics, caregiver behavior) that relate to child and family well-being. The NSCAW also documents experiences of children and parents with the child welfare system, other concurrent life experiences, and outcomes by developmental stage to demonstrate how these factors affect children's well-being.

Limitations

The research literature reporting health disparities for different racial/ethnic groups is uneven in part because the available data on these disparities are uneven. For example, data on Asian/Pacific Islander children are sparser than those on African American or Latino children. Only 24 of the 109 race/ethnicity-specific studies in the AAP Technical Report address disparities in Asian/Pacific Islander children (Flores, 2010). Further, current groupings of Latinos or Asian/Pacific Islanders include culturally heterogeneous subgroups with quite different sets of risks and outcomes (e.g., "Latino" may include Mexicans, Puerto Ricans, and Central Americans). These groupings convey a false sense of homogeneity that may mask disparities.

Disparities that arise from differences in access to social and economic resources and networks are difficult to study in large data sets because socioeconomic information is often limited in routine data sources on health. Often when income information is included, the range of income levels reported is too narrow to permit meaningful comparisons across a range of income groups. For example, the highest income category reported is often "$75,000 or higher"; $75,000 is not a high income level when it supports a family of four to six, a common family size. To understand the role of social factors in child health, one must be able to compare not just poor or low-income persons with everyone else (typically the only comparisons that can be made with most routine data sources), but also risk factors and outcomes among poor, near-poor, low-moderate-income, moderate-income, and high-income groups.

Parental education categories also may be too broad to permit meaningful socioeconomic distinctions. Sometimes income and education are included in the data sets but not in routine reports. One study of more than 20 publications from NCHS released in 2009 revealed that fewer than half examined differences by income (with income usually being considered as a percentage of poverty) or education (most using only three categories—did not complete high school, high school graduate, and at least some postsecondary education) (Braveman et al., 2010).

Furthermore, reliable and complete data with which to measure disparities do not exist in some state-level data sets. In some cases, however, these data can be supplied through linkages. For example, application forms for Medicaid and CHIP are a primary source of information on race, ethnicity, and primary language of the child or family at the state level. Data from accepted applications then inform the state's Medicaid or CHIP eligibility files. Parent-provided information on race, ethnicity, and language is, therefore, often considered the best source of demographic information.

Some states link these eligibility files with claims files and rely on the eligibility files for demographic data. They can then use the linked data set to examine services delivered to children with given diagnoses by racial, ethnic, or language groups. Hence, the eligibility files are an important platform for measuring disparities in health care. Yet these data are collected in varying, nonstandard ways across states, making the development of a national picture of disparities difficult or impossible. For example, only 18 states include Hispanic/Latino ethnicity as a separate category, while 19 merge ethnic and racial categories. Of these, 7 allow the applicant to choose more than one "race"; hence, an individual could select both black and Hispanic. Eight states have no race/ethnicity categories, instead leaving a blank for applicants to fill in. With respect to primary language, 14 states offer the choice of English, Spanish, and either "other" or specific other languages; however, 21 states have only a blank space in which applicants are to fill in their primary language. The nonstandard way in which race, ethnicity, and language data are collected in eligibility files hinders comparisons of data across states for purposes of monitoring disparities in service delivery (IOM, 2009d). It should be noted that these variations are the result of the uniquely diverse and increasingly multiracial makeup of the United States. It should not be surprising if challenges related to nonresponse and changes in response over time regarding race and ethnicity continue to occur when individuals are asked to self-identify in one category.

Access to NSCAW data is limited, and the data are unavailable for use by potential stakeholders, including, notably, employees at child welfare agencies. The sample size is too small for adequately assessing certain subpopulations of interest, including American Indians/Alaska Natives. Finally, bias due to selection into services could play a significant role in the NSCAW. For example, more challenged children and families receive more services but may still fare worse.

Social Determinants of Health

Studies of the health and wellness of children in vulnerable circumstances have placed particular emphasis on the importance of measuring events, exposures, relationships, or experiences that are present or absent within the child's or youth's physical and social environments, particularly those interactions and relationships that support or disrupt bonds essential to healthy development. In the field of youth development, a particular focus is on assessing the presence of caring adults and prosocial relationships that support adolescents and young adults during difficult transitions in life. For children and youth with special health care needs, the emphasis has been on the creation of medical homes that can coordinate and monitor their health care across multiple settings and providers. For children and youth with serious emotional disorders, the Substance Abuse and Mental Health Services Administration funds the System of Care initiative to provide supportive settings for limited communities.

This interest in assessing the impact of the physical environment, the health care delivery system, and social contexts on the current health status and healthy development of young people has generated several key studies aimed at linking specific childhood experiences, events, or relationships with selected health behaviors and health outcomes. Yet few population health databases include data on indicators of positive health (e.g., self-esteem, resiliency, and social support) for children and adolescents. Furthermore, few sources of data on the health indicators discussed in the preceding sections support examination of the relationships among these indicators, the social contexts of children and youth (including family, peer, and community relationships), and their health care services and settings.

The YBRSS and NSCH, discussed above, provide data relevant to social determinants of child and adolescent health. A third source of such data is a new initiative, the National Children's Study (NCS). As discussed in Chapter 3, the NCS is the largest long-term study of environmental and genetic effects on children's health ever undertaken in the United States. It will examine the effects of environmental influences on the health and development of approximately 100,000 children across the United States, following them from before birth until age 21 (NRC and IOM, 2008). Data collected by the NCS will be archived over time and are intended to serve as a valuable resource for analyses many years into the future.[2] This ambitious undertaking has the potential to provide much-needed insights into nonmedical determinants of health, among other critical aspects of child and adolescent health. In 2008, the National Research Council (NRC) and the IOM conducted an in-depth review of the NCS study design and research plan (NRC and IOM, 2008). The strengths and weaknesses of the study are described briefly below.[3]

Strengths

Two of the greatest strengths of the NCS are its large sample size (100,000), which will facilitate analyses of both common and rare con-

---

[2] As of early 2011, the NCS was in its pilot phase (NIH, 2010c).
[3] For a more in-depth review, see The National Children's Study Research Plan: A Review (NRC and IOM, 2008).

ditions, and its longitudinal design (preconception through age 21). The probability sample also was notably well designed (NRC and IOM, 2008). The prospective data collection should minimize the effect of potential recall errors.

Limitations

Questions remain regarding the feasibility of the NCS recruitment strategy (specifically with respect to enrolling women in their homes who are likely to become pregnant, as opposed to recruiting pregnant women from prenatal sites of care) (Savitz and Ness, 2010), as well as plans for managing the data collection and participant retention (NRC and IOM, 2008). The NRC and IOM (2008) report also raises concerns regarding the adequacy of the study's pilot phase. Aside from asthma, the NCS does not have a sufficient number of children with specific conditions to permit detailed analyses of the quality of care. It should be noted that in August 2008, those responsible for the NCS issued an extensive response to the NRC/IOM review, and in the intervening years they have worked to address several of the report's recommendations.[4] The ultimate value of the study, however, is unknown, and will depend on its ability to address the shortcomings identified in the present report.

A Life-Course Approach

The life-course approach helps explain patterns of health and disease across populations and over time. Chapter 2 describes the growing recognition of the ways in which health influences occurring during early childhood—and even interactions with maternal health during the prenatal and preconception stages—lay the foundation for health throughout the lives of children, adolescents, and adults (Ben-Shlomo and Kuh, 2002; Halfon and Hochstein, 2002; Kuh and Ben-Shlomo, 1997).

Fine and Kotelchuck (2010) identify four key life-course concepts:

- Today's experiences and exposures influence tomorrow's health. (Timeline)
- Health trajectories are particularly affected during critical or sensitive periods. (Timing)
- The broader community environment—biologic, physical, and social—strongly affects the capacity to be healthy. (Environment)

---

[4] For additional information, see http://www.nationalchildrensstudy.gov/newsannouncements/announcements/Pages/ncs_response_NAS_review_082608.pdf.

- While genetic make-up offers both protective and risk factors for disease conditions, inequality in health reflects more than genetics and personal choice. (Equity)

Existing measurement efforts are limited in their ability to provide complete information related to timeline, timing, environment, and equity. However, these four concepts are drawing growing attention and provide a basis for the development of new approaches in measuring child and adolescent health.

One aspect of the life-course perspective that has drawn particular attention is the proposal that broad social, economic, and environmental factors may affect health during critical periods of development (e.g., factors associated with the childhood antecedents of adult disease, including those that emerge during fetal development, childbirth, early infancy, and the transition into adulthood). For example, numerous studies have demonstrated an association between negative stimuli, such as undernutrition during fetal development, and lasting or lifelong consequences for health (Alexander, 2006; Barker, 2002; Godfrey and Barker, 2001). Disruptions in fetal and organ development, known as "fetal programming," may increase vulnerability to environmental stressors later in life and have been observed to be associated with coronary heart disease (Barker, 2002) and hypertension (Alexander, 2006). Poor health in childhood also can have significant and long-term implications for educational attainment, socioeconomic status, and productivity. As noted in Chapter 2, for example, analyses of the Panel Survey of Income Dynamics (PSID) reveal that low birth weight has the effect of "aging" an individual by 12 years (Johnson and Schoeni, 2007).

Because the life-course perspective is inherently based on the idea that health is more than the absence of disease, it aligns well with the expanded definition of health adopted by the committee. Moreover, the life-course perspective provides a dynamic approach to monitoring and measuring child and adolescent health and encompasses the seven priority areas for child and adolescent health outlined earlier. Therefore, the committee regards the life-course perspective as an overarching area of focus for measurement.

In addition to life-course indicators, interest has grown in looking beyond the measurement of specific health conditions to focus on positive states of health, wellness, functioning, and health potential during important transition periods, especially early childhood and adolescence. Attention is increasingly being paid to the importance of monitoring the presence of healthy behaviors, such as adequate sleep, good dietary habits, and physical activity. Attention is being focused as well on assessing the mental and emotional status of children and youth, including their safety, resiliency, and capacity to deal with the stresses of daily life, as well as the challenges of certain health conditions, harsh environments, or traumatic experiences. Moreover, many experts in child health and development have emphasized the importance of assessing the functional and developmental status of children and adolescents, focusing on measures that describe their language and motor skills, as well as their capacity to self-regulate their emotions, interact with peers and adults, and perform age-appropriate tasks. Such measures are not commonly viewed as health measures, but they are included in several child and adolescent health surveys and provide indicators of the functional or developmental status of general and selected populations of children and youth.

Currently, the concept of indicators of positive states of health, functioning, and development is relatively new, and a coherent set of priority indicators in these areas is lacking. *Children's Health, the Nation's Wealth* (IOM and NRC, 2004) focuses particular attention on the interactions among children's health; health care services; and health influences, such as poverty and the physical environment. The report recommends several steps, such as integrating existing data sets and offering a conceptual framework that could make better data on these interactions available at the national, state, and local levels (IOM and NRC, 2004).

The literature on developmental milestones is complex since certain behaviors or conditions emerge over several months or years. As a result, it is often difficult to assess developmental status at a specific point in time; such measures require iterative assessments that may involve lengthy intervals and periods of observation. Measures of developmental status may also be subject to extensive bias or variation since they frequently rely on parental reports rather than observation by practitioners who are experienced with the behaviors of large groups of children. Indeed, because many behaviors indicative of poorer functioning or illness cannot be observed during a standard pediatric exam (e.g., sleep, feeding, and behavioral problems), clinicians also must frequently rely on parental reports. Thus there is a clear need to devise better ways of obtaining these data from parents (e.g., questions framed in ways that require less parental inference and more objective behavioral accounts).

Children's Health, the Nation's Wealth (IOM and NRC, 2004) calls particular attention to the need for measures focused on resources that contribute to health and well-being, especially in describing a child's ability to deal with and bounce back from adversity. It defines health potential as "health assets that provide the capacity to respond to physical, psychological, and social challenges and risk states that increase vulnerability to other aspects of poor health" (IOM and NRC, 2004, p. 37). The report distinguishes measures of health potential from measures of child functioning "because of the inherent bias toward defining functioning only as normal or deficient":

> The domain of health potential measures includes positive developmental assets and health capacities that provide and indicate ability to form positive relationships, regulate emotional and cognitive states, and respond to multiple challenges, including exposures to disease and psychological and physical stress, among others. . . . Other characteristics described as resilience factors that fall within this domain include curiosity, responsiveness, reflection, imagination, self-efficacy, problem-solving ability, self sufficiency, optimism, and disease resistance and recovery. (IOM and NRC, 2004, p. 37; see also Starfield et al., 1993)

Two data sources are particularly relevant to a life-course perspective on child and adolescent health: Add Health (discussed above) and the Adverse Childhood Experiences (ACE) study. The ACE is an ongoing collaboration between CDC and Kaiser Permanente's Health Appraisal Clinic in San Diego, designed to assess associations between a range of adverse childhood experiences and health behaviors, health outcomes, and health care use later in life (Felitti et al., 1998). With more than 17,000 participants, the ACE is considered one of the largest studies of its kind (CDC, 2010b). It has produced numerous publications suggesting that certain experiences—including childhood abuse, neglect, and exposure to other traumatic stressors—are risk factors for some of the leading causes of morbidity and mortality in the United States (Anda et al., 2008; Brown et al., 2010; Corso et al., 2008; Dong et al., 2004; Dube et al., 2001; Edwards et al., 2004; Felitti et al., 1998). In addition to Add Health and the ACE, in 2008 five states collected data on adverse childhood experiences as part of the Behavioral Risk Factor Surveillance Survey (BRFSS). The BRFSS is a state-based telephone health surveillance survey conducted by state and local health departments under the guidance of CDC. The survey collects data on health risk behaviors, preventive health practices, and health care access. It is used by all 50 states, the District of Columbia, Guam, Puerto Rico, and the U.S. Virgin Islands; more than 400,000 interviews are conducted each year. BRFSS data can be used to identify and track emerging health problems (e.g., the H1N1 influenza pandemic) and monitor progress toward health objectives (e.g., those of Healthy People).

Strengths

The ACE provides insight into the long-term and potentially multigenerational impacts of adverse childhood experiences. The study, now in its thirteenth year, continues to gather data prospectively on participants from a variety of sources (e.g., outpatient medical records, pharmacy use records, hospital discharge records) to follow their health outcomes and use of health care services (CDC, 2010c).

Limitations

The retrospective reporting of childhood experiences is a potential limitation of the ACE. Respondents may find it difficult to recall specific events. In cases in which childhood abuse has been documented, for example, adult respondents are likely to underestimate the actual occurrence of the abuse upon follow-up (Femina et al., 1990; Williams, 1995). Another limitation relates to the sample included in the ACE. The majority of ACE participants are white (74.8 percent), middle-class adults, the overwhelming majority of whom have completed high school, attended college, or completed college and/or beyond (92.8 percent) (CDC, 2010a). These demographic characteristics limit the extent to which the findings of the study can be generalized.

TIMELINESS, QUALITY, PUBLIC TRANSPARENCY, AND ACCESSIBILITY OF DATA ON CHILD AND ADOLESCENT HEALTH

In its charge, the committee was asked to focus particular attention on the timeliness, quality, public transparency, and accessibility of data on child and adolescent health. Timeliness is a critical element in the assessment and development of measures, as more rapidly released public-use files provide a far more accurate picture of existing conditions than those released long after data collection (NRC, 2010). Public transparency depends on the timely availability and accessibility of quality data to reinforce accountability on the part of responsible agencies (Beal et al., 2004; IOM, 2001a).

A number of online sources are designed to advance the timely and effective use of public data on children, youth, and families in the United States. Box 4-2 includes examples of accessible data sets across the seven priority areas for child and adolescent health that can be used by families, researchers, insurers, policy makers, and advocates to assess the health and mortality experiences of children and adolescents. These include public data sets, aggregations and syntheses of public data (see the next section), and sources that integrate public and private data.

AGGREGATING, SYNTHESIZING, AND LINKING MULTIPLE DATA SOURCES

Title V of the Social Security Act requires annual reporting of state performance and health outcome measurement data, fiscal data and numbers of clients served (individual, source, and service type), screening and treatment data, state priority needs, state Title V initiatives, maternal and child health (MCH) toll-free hotline data, and CSHCN service system data (MCHB, 2010). Although these data are posted in a timely fashion to the Title V Information System website, the data collected on child and adolescent health exist largely in individual silos and are not readily translatable to the seven priority areas discussed above.

In the absence of population or administrative data sources that can link specific experiences or events to selected health behaviors in individual children, many researchers rely on linking selected data sources at the geographic level—for example, census tracts, counties, or states. Typically they link one of the individual-level data sources discussed above with another data source describing the social contexts of children and youth as proxy measures for adverse or supportive environments in a child's census tract, county, or state. Such data include measures describing education, employment, income, and community crime trends for national or regional populations of children and youth.

Box 4-3 provides examples of efforts to aggregate, synthesize, and link data from multiple sources. These include state, local, and national efforts using both publicly and privately collected data. Key sources of data for these efforts include the Current Population Survey (CPS), the American Community Survey (ACS), the National Survey of American Families (NSAF), the National Center for Education Statistics (NCES) surveys, the NVSS, and the BRFSS, among others.

Strengths

Aggregating, synthesizing, and linking data from multiple data sources allows agencies and organizations to convey trends in child and adolescent health to policy makers and the general public. These efforts often generate easy-to-understand reports, fact books, and online tools.

Limitations

Unfortunately, linking multiple data sources cannot capture the dynamics of child and adolescent health and does not provide insight into the interactions among various influences on child and adolescent health. The data sets are frequently based on cross-sectional data, a disadvantage for any effort to link multiple data sources. At present, moreover, financial barriers hinder the ability to access deidentified Medicaid files for purposes of cross-state quality measurement. As a result, current efforts to aggregate, synthesize, and link data result in something more akin to a mosaic than a snapshot of child and adolescent health, falling short of the goal of provid-

BOX 4-2
Selected Online Sources of Data on
Child and Adolescent Health

- **Behavioral Risk Factor Surveillance System (BRFSS) Interactive Databases** provide online access to the state-based system of health surveys that collects information on health risk behaviors, preventive health practices, and health care access primarily related to chronic disease and injury (http://www.cdc.gov/brfss/).
- **CPONDER** is a web-based query system created to access data collected through Pregnancy Risk Assessment Monitoring System (PRAMS) surveys. Users have the ability to design their own analysis by choosing from an indexed list of available categorical variables. Descriptive statistics in the form of proportions are included in the resulting report and corresponding graph. CPONDER contains PRAMS data from 2000 through 2006 for state/year combinations that achieve at least a 70 percent response rate. CPONDER contains 2007 data for PRAMS state/year combinations that achieve at least a 65 percent response rate. As additional years of data are weighted, they will be added to the system (http://www.cdc.gov/prams/cponder.htm).
- **DATA2010** is an interactive database system developed by staff of the Division of Health Promotion Statistics at the National Center for Health Statistics, and contains the most recent monitoring data for tracking Healthy People 2010. Data are included for all the objectives and subgroups identified in the Healthy People 2010: Objectives for Improving Health. DATA2010 contains primarily national data. However, state-based data are provided as available (http://wonder.cdc.gov/data2010/).
- **The Data Resource Center for Child and Adolescent Health (DRC)** provides online access to the survey data that allows users to compare state, regional, and nationwide results for every state and HRSA region as well as resources and personalized assistance for interpreting and reporting findings. DRC includes data from the National Survey of Children's Health (NCHS) and the National Survey of Children with Special Health Care Needs (NS-CSHCN) (http://www.childhealthdata.org/content/Default.aspx).
- **HCUPnet** is a web-based interactive service for identifying, tracking, analyzing, and comparing statistics on hospital care. HCUPnet was created with the intention to make health care data available to the public. HCUPnet allows anyone to access aggregate statistics from these data sets to generate descriptive statistics on many topics of interest, including, for example, the percentage

of hospitalizations for children who are uninsured by state, trends in hospital admissions for specific conditions, quality indicators and information on the expenses of conditions treated in hospitals (http://hcupnet.ahrq.gov/).

- **Health Data Interactive** presents tables with national health statistics for infants, children, adolescents, adults, and older adults. Tables can be customized by age, gender, race/ethnicity, and geographic location to explore different trends and patterns (includes the following data sources: Current Population Survey [CPS], National Ambulatory Medical Care Survey [NAMCS], National Health and Nutrition Examination Survey [NHANES], National Health Care Survey [NHCS], National Health Interview Survey [NHIS], National Home and Hospice Care Survey [NHHCS], National Hospital Ambulatory Medical Care Survey (NHAMCS), National Hospital Discharge Survey [NHDS], National Vital Statistics System [NVSS] [mortality and natality], and population estimates) (http://www.cdc.gov/nchs/hdi.htm).

- **MEPSnet/HC** is an interactive query tool that generates statistics of health care use, expenditures, sources of payment, and insurance coverage for the U.S. civilian noninstitutionalized population. However, none of the *Child Health and Preventive Care* section variables are available on MEPSnet/HC (http://www.meps.ahrq.gov/mepsweb/data_stats/MEPSnetHC.jsp).

- **National Center for Health Statistics**. Data files for the National Survey of CSHCN can be downloaded in SAS file format at no cost from the National Center for Health Statistics website (http://www.cshcndata.org).

- **National Immunization Survey Public Use Data Files** are available for statistical analysis or reporting purposes through the National Center for Health Statistics (http://www.cdc.gov/nis/data_files.htm).

- **WISQARS™** (Web-based Injury Statistics Query and Reporting System) is an interactive database system that provides customized reports of injury-related data (http://www.cdc.gov/injury/wisqars/index.html).

- **Youth Online** is an online database allows users to analyze national, state, and local Youth Risk Behavior Surveillance System (YRBSS) data from 1991-2009. Data from high school and middle school surveys are included. Users can filter and sort on the basis of race/ethnicity, sex, grade, or site, create customized tables and graphs, and perform statistical tests by site and health topic (http://apps.nccd.cdc.gov/youthonline/App/Default.aspx?SID=HS).

NOTE: Descriptions are verbatim from source websites.

BOX 4-3
Examples of Efforts to Aggregate, Synthesize,
and Link Multiple Data Sources

State and Local Governments/Health Departments

California Report Card (Children Now)
The Children's Agenda (Montgomery County, Maryland)
Children's Score Card (Los Angeles County)
Delaware Children's Health Chartbook (Nemours)
MassCHIP (Massachusetts Department of Public Health)
North Carolina Child Health Report Card (Action for Children North Carolina, NC IOM)

National

America's Children: Key National Indicators of Well-Being (Federal Interagency Forum on Child and Family Statistics)
America's Health Starts with Healthy Children: How Do States Compare? (Robert Wood Johnson Foundation)
The Child and Youth Well-Being Index (The Foundation for Child Development)
Child Health USA (Health Resources and Services Administration/ Maternal and Child Health Bureau)
Child Trends DataBank (Child Trends)
The Child Well-Being Index (The Foundation for Child Development)
Indicators of Youth Health and Well-Being: Taking the Long View (Stagner and Zweigl, 2007)
Key Indicators of Health and Safety: Infancy, Preschool, and Middle Childhood (Hogan and Msall, 2008)
Kids Count (Annie E. Casey Foundation)
Appendix A: Datasets for Measuring Children's Health and Influences on Children's Health, in *Children's Health, the Nation's Wealth* (IOM and NRC, 2004)
Appendix B: Gaps Analysis of Measures of Children's Health and Influences on Children's Health in Select National Surveys, in *Children's Health, the Nation's Wealth* (IOM and NRC, 2004)
Appendix C: Selected Indicators from National Children's Data Syntheses, in *Children's Health, the Nation's Wealth* (IOM and NRC, 2004)

---

ing a complete and accurate picture. Technology may make it possible to achieve this goal in the near future. Chapter 2 provides a brief overview of the implications of health information technology (HIT) for child and adolescent health. A more in-depth analysis of future implications of HIT for health and health care services is provided in Chapter 6.

EFFORTS TO MAKE DATA MEANINGFUL BY LINKING POPULATION HEALTH INDICATORS AND PUBLIC HEALTH INTERVENTIONS

During the past three decades, efforts have been undertaken within public health and child advocacy centers to link population health data with national, state, and local initiatives designed to ameliorate those factors that contribute to adverse health outcomes for children and youth. These efforts have emphasized identifying health conditions and behaviors that would benefit from public health interventions, as well as changes in social and economic settings, as opposed to medical treatments. Three such efforts are the Healthy People program, administered by CDC; *County Health Rankings*, developed within several states and published by The Robert Wood Johnson Foundation; and the Kids Count initiative, funded through the Annie E. Casey Foundation.

The Healthy People 2010 and forthcoming Healthy People 2020 objectives provide a comprehensive agenda for nationwide health promotion and prevention of disease, disability, and premature death; they serve as a road map for improving the health of all Americans during the first decade of the 21st century. CDC relies extensively on health measures drawn from the NHIS and other data sources in the implementation of the Healthy People initiatives (HHS, 2000a).

Healthy People 2010 includes 28 focus areas with 467 specific objectives. One of the 28 focus areas is maternal, infant, and child health, and 107 of the objectives pertain to adolescents and young adults. The two overarching goals of Healthy People, which are applicable across the life course, are to increase quality of life and years of healthy life and eliminate health disparities. A recent report on progress toward the Healthy People 2010 objectives describes mixed results for child and adolescent health. On the one hand, between 1996 and 2008, exposure of children to tobacco smoke at home and exposure to environmental tobacco smoke showed significant progress (reductions of 69.2 percent), and immunization of children aged 19–35 months increased by 10.9 percent. On the other hand, overweight in children and adolescents increased by 58.7 percent (Sondik et al., 2010).

Efforts to finalize the Healthy People 2020 objectives have been under way since December 2010. Early indications point to a continued commitment to eliminating health disparities and a greater focus on the social determinants of health that have a disproportionate impact on specific racial/ethnic populations (Sondik et al., 2010). Two new overarching goals will be added: "promoting quality of life, healthy development, and healthy behaviors across life stages; and creating social and physical environments that promote good health" (Koh, 2010, p. 1656).

The Robert Wood Johnson Foundation's *County Health Rankings* ranks the overall health of every county in all 50 states. The rankings are based on a model of population health that includes health outcomes (based on equal weighting of length and quality of life) and health factors (weighted scores for health behaviors, clinical care, social and economic factors, and the physical environment) (see Figure 4-1) (Booske and UWPHI, 2010). The rankings are based on data from multiple sources, including

- the BRFSS;
- the NCHS;
- the National Center for Chronic Disease Prevention and Health Promotion (Division of Diabetes Translation);
- the National Center for Hepatitis, HIV, STD, and TB Prevention;
- the Environmental Protection Agency (EPA) Collaboration;
- the Health Resources and Services Administration;
- the CPS;
- the Federal Bureau of Investigation;
- Medicare claims; and
- the National Center for Education Statistics.

Bethell (2010) has identified four key questions to be considered in aligning population health indicators with efforts to improve the quality of health care services for children and youth:

- Should the emphasis be on leading causes of death and most common reasons for using medical care or on the prevalence of ongoing health conditions (also described as the low-volume/high-cost versus high-volume/low-cost trade-off)?
- Should the population health measures be condition-specific (e.g., reflect the ICD categories), or should the broad-based, consequences-focused definition used in the survey of children with special health care needs (NS-CSHCN) be adopted?
- What effort should be directed toward indicators of risk versus established conditions (e.g., overweight and obesity, or risks for developmental delay or substance use)?
- Should population health indicators aim to address categories of conditions (e.g., mental and behavioral health, oral health, injuries)?

SUMMARY

This chapter has reviewed the relative strengths and limitations of measures of the health of children and adolescents based on population

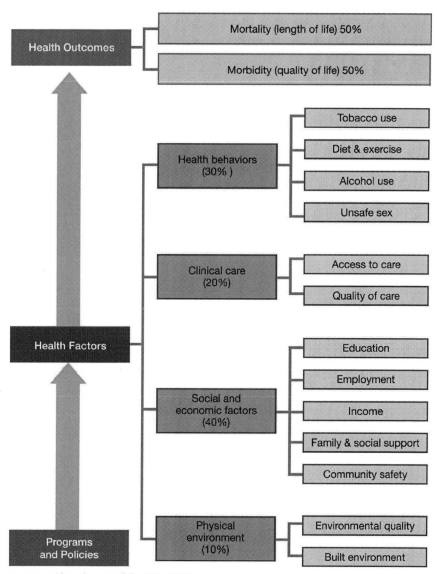

County Health Rankings model ©2010 UWPHI

FIGURE 4-1 *County Health Rankings* model.
SOURCE: Booske and UWPHI, 2010.

health and administrative data sources. This review has highlighted the diversity and complexity of existing measures while calling attention to areas in which existing data systems are insufficient to address key topics of interest. For example:

- A lack of standardization in the measurement of disparities in health limits the ability to identify, monitor, and address persistent health disparities among children and adolescents.
- Current child health measures lack the capacity to capture important functional data and developmental stages; valid measures in these areas that have been tested across diverse populations do not yet exist.
- Most child and adolescent health data sets lack the capacity to support efforts to track the life-course implications of child health events, especially those that occur in early stages of development.

The committee has identified seven priority areas for future measures that could provide relevant information on the health of children and adolescents for policy makers, service providers, and the general public and also inform quality improvement efforts within public and private health plans. The committee also has emphasized the importance of using a life-course approach, which may require changes to current public- and private-sector criteria and methods for the selection of existing and the development of new health quality measures. Indicators generated from data acquired with a life-course perspective in the seven priority areas should make it possible to examine specific conditions and issues of particular importance to vulnerable and underserved children and adolescents, especially those served by Medicaid and CHIP programs. Such conditions and issues might include

- gestational and perinatal issues that impact child health, such as prenatal care;
- unique neonatal issues, such as prematurity and low birth weight;
- health issues in the transition of those with chronic illnesses from adolescence to young adulthood (particularly in light of health reform changes that include coverage of children under their parents' health insurance until age 26);
- chronic childhood conditions that impact adult health, such as Down syndrome, cystic fibrosis, childhood cancer, and congenital heart defects; and
- opportunities presented by the NCS, which will follow subjects from preconception to age 21.

Ideally, child and adolescent health quality measures should support analyses that can demonstrate how changes in funding levels for public insurance programs (such as Medicaid or CHIP) or changes in eligibility requirements, enrollment levels, or service procedures would affect child health outcomes, school achievement, and health care costs. Such measures should also be useful in assessing whether and how the organization and delivery of health care achieve public goals of effectiveness, efficiency, safety, timeliness, equity, and patient satisfaction. Realizing these goals will require capacity for state-level analyses because Medicaid and CHIP are executed and managed at the state level, and there has historically been significant state-level variation in eligibility, coverage, and access to providers.

Additional themes that deserve attention include the following:

- the distinction between low-incidence/high-cost conditions and those that reflect the most common child and adolescent health disorders;
- significant trends in child health, health care access and quality, and outcomes (e.g., immunization coverage rates);
- indicators of resilience and protective factors/effects; and
- comorbidities (because of their potential multiplier effects).

Finally, the seven priority areas, as well as a life-course perspective, should be used to direct analysis toward possible emerging threats to child health as a test of how comprehensive and useful this taxonomy can be in generating priority indicators for child and adolescent health.

5

Measures of Quality of Child and Adolescent Health Care

Summary of Key Findings

- The prevalence and the aggregate cost of treatment of complex health conditions are lower for children and adolescents compared with the high cost of hospital care for adults and older adults.
- Measurement of health care quality for children and adolescents serves the same purposes as that for adults—accountability, quality improvement, and population health. However, the development of quality measures for child and adolescent populations has been slow to emerge from the private sector because enhanced quality is unlikely to produce short-term reductions in health care costs (in contrast to the results associated with quality improvement efforts for adults and older adults).
- The Centers for Medicare and Medicaid Services uses only seven standardized measures to assess care for children and adolescents enrolled in Medicaid programs, and these measures apply only to those who are enrolled in Medicaid managed care plans. These measures involve some of the most common chronic medical conditions, preventive services, and acute care. However, they generally measure specific elements of care rather than serving as comprehensive measures, and they miss

important areas of health (mental health, oral health, and in-patient care) and care processes (particularly care coordination across multiple settings).

- The effectiveness of preventive services is particularly difficult to measure because the outcomes may not be known for many years, and the impact may vary according to the risk profile of the patient population. Current preventive measures are largely process focused, and do not consider the outcomes of screening efforts or whether recommended treatment services were actually provided in an effective, evidence-based, equitable, family-centered, or timely manner. This is the case largely because the measures are derived from the claims data generated by a single visit.

- The number of children and adolescents who live in poverty or in low-income families (generally considered to be below 200 percent of the federal poverty level) is higher relative to adults, a fact that has a significant influence on their health outcomes. For example, high-quality asthma care may produce marginal outcomes for children and adolescents whose housing conditions create persistent risk factors for this condition.

- The measurement of quality of care for children with special health care needs requires attention to their functional status and care transitions as well as their health conditions. Functional status measures for children and adolescents are not standardized, however, and frequently rely on parental reports rather than comparison of a child's behavior or skills with those of others with similar health conditions.

- Variations in the definitions of race, ethnicity, and primary language in state databases are major obstacles to the development and use of heath care quality measures for children and adolescents. A few states have made efforts to gather demographic data by linking their Medicaid or CHIP eligibility files to their claims data sets, but such strategies are not in common use.

- Many states and some local districts have demonstrated interest in expanding the number and types of measures used to assess quality of care, as well as in applying the measures to children and adolescents enrolled in public and private health plans. Several states and local districts already collect data that can identify early antecedents of unhealthy behaviors that may have lifelong and communitywide consequences.

In September 2010, the Secretary of Health and Human Services (HHS) released the first annual report on the quality of care for children in Medicaid and the Children's Health Insurance Program (CHIP), as required by the Children's Health Insurance Program Reauthorization Act (CHIPRA) of 2009 (HHS, 2010c). The report notes that nearly 40 million infants to young adults are now enrolled in these public health insurance plans, representing about half of this population in the United States.[1] In addition, Medicaid pays for nearly half of the annual births nationwide.

Although the Secretary's report provides an important benchmark for assessing the current status of quality measurement of child and adolescent health care services, it also highlights key barriers and challenges that have yet to be resolved. In summary, the Secretary's report offers the following key findings:

Measurement and Reporting

- A lack of uniformity and substantial variation in data reliability exist in state-based quality metrics, demonstrating a need for standardized data collection formats.
- Medicaid managed care plans have developed an infrastructure and processes to support external quality reviews, but these efforts do not include information on children in fee-for-service payment arrangements, and they have not yielded statewide information.
- Many state officials welcome the opportunity to create more meaningful and useful measures, and they recognize that current performance measures are inadequate.

Quality of and Access to Care

- A report on the seven quality-of-care effectiveness measures in Medicaid managed care plans from 34 states showed mixed performance: three of the seven measures had relatively high 2008 performance rates, while four of the seven had relatively low performance rates for the same period (see Box 5-1 for a list of the seven measures).
- Children enrolled in Medicaid/CHIP have much better access to primary care services than uninsured children and access com-

---

[1] Estimates of the rates of coverage of children in public health insurance plans may vary according to the source and method of data collection. The 2010 HHS Secretary's report draws on administrative data from the Centers for Medicare and Medicaid Services (CMS). Other data sources, such as those collected by the Census Bureau and those based on parental reports, estimate that about 30–35 percent of children and adolescents are covered by public health insurance plans (HHS, 2010a).

BOX 5-1
Quality-of-Care Effectiveness Measures
(Reported by the National Committee for Quality Assurance
for Children in Medicaid Managed Care Plans)

- Use of appropriate medication for asthma
- Appropriate treatment for upper respiratory infection
- Childhood immunizations
- Lead screening
- Chlamydia screening in 16- to 20-year-olds
- Follow-up care for children prescribed medication for attention-deficit/hyperactivity disorder
- Appropriate testing for children with pharyngitis

SOURCE: NCQA, 2009.

---

parable to that of privately insured children. However, access to specialty care services (e.g., dental, mental health) needs substantial improvement.

- Once enrolled in Medicaid or CHIP, racial/ethnic minority children and children with special health care needs experience improved access to care, but disparities in access to and quality of care persist despite these gains.

This chapter reviews how efforts to improve the measurement of health care quality for children and adolescents have evolved in public and private health care settings. The analysis considers how these efforts compare against a vision of an optimal system of health care quality measurement for younger populations. The review highlights how the findings from the 2010 HHS Secretary's report might be considered in light of persistent areas of need and emerging opportunities for improving the measurement of health care quality, particularly for children and adolescents enrolled in Medicaid and CHIP health plans. The focus is on five key questions:

- What is the purpose of health care quality measurement for children and adolescents?
- What are the critical features of an optimal health care quality measurement system for children and adolescents?
- What steps have been taken to develop such a high-quality measurement system?

- What are examples of current efforts to improve the system?
- Are these efforts sufficient to achieve the vision of an optimal system?

The chapter also highlights promising state and local initiatives.

PURPOSE OF QUALITY MEASUREMENT

Measuring the quality of health care services overall fulfills three major purposes: accountability, quality improvement, and population health (IOM, 2006b):

- *Accountability*—Quality measures provide a basis for assessing and comparing the performance of selected components of the health care system, including individual professionals, provider groups, hospitals, health plans, and states. Quality measures can identify differences in health care practices or processes, service delivery settings, health plans, and state programs and policies, as well as the outcomes associated with these differences. They provide a basis for determining whether the care patients receive from specific providers is consistent with evidence and professional standards. Such information can assist multiple stakeholders in making choices about providers, about plans, and about state policies and programs. These stakeholders include, among others, patients deciding on a clinician, hospital, or other provider from which to seek services and a health plan from which to obtain coverage; purchasers and health plans selecting providers to include in their health insurance networks; and quality oversight organizations making accreditation and certification decisions. Quality measures facilitate assessment and monitoring of the overall functioning of the health insurance and care delivery system over time, demonstrating who is being reached and who is not. Thus they provide the ability to hold health care state systems and health plans accountable for their performance.
- *Quality improvement*—Quality measures can be useful for providers and others who are seeking to improve the quality of care. Such measures can identify gaps in performance that merit attention and can also be used to track progress as individuals and organizations undertake changes to improve care. Key users of such data for improvement include clinicians, quality improvement staff, and managers and members of health care organizations.
- *Population health*—Quality measures must be able to identify gaps in population health, as well as in the clinical care of individuals,

and to track progress in addressing these gaps. Stakeholders include those with specific responsibility for broad population health, as well as those involved in the delivery of health and public health services, such as communitywide programs and efforts to address racial and ethnic disparities and promote healthy behaviors.

The creation, selection, and certification of quality measures are driven by multiple public- and private-sector efforts aimed at accomplishing one or more of the above three objectives. Providers have tended to focus on opportunities for clinical improvement, while employers and other private payers have tended to place more emphasis on improving the effectiveness and efficiency of clinical services for prevalent, high-cost conditions that often require interactions with multiple health care providers and health care settings. As a result, many quality measures include an emphasis on procedures or settings associated with effective and timely clinical care, such as the use of specific treatments or the performance of specific tests and monitoring procedures. Public payers have placed more emphasis on broader population-level measurement, such as rates of hospitalization for preventable conditions or rates of rehospitalization.

As noted in earlier chapters, younger populations tend to be relatively healthy, and the frequency of high-cost conditions is much lower among children compared with adults. Given these characteristics and the increasing numbers of children insured through public payers, the public sector has demonstrated far greater interest to date, relative to the private sector, in the development and use of health care quality measures for children and adolescents.

Solid reasons exist for the lag in development and use of measures of health care quality for children and adolescents:

- The relatively low cost of child health care and the rarity of many child health conditions have impeded clinical research into many of these conditions, limiting the quality of evidence underlying the effectiveness of treatment for younger populations. Without strong evidence linking care processes and outcomes, performance measurement (at least in the domain of effectiveness) is difficult.
- Prevention is particularly important for children, but proving the effectiveness of many clinical preventive services in children is difficult. There is a long lag time between many of these preventive interventions and potential outcomes, and the determinants of these outcomes are complex—health care may be but one of many inputs. Consensus guidelines for preventive services in childhood are now available and widely used (e.g., *Bright Futures* or the Promoting Healthy Development Survey [PHDS]) but the effectiveness

of these services in improving health outcomes for children has not yet been demonstrated (Bethell et al., 2001).

- The processes of care associated with many health services for children and adolescents involve detailed clinical information that may be included in medical records but is not easily accessible from claims-based or other administrative databases. The time and costs associated with abstracting clinical data (such as the results of routine clinical exams and screening tools associated with well-child care) impede the use of these data in large data collection efforts.

- Because many important services and conditions other than health care, such as educational services and community nutrition programs, contribute to child health outcomes, a framework that explicitly acknowledges this shared accountability is especially important for child health. Measures that reflect this shared accountability, such as school readiness, can be constructed and used for quality improvement programs, but they are more difficult to apply within the narrow context of health care accountability. A more popular approach has been the use of a process measure, such as access to a medical home (or health home) for children and adolescents, especially those who have a complex or chronic health condition.

CRITICAL FEATURES OF AN OPTIMAL HEALTH CARE QUALITY MEASUREMENT SYSTEM FOR CHILDREN AND ADOLESCENTS

In considering the features of an optimal health care quality measurement system for children and adolescents, the committee took into account the charge for this study from the Congress; the principles underlying performance measurement as articulated in earlier Institute of Medicine (IOM) studies on performance measures (IOM, 2006b); the family/patient focus expressed in the IOM report *Crossing the Quality Chasm: A New Health System for the 21st Century* (IOM, 2001a); and the committee's own deliberations, which were strongly influenced by another earlier IOM study, *Children's Health, the Nation's Wealth* (IOM and NRC, 2004). The optimal features thus identified are as follows:

- Measures should address those topics that (1) are associated with the greatest burden of mortality and morbidity during childhood, (2) have the greatest potential impact over the life span, (3) address the drivers of high child health care costs, (4) are most sensitive to the quality and safety of services, and (5) are of greatest concern to patients/families.
- Measures should be based on the best available evidence.

- Measures should recognize the unique characteristics of the child and adolescent population, often termed "the four D's" (differential epidemiology, developmental focus, dependent status, and different demography) (Forrest et al., 1997).
- Measures should apply to the whole population of children and adolescents, not just those in specific health plans or states.
- Measures should be capable of aggregation at multiple levels (provider, organization, community, state, nation).
- Measures should take account of the social environment in which children live to allow assessment of how health care services interact with conditions of adversity to influence health outcomes.
- Measures should be broader than the presence or absence of disease.
- Measures should minimize the burden and cost of collection.
- Measures should be able to generate data to drive action and quality improvement at the program (provider) and policy levels.
- Measures should be readily available to all (transparent).
- Measures should be available in a timely manner.
- Measures should reflect patient, family, and community perspectives on quality.

The contrast between these features and the quality measures that are cited in the 2010 HHS Secretary's report is remarkable. Only seven quality measures for children and adolescents are reviewed in that report, and those measures are used in only 30 states and only for those enrolled in Medicaid managed care programs. As a result, the nation is far from having a performance measurement system that can foster the incorporation of the above features into the development and use of quality measures for child and adolescent health care.

INITIAL EFFORTS TO DEVELOP A MEASUREMENT SYSTEM FOR QUALITY OF CARE FOR CHILDREN AND ADOLESCENTS

Initial efforts to improve the measurement of health care quality for the general population include reports by the IOM and initiatives by such groups as the National Committee for Quality Assurance (NCQA) and the National Quality Forum (NQF) (see Appendix C). More recently, the National Initiative for Children's Healthcare Quality (NICHQ) and the Child and Adolescent Health Measurement Initiative (CAHMI) have sought to emphasize the need for consumer-driven measures of health care quality for children and adolescents, as well as to develop approaches for encouraging the use of available measures. These various efforts were encouraged and supported through congressional guidance in the CHIP (1997) and CHIPRA (2009) legislation, which stimulated national leadership and research support by the Agency for Healthcare Research and Quality (AHRQ), as well as demonstration and state-based coordination efforts within the Centers for Medicaid and Medicare Services (CMS).

Initial Congressional Guidance and Federal Leadership

In 1997, Congress created the State Children's Health Insurance Program (SCHIP), one success resulting from the earlier, intense, but ultimately unsuccessful battle over health care reform (Iglehart, 2007). The legislation proved to be a major advance for children and families in terms of expanding health plan coverage and access to services and reducing disparities in these two areas. In addition, the 1997 SCHIP legislation required that state annual reports include for the first time information on quality—a requirement that did not exist in Medicaid. HHS developed a standardized template for these state reports emphasizing the use of Healthcare Effectiveness Data and Information Set (HEDIS©) measures that had been developed as part of quality improvement efforts among private health plans—efforts focused largely on adult health care quality.

During the past two decades, CMS worked with multiple partners to develop quality measures that could be used to assess and improve health care services for children and adolescents enrolled in Medicaid and CHIP health plans. These efforts focused initially on use of the HEDIS measures and collaboration with NCQA. In 1996, for example, prior to passage of the CHIP legislation, Medicaid HEDIS was developed, incorporating standards specific to Medicaid populations (MacTaggart, 2010). Although the use of such measures was voluntary, more than 30 state Medicaid agencies were using at least portions of Medicaid HEDIS within a year. Further collaboration with NCQA, the American Public Human Services Association, and the Commonwealth Fund led to a 2002 report that covered 13 HEDIS measures, 5 of which were child-specific, from 176 managed care organizations in 33 states plus the District of Columbia and the Commonwealth of Puerto Rico (MacTaggart, 2010). One year later, HEDIS 2003 contained 23 measures designed for or applicable to children and adolescents, including child and adolescent immunization status, chlamydia screening for women, use of appropriate medications and follow-up care for people with asthma, and experience of care (based on responses to the Consumer Assessment of Healthcare Providers and Systems [CAHPS] 3.0H Child Survey, which included a screener for children with chronic conditions) (MacTaggart, 2010).

Early Attributes of Quality Measures for Children and Adolescents

In 2004, the Commonwealth Fund examined existing child health care quality measures within 19 different data sources or measurement sets (Beal et al., 2004; Leatherman and McCarthy, 2004). This analysis identified 396 quality measures for children within the 19 data sources, 10 of which relied on administrative or medical record data and 9 of which used survey data.

In categorizing these measures according to the six aspects of quality care identified in *Crossing the Quality Chasm* (IOM, 2001a)—safety, timeliness, effectiveness, equity, efficiency, and patient-centeredness—the authors found that more than half (59 percent) of the measures involve indicators of effectiveness, while about one-sixth (14 percent) are relevant to the safety domain (Beal et al., 2004). The safety measures involve primarily serious errors in health care delivery, especially medical and surgical errors during hospitalization. The authors also examined how existing health care quality measures are distributed across the different purposes of health care—acute care (getting better), preventive care (staying healthy), and chronic care management (living with illness). They found that a large proportion of the measures (40 percent) could be categorized under getting better, about 24 percent under staying healthy, and 17 percent under living with illness. There were no measures related to end-of-life care. Nearly one-fourth of all measures were not classifiable by the six aspects of quality care (Beal et al., 2004).

In addition, some efforts have focused on developing quality measures that would apply to children of all ages, as well as measures that would have specific application to selected age groups—infants, toddlers, children, and adolescents. Analyses of these efforts have shown that the majority of measures they produced can be applied to children across all age groups; however, there are no unique measures for school-aged children (aged 5–18) (Beal et al., 2004).

Despite the advances achieved through the above efforts, studies have revealed many areas in which quality measures fall short (Landon et al., 2007; Leatherman and McCarthy, 1999; Mangione-Smith et al., 2007; Thompson et al., 2003). In particular, measures fail to capture aspects of care that are relevant for low-income, Medicaid-insured children. Moreover, quality measures are lacking for many important areas of health care, even though major studies have demonstrated significant shortcomings in these areas both for the general population (such as inpatient care or mental health services) and with respect to disparities in access to and use of services (such as oral health care).

CURRENT EFFORTS TO IMPROVE THE
MEASUREMENT OF QUALITY OF HEALTH CARE
FOR CHILDREN AND ADOLESCENTS

Recognizing the shortcomings detailed above, recent health care legislation places new emphasis on the importance of measuring health care quality for younger populations. This legislation includes CHIPRA (especially Title IV), the Patient Protection and Affordable Care Act (ACA), the American Recovery and Reinvestment Act (ARRA), and the Health Information Technology for Economic and Clinical Health (HITECH) initiative included in the ARRA.

2009 Congressional Action and Title IV of CHIPRA

In reauthorizing the CHIP legislation in 2009, Congress renewed its initial efforts to foster the use of health care quality measures for Medicaid and CHIP populations, adding new dimensions that had emerged as major concerns. The new legislation required that quality measures specifically address three broad types of care (prevention, acute care, and chronic care) and specific elements of clinical quality (effectiveness, safety, patient and family experience, and equity [disparities]). Congress also directed that child health care quality measures specifically address mental as well as physical health care, care across the full spectrum of child development, care integration and access as reflected by accessibility of care in inpatient and outpatient settings, and the duration and stability of health insurance coverage.

Title IV of CHIPRA (P.L. 111-3) significantly expanded various child health care quality improvement initiatives and authorized several new efforts, including

- development of an initial core set of health care quality measures for children enrolled in Medicaid or CHIP, to be supplemented by research grants to address incomplete or missing measures (known as the U18 awards);
- a new program of 10 quality demonstration grants to states as the basis for a future national quality system for children's health care;
- creation of the Medicaid and CHIP Payment and Access Commission (MACPAC) to review Medicaid and CHIP access and payment policies and report recommendations to Congress;
- creation of a Federal Quality Workgroup of the CHIPRA Steering Committee to ensure that the expertise of key HHS entities is brought to bear on improving quality measurement and the quality of health care for all children;

- authorization of a $20 million program for the Census Bureau to improve state-specific estimates of the child population;
- encouragement of collaboration between AHRQ and CMS to develop an electronic health record (EHR) format for children;
- an AHRQ research program to develop, validate, and improve a final core set of pediatric quality measures, to be completed by January 1, 2013; and
- technical support from AHRQ to CMS, including content for best practices related to the implementation of core measures, and an evaluation of outcomes of child health care quality demonstration projects.

Title IV also mandated a study by the National Academies "on the extent and quality of efforts to measure child health status and the quality of health care for children across the age span and in relation to preventive care, treatments for acute conditions, and treatments aimed at ameliorating or correcting physical, mental, and developmental conditions in children." That study is the subject of this report.

The CHIPRA legislation represents a landmark in its emphasis on quality of care for the nation's children, reflecting a drive toward achieving quality measures that can provide common data elements and facilitate consistent reporting by the states, with allowance for flexible use to address each state's individual needs. Of importance, the legislation established that these provisions apply to both Medicaid and CHIP, moving toward a consistent strategy across both programs nationally and at the state level. It is important to note as well that CHIPRA included provisions calling for identification of existing quality measures in use by public and privately sponsored health care coverage arrangements, as well as provisions around guidance for reporting performance by the states and demonstration programs to showcase and test child health care quality measures. As noted above, CHIPRA also contained a provision and funding ($5 million) for development of an EHR format for children to support quality reporting. While the inclusion of this provision was important, the subsequent passage of the ARRA (discussed below) sharply enhanced the ability of the health care system (ambulatory care providers and hospitals) to implement EHRs through a $19 billion investment, although not as tightly focused on children.

The CHIPRA legislation recognized that stability of coverage is integrally linked to program quality overall. States are now required to report on eligibility criteria, enrollment, retention, use of simplification measures, access to care, and care coordination, among other aspects of coverage. Furthermore, reporting on these dimensions of coverage is required, whereas reporting on quality remains voluntary.

Other Recent Relevant Legislation

The CHIPRA legislation was soon followed by additional laws that lent further momentum to quality improvement efforts and the development of the next generation of health care quality measures. None of these more recent initiatives address the unique needs of children and adolescents, raising concern that the distinct demographic, developmental, epidemiological, and dependency characteristics of younger populations may once again be sidelined in the evolving national infrastructure for quality improvement in the health care system. The recent legislative initiatives include

- the ACA (P.L. 111-148),
- the ARRA (P.L. 111-5), and
- the HITECH Act, part of ARRA.

These additional pieces of legislation placed further emphasis on issues of access (to both insurance coverage and health care services), quality, and cost in the health care system. Together, they have major implications for the future health of America's children and adolescents. The expanded federal efforts also reflect the recognition that improving the quality and affordability of health care is an enterprise that requires strong collaboration between the private and public sectors at all levels of government. The ARRA legislation, for example, offers substantial incentives for physicians and hospitals to adopt EHRs to improve the quality and safety of care.

The structure of health care organizations and the financing of health care are currently in flux, with the pace of change accelerating as a result of numerous provisions in the ACA that encourage coordination within the health care delivery system and a payment structure that rewards quality and outcomes. These provisions include the creation of accountable care organizations (ACOs); the promotion of medical homes for Medicaid enrollees with chronic conditions; and various efforts to improve health care quality and reward better outcomes, such as lowering rates of hospital readmissions and hospital-acquired conditions.

With few exceptions, such as the Pediatric ACO Demonstration project, these payment reforms do not focus on children. Indeed, much of the push for payment reform is embedded in the Medicare program—the other end of the age spectrum. While few efforts to reform payment and delivery systems target children, other, broader changes that are slated for implementation under health care reform will certainly have an effect on children's care.

The ACA includes a number of other provisions that are likely to have profound effects on children's health and quality of care, including the development of a National Health Care Quality Strategy (National Quality

Strategy) and an associated strategic plan that will identify priorities for improving the "delivery of health care services, patient health outcomes, and population health," as well as introduce new reporting requirements for health insurance plans that will lead to greater transparency and accountability (P.L. 111-148). The legislation also establishes the Center for Medicare and Medicaid Innovation, whose efforts could include the evaluation of new payment and delivery models for delivering care to children in Medicaid and CHIP.

The Obama Administration's National Quality Strategy, announced by the Secretary of HHS, strives to align federal efforts with those of the states and the private sector and to foster collaborative partnerships wherever feasible. The ACA directs the Secretary of HHS to integrate these efforts into a cohesive strategic plan with priorities for improving the delivery of health care services, patient health outcomes, and population health. This strategic plan is due to Congress by January 1, 2011, and must include provisions for (1) agency-specific plans and benchmarks, (2) coordination among agencies, (3) strategies to align public and private payers, and (4) alignment with meaningful use of health information technology (HIT). The plan is to be updated and refined periodically through annual reports to Congress to accommodate emerging issues. Most notably, the National Quality Strategy, required by the ACA, strives to link improvements in health care quality and health outcomes and reduced costs. The draft strategy (not yet finalized) does not specifically use a life-course framework (as detailed in Chapter 2) in considering priorities; a life-course approach may be appropriate for future reports to Congress.

The ACA also calls for the development of a National Prevention and Health Promotion Strategy (National Prevention Strategy) that is scheduled to be released in March 2011. The National Prevention Strategy focuses attention on the need for community-based efforts emphasizing prevention to reduce the incidence of the leading causes of death and disability (Bilheimer, 2010).

Both the National Quality Strategy and the National Prevention Strategy are aimed at strengthening collaboration among public- and private-sector partners. The National Prevention Strategy will also be developed by consultation across the federal government. The two strategies will share common goals and priorities for healthy people and communities. Both will include an explicit focus on goals that require close collaboration between clinical and community partners (HHS, 2010d). These two initiatives will have a broad impact on the design of measures of health and health care quality for children and adolescents, highlighting the importance of improvements in the health care system and the social and economic environments of children and their families that can lead to better health outcomes for all.

While the legislation passed since the beginning of 2009 collectively advances opportunities to improve quality measurement dramatically for adults, the impact on children remains uncertain. The ACA extended the emphasis on quality and added a heavy emphasis on cost containment, value, and accountability, while the ARRA provided unprecedented funding for HITECH and a fresh emphasis on HIT for quality improvement. These legislative initiatives, especially those efforts authorized under CHIPRA, offer opportunities for significant improvement in the state of measurement of health care quality for children and adolescents. But realizing this potential depends not only on improving the inventory of quality measures and developing measures for priority health conditions, but also on creating data systems that can reduce the variability and inconsistency in the quality of state-level Medicaid databases, as well as on developing strategies that allow the states to use the data to improve system performance and health. Such strategies may require collaboration with other service settings so as to look beyond the health care system for environmental factors, such as poverty, stress, and inadequate nutrition that significantly influence the health status of children and adolescents.

Implementation Efforts of the Agency for Healthcare Research and Quality

The recent emphasis on health care quality for children and adolescents needs to be considered within the broader context of other quality improvement efforts at AHRQ. For example, Title IX of the Healthcare Research and Quality Act of 1999 (P.L. 106-129) required AHRQ to issue an annual public report on health care quality, beginning in 2003 (U.S. Congress (106th), 1999). In preparation, AHRQ funded the first in a series of IOM studies to produce recommendations for the selection of measures for this annual report, which has included a report on children's health care quality even though such measures for children have not been as well developed as those for adults (Halfon et al., 1998; Homer et al., 1998; IOM, 2001b; McGlynn et al., 2000; Szilagyi and Schor, 1998).

In April 2009, AHRQ and CMS executed a Memorandum of Understanding (MOU) outlining which agency will take the lead role for various provisions in Title IV of CHIPRA. According to the MOU, AHRQ is leading the implementation of four provisions: the identification of the initial core measure set, the establishment of a quality measures program, the development of a model EHR, and the IOM study that is the basis for this report.

In responding to congressional guidance, AHRQ formed an expert advisory panel, the AHRQ National Advisory Council for Healthcare Research and Quality's Subcommittee on Children's Healthcare Quality Measures for

Medicaid and Child Health Insurance Programs (SNAC). The SNAC was charged with providing guidance on measure evaluation criteria to be used in identifying an initial core measure set for health care quality for children and adolescents and on a strategy for gathering additional measures and measure information from state programs and others. The SNAC's recommendations were to be provided to CMS and the AHRQ National Advisory Council, which in turn would advise the director of AHRQ. The directors of AHRQ and CMS would then review and decide on the final core set to be presented to the Secretary of HHS for consideration.

The SNAC solicited proposals for candidate measures that were assessed by the subcommittee members according to three key evaluation criteria—validity, feasibility, and importance—using an adaptation of the RAND-University of California, Los Angeles (UCLA) modified Delphi process (a structured method of creating consensus through anonymous evaluations). The candidate list was reduced to a group of 25 core measures through a series of deliberations and panel discussions. The SNAC process gave immediate priority to the validity, reliability, and feasibility of the measures over the comprehensiveness of the set. All but three of the proposed core set of measures were recommended by the HHS Secretary. The deleted measures include child and adolescent suicide risk assessment, the CAHPS Clinician and Group Survey, and the NCQA HEDIS annual dental visit measure. Furthermore, the HHS Secretary chose to list the three separate well-child visit measures individually, resulting in a total of 24 measures.

The initial set of core measures proposed by the SNAC is well balanced across developmental stages. The measures are heavily weighted to address prevention and strongly oriented toward ambulatory settings in general and primary care in particular. Physical health is emphasized to a much greater extent than developmental, social, emotional, or mental health.

The core measures recommended by the SNAC, and ultimately revised and then adopted by the Secretary of HHS, set the stage for the development of a state-based measurement system that can be used to examine and compare the performance of different health plans in serving the needs of vulnerable children and adolescents (see Box 5-2). The ultimate goal is to support states in their efforts to adopt consistent, standardized statewide health and health care quality measures; encourage the use of existing data sources, including both population health surveys and administrative records; and provide a basis for comparing provider and health plan performance in contributing to the achievement of national and statewide health goals for children and adolescents.

AHRQ has begun the process of expanding the core measure set and has called for the development of new measures (AHRQ, 2010f). AHRQ also has funded 10 Centers of Excellence and demonstration projects, three of which include significant efforts to develop new measures. These grant programs are designed to showcase best practices for improving care; some have developing measures, particularly for behavioral health, as part of their mandate (AHRQ, 2010d).

As noted in Chapter 2, different data sources are used for different objectives, and the nation lacks effective mechanisms that can link the health indicators generated by population health surveys to privately and publicly funded quality improvement efforts focused on measuring health care processes and outcomes in clinical care settings. Health care providers and organizational units such as hospitals, group practices, and health plans are especially concerned about being held accountable for the health of underserved populations when they cannot control all the factors that influence the health outcomes of these groups.

As federal, state, and local health and health care agencies move toward greater reliance on using data and indicators to drive improvements in the performance of the health care system, opportunities will emerge to align disparate interests and to develop standards of shared or partial accountability for the health status of selected populations. Inevitably, these efforts will require collaboration and discussion of shared goals, the creation of mechanisms to set benchmarks and timelines for achieving these goals, the designation of entities that can be held responsible for contributing to these efforts, and consideration of the extent to which public and private data sources created for specific aims can be used for other purposes.

Initiatives of the Centers for Medicare and Medicaid Services

Following the passage of the CHIPRA legislation in 2009, CMS accelerated its efforts to work with public- and private-sector organizations on improving quality-of-care measures that could be used within both Medicaid managed care organizations and primary care settings that serve Medicaid and CHIP populations. These efforts included the identification of a core set of measures for voluntary reporting by the states, as well as a comprehensive technical assistance plan that could be applied for states across all of the CHIPRA provisions. CMS also placed a new emphasis not only on supporting state efforts to improve Medicaid and CHIP programs with respect to the delivery of care, but also on encouraging the states to identify actual improvement in health outcomes as a major focus of these efforts. These initiatives have led to a close partnership with AHRQ and other federal agencies in support of the general vision of HHS of providing the right care for every person every time.

The 2010 HHS Secretary's report also described emerging investments in building the infrastructure within federal and state agencies needed to assess the quality of care received by children and adolescents under Medicaid and CHIP (HHS, 2010c). These efforts include individualized support

BOX 5-2
Final Core Set of Measures for Children's Health
Care Quality Recommended by HHS Secretary*

Prevention and Health Promotion
- Prenatal/Perinatal
  —Frequency of ongoing prenatal care (National Committee for Quality
   Assurance [NCQA] measure)
  —Timeliness of prenatal care (NCQA measure)
  —Percent of live births weighing less than 2,500 grams
  —Cesarean rate for low-risk first-birth women
- Immunizations
  —Childhood immunization status (NCQA measure)
  —Adolescent immunization (NCQA measure revised for 2010)
- Screening
  —Body mass index (BMI) documentation ages 2–18
  —Rates of screening using standardized screening tools for potential
   delays in social and emotional development (ABCD)
  —Chlamydia screening for women
- Well-Child Care
  —Well-child visits in the first 15 months of life
  —Well-child visits in the third through sixth years of life
  —Well-child visits for ages 12–21 with primary care provider (PCP)
- Dental
  —Total eligibles receiving preventive dental care (EPSDT)

Management of Acute Conditions
- Pharyngitis-appropriate testing (NCQA measure)

for and feedback to states with respect to the performance of managed care organizations that serve children and adolescents enrolled in Medicaid and CHIP plans and external quality reporting. CMS has piloted a pediatric measure program to develop and evaluate the core quality measures, as well as created a strategy for states' voluntary collection and reporting of data on the performance measures. CMS also has developed a compendium of quality measures to give states options to consider in identifying quality measures that best support their specific quality strategies and address the needs of their populations.

A major challenge persists in the nature of collaboration between CMS initiatives and data collection and reporting practices within individual states: how to achieve and accelerate consistency across state quality reporting while allowing for states' flexibility and innovative practices. In addressing this challenge, CMS has developed a national patient-centered

- Otitis media effusion—avoidance of inappropriate use
- Total Early Periodic Screening, Diagnosis, and Treatment (EPSDT) eligibles who received dental treatment
- Emergency department (ED) utilization—average of three ED visits per member
- Pediatric catheter-associated blood stream infection rates (pediatric intensive care unit [PICU] and neonatal intensive care unit [NICU])

Management of Chronic Conditions
- Annual number of asthma patients with one or more asthma-related ED visits
- Follow-up care for children prescribed attention-deficit/hyperactivity disorder (ADHD) medication
- Annual hemoglobin A1C testing

Family Experiences of Care
- Consumer Assessment of Healthcare Providers and Systems (CAHPS) Health Plan Survey 4.0, Child Version
- Survey for families of children with special health care needs

Availability of Services
- Access of children and adolescents to a PCP

---

* Based on recommendations by AHRQ National Advisory Council for Healthcare Research and Quality Subcommittee on Children's Healthcare Quality Measures for Medicaid and CHIP Programs (SNAC).
SOURCE: HHS, 2009.

framework (focused on the "beneficiary") that combines the efforts and successes of national initiatives with the multiple types of activities that are occurring at the state level (AHRQ, 2010e). Further opportunities to address this challenge include expanding and improving states' access to encounter data (e.g., Medicaid Statistical Information System [MSIS] encounter data); resolving anomalies in state-level claims and enrollment records; and encouraging states to link to other databases, including the National Vital Statistics System (NVSS).

The annual report to Congress mandated by CHIPRA may eventually provide an opportunity for CMS to integrate the successes of both national and state efforts through the development of a menu of national and state-specific goals; public reports that describe progress toward meeting those goals; and reports on progress toward achieving consistent, standardized measures that can be used in both national and state-level data collection and reporting efforts. In supporting these objectives, CMS is working with the states to develop an annual reporting template to facilitate the annual submission of publicly available information on the quality of pediatric care (AHRQ, 2010e). As authorized under CHIPRA, AHRQ and CMS also are collaborating to develop an EHR format for children and adolescents to standardize and facilitate reporting of quality indicators.

ADEQUACY OF THESE EFFORTS TO ACHIEVE AN OPTIMAL SYSTEM

The reporting specifications initiated by the CHIPRA legislation and states' ability to respond to them are extremely important. It remains uncertain whether voluntary reporting will be an effective means of securing data from all states, and states have not yet demonstrated their capacity to report on *all* Medicaid and CHIP children and adolescents, not just those enrolled in managed care plans. Finally, it will be necessary to determine how states use health care quality measurement to improve outcomes for these children and adolescents, and how these outcomes compare with those of other populations of children and adolescents, such as those who are uninsured or are enrolled in private health plans.

The process initiated by AHRQ and CMS in identifying a small set of core measures for use by the states is an important beginning. Other key areas, including but not limited to the dimensions specified in the legislation, such as fostering greater consistency in the collection of racial and ethnic data or the collection of data on prevalent health conditions that involve mental health or substance abuse services, were not addressed in the initial core set either because no current measures existed or if they did, they did not pass the process established by the SNAC. Several additional key issues require attention in improving the usefulness of health care quality data now available in national and state-level data sets. Some of these issues involve improving the validity and reliability of data sources through consistent definitions and standardized criteria. Others pose greater challenges, requiring the collection of data across different care settings and time periods, or the collection of data in areas that involve difficult-to-measure or difficult-to-reach populations, especially with respect to preventive and mental and behavioral health services. Still others require new data sources and new data collection methods that can provide information about the social environments of populations enrolled in Medicaid and CHIP health plans, as well as the relationship between their health status and other measures of child well-being, such as educational achievement.

Need for Additional Work on Core Measures

The legislation required that the initial core set be drawn from existing measures, that these measures be improved, and that new measures be developed. The SNAC explicitly conceptualized and reached consensus on its approach by dividing possible measures into three categories: grounded, intermediate, and aspirational. *Grounded* measures were defined as currently feasible; many such measures were already in widespread use. *Intermediate* measures were defined as having good specifications with some isolated examples of use; however, they lacked broader established validity and existing widespread implementation. *Aspirational* measures were defined as those that were needed to fill an important gap but did not yet exist as valid or feasible measures. The consensus of the committee was to focus on identifying and choosing from the most grounded measures (AHRQ, 2010f).

Ultimately, the process used by the SNAC members to identify the initial core set of measures took into account validity, feasibility, and importance (AHRQ, 2010g). *Validity* was defined as being supported by scientific evidence or expert consensus. A measure considered to be valid supported a link between structure and outcomes, structure and processes, and processes and outcomes. In addition, the measure must have been judged to measure what it purported to measure. Finally, for a measure to meet the criteria for validity, it had to relate to an aspect of health that was thought to be impacted primarily by health care providers or the health care system. Although the strict accountability approach used by the SNAC is traditionally applied in quality measurement, this criterion has been challenged in a previous IOM report (IOM, 2006b) as well as the present report with respect to the need for shared accountability.

The *feasibility* criterion required that the data necessary to score a measure be available to organizations from administrative records, medical records, and/or surveys. The SNAC looked for existing detailed specifications that would allow for "reliable and unbiased" scoring of measures across government levels and health care organizations. To be ranked highly on feasibility, a measure also had to be in current use as mandated by legislation (AHRQ, 2010e).

In the refinement of the SNAC methodology for the second Delphi evaluation, a third criterion for evaluation, *importance*, was also applied. For a measure to be considered important, it needed to be deemed "actionable" in that there should be a clear intervention that could be undertaken to impact the measure. The definition and scoring of importance also included estimation that the cost of the condition measured was a significant burden on the American health care system, that there was evidence that the measure was indicative of a substantial quality problem, and that an assessment of accountability for the problem was possible. Finally, a consideration in evaluating importance was that there should be documented variation in performance by socioeconomic factors, specifically race/ethnicity or insurance type (AHRQ, 2010h). The overall goal of the importance criterion was to identify "sentinel" measures for prevention and care that would signal the status of a substantial quality problem for which accountability could be assigned and action taken for improvement.

However, in accordance with the SNAC's legislative mandate, the importance of a particular type of measure was not the driving force behind the identification of the core set. Thus the SNAC evaluated the current validity, feasibility, and importance of measures that could be improved upon directly by a change in health care services only. Now that the initial core set of measures has been developed, AHRQ and CMS are moving into the next phase of development for the core set of pediatric quality-of-care measures under a Pediatric Quality Measures Program. This program is charged with improving and strengthening the initial core set of measures by continuing to evaluate those measures, as well as increasing the portfolio of evidence-based measures that can be used by purchasers, providers, and consumers of health care for children (AHRQ, 2010c). This is being accomplished through awards totaling $55 million over a 4-year period for demonstration research and dissemination projects designed to implement and improve upon the core set of children's health care measures (AHRQ, 2010c).

Gaps in Mental Health and Substance Abuse Measures

As noted in Chapter 4, nearly 20 percent of children and adolescents experience some type of mental health or substance abuse disorder (IOM, 2009c). The development of health care quality measures for these conditions for children and adolescents lags far behind that for adults. The measures used most commonly in Medicaid managed care plans involve two HEDIS indicators: one focused on attention-deficit/hyperactivity disorder (ADHD) medication and the other on psychiatric hospital follow-up.

A recent review by Bickman and colleagues (Bickman et al., in press) found little value for quality improvement from these two indicators, but there are reasons to pursue both. The low rate of follow-up by parents for ADHD medication has been well documented. For ADHD, the potential loss of benefit due to unfilled prescriptions or negative experiences with a given medication suggests the importance of further contact to reassess the reasons for nonadherence and consider alternative medications. With regard to posthospital follow-up for a psychiatric admission, the limited studies are equivocal. Attention might be given to a recent longitudinal study by James and colleagues (James et al., 2010) that documents significantly lower rates of rehospitalization when community mental health resources are utilized.

The committee has identified opportunities to develop new priorities in considering the quality of mental health services for children and adolescents, as well as other types of care, within the framework recommended by the IOM for the AHRQ annual report on health care quality (Table 5-1) (IOM, 2001b). Under care coordination, for example, combining treatment plans for a parent's mental health disorder with preventive services for the parent's child(ren) is recommended in cases such as parental depression (IOM, 2009c). Second, a focus on disruptive behavior disorders (oppositional defiant and conduct disorders) is particularly important given their well-documented relationship to poor outcomes in childhood and adulthood and significant comorbidities (ADHD, trauma, and substance abuse). The prevalence of these disorders is high among adolescents in the general population and much higher among adolescents in juvenile justice and child welfare systems, and they are among the most frequent reasons for mental health specialty treatment. Evidence-based interventions to address these disorders have been developed for all age groups, although these interventions are not necessarily available in usual practice. Finally, this clinical group exhibits the highest risk of out-of-home placement—hence the focus on indicators related to residential treatment. According to parental reports, 628,000 adolescents had experienced care for emotional and behavioral problems under out-of-home placement in the past year: 510,000 in a hospital, 199,000 in a residential treatment center, and 112,000 in treatment foster care (SAMHSA, 2007). According to other surveys, 93,000 adolescents were in juvenile detention in 2006 (OJJDP, 2008), and 748,000 were in the foster care system in 2008 (ACF, 2010). This national estimate of nearly 1.5 million youth in such placements is astounding, and although not broken out by diagnosis here, suggests the need for attention to the quality of care for these high-risk adolescents (many of whom may already be enrolled in Medicaid or CHIP plans), as well as relevance to their extensive use of the health care system.

To the extent that the health care system routinely screens for mental health problems among children and adolescents, the focus is on cognitive and motor delays and autism. Screening for other mental health problems in children or their parents is much more limited, and the prevalence of selected disorders is not readily available in administrative data or national surveys. There is much evidence that the system is not detecting or dealing with mental health issues (Fairbrother et al., 2010). Furthermore, there is increasing concern regarding the treatment of certain highly prevalent mental health issues in children, including a lack of follow-up (Gardner et al., 2004) and an increase in off-label prescribing (Zito et al., 2008).

Routine screening for mental health and behavioral problems would

TABLE 5-1 Opportunities to Adapt the Priorities of the AHRQ Annual Report to Address the Quality of Services for Children and Adolescents

Component of Quality	Type of Care			
	Preventive Care	Acute Treatment	Chronic Care Management	End-of-Life Care
Effectiveness	Prevention: immunizations, prenatal care, programs for improved nutrition and exercise Screening for physical and learning disabilities, mental health, substance abuse, and parental depression; nurse home visitation for high-risk infants	Appropriate care for various common conditions, evidence-based practice (EBP) for behavioral disorders in young children (e.g., parent management training), parental treatment for psychiatric diagnoses	Appropriate follow-up, early intervention and supportive services for disability (physical, learning, etc.) and early-stage mental disorders; in-home EBP treatment (e.g., multisystemic therapy [MST]) for serious behavioral disorders; monitoring of rate of treatment completion	Adequate education for patient and family about palliative care options to prevent imprudent use of aggressive treatments where risks of complications (including inadequate pain control) outweigh benefits at this stage of care
Safety	Parent education about environmental hazards; assurance that contraindicated vaccines are not administered; developmentally appropriate screening for trauma, truancy, bullying, suicidality, and domestic violence; sex education	Use of practices known to reduce hospital complications, including iatrogenic pneumothorax, decubitis ulcer, postoperative sepsis, inadvertent retention of a foreign body; monitoring of medications for evidence and off-label use; monitoring of iatrogenic treatment (e.g., group therapy for eating disorders)	Medication management system to reduce adverse events due to known drug interactions; monitoring of psychotropic polypharmacy (3+ or 2 in one class); monitoring of seclusion/restraints in institutional and other placements	

continued

Timeliness	Prevention and screening; immunizations and screening exams on schedule	All-hours access for childhood diseases; timely referral	
Patient/ Family-Centeredness	Parent and adolescent assessments of communication of information about child's developmental status, child's needs to maintain healthy development; parent education at each developmental stage to foster cognitive, emotional, and social functioning	Parent and adolescent assessments of communication, responsiveness to preferences, etc. in acute care; child/parent participation in decisions about treatment type	Supports to children with special health care needs and their parents/caregivers; communication of treatment plans and prognosis; child/ parent participation in treatment planning, implementation, and monitoring
Access	Regular source of care; primary care and schools as portals of entry to care; primary care providers trained to assess mental health/ substance abuse	Ability to obtain treatment for acute illness; insurance coverage for all youth; support for access to care (transportation and child care); access to a full continuum of care	Availability of needed services for children with special health care needs; access to specialty care for major depression, including medication and psychosocial treatment; appropriate access for all age and racial/ethnic groups

TABLE 5-1 Continued

Component of Quality	Type of Care			
	Preventive Care	Acute Treatment	Chronic Care Management	End-of-Life Care
Efficiency	Ratio of positive screen for mental health and referral to appropriate care setting	Reimbursement linked to evidence; appropriate assessment and follow-up for prescriptions for attention-deficit/hyperactivity disorder (ADHD)	Link to community care after psychiatric hospitalization or other residential care	
Care Coordination	"Medical home" measures; comprehensive developmental and treatment plans; integration of information and treatment among health care providers, schools, other institutions involved in child welfare			
	Coordination of child and parent treatment in "medical home" (e.g., treatment of a parent's depression should be coordinated with preventive services for the parent's child(ren))			
	Individualized team-developed care plans, tracking of modifications, and family input			
	Integration of information and treatment among health care providers, schools, and other human services, especially child welfare and juvenile justice			
Infrastructure	Integration of data systems across all systems of care, comprehensive medical/developmental record; systems for referral			
	Mental health content in electronic and medical records			
	Feedback systems that report reduction in symptoms, improved functioning, and corrective actions			
	Measurement of outcomes by child's age and race/ethnicity, including family indicators and family experience with treatment			

require closer adherence to guidelines associated with well-child care and would need to include information collected by the child's provider about the parent's mental health as well. These efforts would require additional training of providers as well as appropriate screening instruments for primary care settings. Measurement of the quality of mental health care would also need to go beyond reporting a particular diagnosis and the use of medication. Some states (such as Massachusetts) mandate routine child screening for certain medications, and measures such as the Pediatric Symptom Checklist have been endorsed by NQF. But the use of these measures has not been adopted within Medicaid or CHIP health plans.

As one interviewee stated, "We have a measure of whether kids are being followed; but really, what we really want to know is whether the child needs to be on medication in the first place. What were the symptoms? Was the diagnosis correct? Is someone measuring the symptoms to ascertain that symptoms are improving?" (Fairbrother et al., 2010).

Emerging Signs That States and Clinicians Want to Do More

The goals of quality measurement are to create national benchmarks, highlight areas of performance that need improvement, and implement quality improvement strategies. For this to happen at a national level, states will need to report measures in a consistent way so the measures can be aggregated and compared across states and with national indicators. Achieving this goal will require capacity at the national and state levels to collect, warehouse, and analyze data; the use of standard definitions and selection criteria to guide reporting; and the creation of measures that are valid, reliable, feasible, and cost-effective for use by state agencies. While many states lack these capabilities, a few are taking steps toward building the technical resources and analytical skills that address these objectives.

The use of quality measures in state-level reporting may be enhanced by greater national benchmarking efforts and efforts to achieve more transparency in the state-based reports and other information presented to AHRQ and CMS. A recent IOM report, *Future Directions for the National Healthcare Quality and Disparities Reports*, recommends benchmarking as a strategy to make information more forward-looking and action-oriented, including the use of more creative data display mechanisms and general organization of the data sources (IOM, 2010a).

It is questionable whether the current collection of state-specific measures for assessment and quality improvement constitutes a federal data source. The potential to build a coordinated system through the state-based Medicaid data centers, under the guidance and oversight of CMS, does exist. But if the ultimate goal is for state programs to be able to compare their performance with each other and with national benchmarks, the measures that are used in such assessments must be valid, reliable, and feasible for use. Furthermore, the question of whether CMS can adequately influence state data collection and reporting efforts through its own rule-making authorities or legislative action is required to support such activity must be addressed.

Despite the lack of uniformity across the states in their CHIP reporting, most states appear to be ready to collaborate in efforts to achieve greater consistency. A 2009 survey found that states want to be able to compare their own performance against that of others in a national data set using common metrics and methodologies (Smith et al., 2009). The survey also found that states want to enhance their quality improvement efforts by incorporating data on quality and performance into reimbursement methodologies for health plans and individual providers (Smith et al., 2009). It is important to note that this survey found that CHIP directors were more ready to move forward than were Medicaid directors, possibly reflecting the fact that most CHIP children are enrolled in managed care plans and that HEDIS specifications exist for this population, while children enrolled in Medicaid plans are more likely to receive care through fee-for-service and primary care case management arrangements.

At the clinical level, there is growing experience with examining quality and requirements for quality improvement as part of training. Clinicians are being asked to examine their practice against national or regional benchmarks. This focus on quality improvement as part of clinical practice offers fertile ground for the introduction and use of relevant quality measures.

Monitoring of Care Transitions and a Life-Course Perspective

Understanding of child and adolescent health has evolved to embody a life-course perspective, as discussed in Chapter 2, an approach that recognizes that children are in a constant state of development; that they have different needs from health care providers at different points in their development; that disease prognosis and treatment are affected by developmental factors; and that in this unique stage of life, children are perhaps even more susceptible to environmental influences on their health and well-being than are adults (IOM and NRC, 2004) (see also Chapter 4). Yet measures of child health care are not yet capable of monitoring services within a life-course perspective.

Linking Prenatal and Pediatric Care Data

One gap that results from failing to take a life-course perspective occurs during the transition from prenatal to pediatric health care. This gap stems from both the conceptualization of what is included in the measurement of child health and the logistics of linking medical records across systems (for example, linking hospital records with primary care records, or obstetric records with pediatric records). Complications at birth, handled by the obstetrician and hospital physicians, are not always reported to the infant's future pediatrician or family physician. The result is that pediatricians do not always know about pregnancy complications or birth issues that could have implications for the child's current or future health and development.

Managing and Measuring Care Transitions for Chronic Disorders

The 2006 IOM report *Performance Measurement: Accelerating Improvement* (IOM, 2006b) identifies multiple difficulties associated with the management and measurement of care transitions, including "the misalignment of financial incentives, the unexplored accountability, the difficulty sorting out failed 'hand-offs' from worsening illness, the limited utility of administrative data, and the lack of training and support for clinicians in this area" (IOM, 2006b, p. 268). These issues apply equally to both adult care and care for younger populations of children and adolescents with chronic or complex disorders. Several efforts have evolved to address these problems, frequently focused on improving the capacity to measure the quality of care for an "episode" of illness as opposed to measuring specific procedures associated with a single office visit. But defects in the transmission of information and the absence of an evidence base regarding practices that contribute to effective care transitions impede the ability to assess high-quality care.

In addition to problems associated with the management of care transitions, there are challenges in measuring the quality of the transition. Most of the existing measures involve the quality of the transition from hospital to home for adults or an elderly population. Similar work is lacking and needs to be developed for children and adolescents, not only for the transition from hospital to home care, but also for the prenatal-to-early childhood transition and the transition from adolescence to young adulthood.

Measuring the Transition from Adolescent to Adult Health Care

Because of the current fragmented system in which coverage rules and health care providers are different for children and adults, the transition from adolescence to adulthood with respect to health care is often difficult. This gap may be especially acute for adolescents with special health care needs or with chronic health care problems, who have a critical need to find new doctors that serve adults, as well as find other forms of insurance coverage (Callahan et al., 2001; Scal et al., 1999). Population surveys shed some light on this issue, showing, for example, that at age 18 or 19, when adolescents typically lose public coverage, they often fall out of the system and experience dramatically decreased care (Adams et al., 2007; White, 2002). However, population surveys are cross-sectional and do not follow the same adolescents through the transition. Further, there is a shift in the methodology used in cross-sectional surveys at this juncture: parents answer for children through age 17, whereas individuals answer for themselves thereafter. Questions are also different on child and adult surveys, hampering comparisons across age ranges.

Measuring Across Settings, Across Multiple Domains of Care, and Across Time

Measurement of quality for a specific hospital stay or given outpatient visit is more straightforward than measurement of the overall quality of care across an episode of illness. New measures of health care quality for children and adolescents will need to track individuals over time and across multiple encounters with different care settings within the health care system. For adults, these episode-of-care measures tend to focus on curative outcomes (such as reduced hospital stays or lower rates of readmission). But this approach may need to be modified when applied to children with chronic conditions, for whom the issues are rehabilitative and functional rather than curative. Emerging work within NCQA and the American Academy of Pediatrics is focused on such efforts, for example, through the use of medical or health home measures or the new NCQA health care supervision measures (AAP, 2002; NCQA, 2010).

Measuring child and adolescent health care requires having the ability to look across visits and services to determine whether all required components of care were delivered for a particular age (Scholle et al., 2009). It also requires the ability to determine whether the appropriate combination of drugs was prescribed for a given mental illness, for example, or whether appropriate care was provided after a hospitalization (not merely whether there was a visit) or whether the child was rehospitalized for the same condition.

Current measurement systems and metrics are not capturing these vital longitudinal dimensions of care. Much of the information on health care quality comes from administrative data that measure services delivered (for example, a lead screening test), but not the outcome of the test or follow-up treatment. While organizations understand the potential for medical record abstraction to create such quality measures, they face numerous barriers (financial, privacy, and infrastructure) to implementation. In addition, rehabilitative and other services are delivered in non–health care settings, such as special education services and social work support services.

Adequate assessment of the quality of care would require capturing these services as well.

Measuring Quality in Preventive Care Services

The conceptualization of "health" for children embodied in *Children's Health, the Nation's Wealth* and elsewhere calls for departure from thinking of health as physical health and absence of illness and extends the concept of prevention into health promotion and well-being (IOM and NRC, 2004). Measurement of this broader concept of "health" is now reflected in cross-sectional population surveys such as the National Survey of Children's Health, but it is generally not present in the design, organization, and financing of the health care system. Significant efforts are now under way, however, to introduce broader concepts of prevention and health promotion into the routine services offered as part of well-child visits, especially through screening and practice changes to promote healthy development for children with or at risk for developmental delays. One such effort is the Assuring Better Child Health and Development (ABCD) initiative, sponsored by The Commonwealth Fund, in which state Medicaid agencies partner with others to increase the use of such screening and practice changes for low-income children (Kaye et al., 2006).

The Child and Adolescent Health Measurement Initiative (CAHMI) conducts two surveys aimed specifically at prevention measures: the Young Adult Health Care Survey (YAHCS) and the Promoting Healthy Development Survey (PHDS). The YAHCS seeks to assess whether young adults (aged 14–18) are receiving preventive services through a 54-question survey, which can be administered via telephone or mail (an online version is in development). The results are scored according to nine measures of care quality, emphasizing preventive screening and counseling on risky behaviors, sexual activity, and emotional health, as well as private and confidential care (CAHMI, 2010). The survey has been adopted by several states (California, Florida, New York, and Washington) for use in their quality improvement efforts (CAHMI, 2010), and its results can be used to create community-specific assessments of adolescent health.

The PHDS is a family-focused survey intended to capture both provider- and parent-based data that can be used during a well-child visit and can then become part of the medical record (Bethell et al., 2001). Parents may fill out the PHDS before the visit (either by mail, in the waiting room, or online), answering questions regarding concerns about the child, anticipatory guidance, and parental education needs and providing a brief assessment of the child's development and family risk factors. If physicians have access to EHRs, they can use a link in the EHR to review the survey results for family risk screening, family risk assessment, and priority educational needs prior to the visit. During the visit, physicians and other clinicians use the results to prioritize and individualize the content of the visit.

The PHDS-PLUS is an adaptation of the PHDS that provides a telephone/interviewer-administered survey for parents of young children (aged 3–48 months). One study indicates that data have been collected using the PHDS-PLUS from almost 14,000 children in Medicaid programs in seven states. These data provide a basis for comparing state-based performance in 11 designated topic areas, such as assessment of concerns about child development, family psychosocial assessment, and help with care coordination (Bethell et al., 2007).

Both the ABCD initiative and the PHDS-PLUS effort have developed quality measures that states can use as baseline information systems to improve their efforts to implement preventive and developmental services for children served through Medicaid managed care plans. These measures allow states to track the use of and experience with such preventive care services (Bethell et al., 2007; Scholle et al., 2009).

In the past, quality measures for preventive care have been largely process focused, examining whether a specific service had been delivered without examining the content of the visit or appropriate follow-up care. For example, there are HEDIS measures for whether a well-child visit has taken place or whether a chlamydia screening has occurred, but such measures do not consider the outcome of the screening procedure, or whether recommended treatment services were provided in a timely and effective manner (Scholle et al., 2009). This is largely because measures are derived from the claims data generated from a single visit. In the absence of EHRs and detailed clinical data on processes of care, efforts to abstract this information encounter major issues related to feasibility and cost.

Recently, important work has been done to expand the scope and flexibility of measurement approaches, particularly with regard to well-child visits (Scholle et al., 2009). New measures have been proposed that go beyond whether a visit has taken place to encompass the content and outcome of the visit. These new proposed measures assess whether all services that are required by age have been delivered across four domains: protection of health, healthy development, safe environment, and management and follow-up of health problems (Scholle et al., 2009). The age groups are infancy to 6 months, by age 2, by age 6, by age 13, and by age 18. Box 5-3 shows as an example the elements of care that need to have occurred by age 6. What is not yet known is the extent to which adherence to these services is associated with child health outcomes.

BOX 5-3
Quality Measures for Well-Child Visits (by age 6)

Protection of Health
- Immunizations
- Vision screening
- Oral health exam
- Blood pressure assessment
- Hearing

Healthy Development
- Developmental screening
- Weight assessment and counseling for nutrition and physical activity
- Counseling on screen time
- Parental competencies

Safe Environment
- Environmental tobacco assessment and counseling
- Domestic violence
- Firearm safety
- Vehicle safety
- Water safety
- Sports safety

Management and Follow-Up of Health Problems
- Individualized care plan

SOURCE: Scholle et al., 2009.

Opportunities to Link National Databases

Improved outcomes for populations of children and adolescents may be monitored through efforts to link to more national databases. The potential to link files across two or more national databases holds promise for providing further insight into contextual factors that constitute important health influences for children and adolescents, demographic variables that may be correlated with the use and quality of health care services, important outcomes for populations of children and/or adolescents, and improvements at the community and national levels.

A National Research Council (NRC) workshop summary reviews the strengths and limitations of key national databases that serve as sources for estimates of insurance coverage for children (NRC, 2010). These databases include data collected by the American Community Survey, the Current Population Survey, the National Health Interview Survey, the Medical Expenditure Panel Survey (Household Component), the Survey of Income and Program Participation, and the National Health and Nutrition Examination Survey. The report notes that "the presenters emphasized conducting targeted methodological research, building bridges between the surveys so that they could benefit from the strengths of each other, and providing data users more information for analyzing and possibly further adjusting data" (NRC, 2010, pp. 3–12).

Jurisdictional Issues Among Federal Agencies

One persistent barrier to efforts to achieve an optimal national measurement system for child and adolescent health and health care quality involves jurisdictional issues among federal agencies. The surveys described in the preceding section, for example, are conducted by separate agencies within HHS as well as other federal departments. Although a coordinating mechanism exists in the form of the Federal Interagency Forum on Child and Family Statistics, no agency is charged with leadership in striving for greater consistency and standardization in such basic areas as definitions of race and ethnicity or the inclusion of common age breaks that could facilitate comparisons across multiple surveys. Furthermore, research on the design and use of innovative measures, especially in such areas as a life-course perspective, social and behavioral determinants of health, and family-focused measures, is limited. Although various coordinating and high-level workgroups have attempted to solve these problems, their efforts have met with little success. The absence of a central registry of all federally supported longitudinal studies of children and adolescents, for example, is a sign of the limited resources and support allocated for efforts to coordinate interagency data sets.

PROMISING STATE AND LOCAL INITIATIVES

In addition to national efforts to do more with existing databases, some states and localities are experimenting with strategies to enhance their use of state and local data sources. These efforts include integrating health care data sets, as well as linking health care information with other data sources. An alternative approach is "layering" data systems through geocode mapping to highlight areas of common interest where problem behaviors tend to cluster. The feasibility of taking these initiatives to scale involves numerous questions around agency lead, infrastructure development, and resources required, among others. The 2011 IOM report *For the Public's Health: The Role of Measurement in Action and Accountability* addresses these linkages in greater detail (IOM, 2011a).

Massachusetts: Pregnancy to Early Life Longitudinal Data System

Massachusetts has developed a linked research database—the Pregnancy to Early Life Longitudinal (PELL) data system. This system links maternal and infant hospital discharge records with birth and fetal death records, and further links these records to additional public health and social services databases, including Early Intervention; the Supplemental Nutrition Program for Women, Infants, and Children (WIC); and birth defects and cancer registry data (BUSPH, 2010). The linkage in the Massachusetts PELL data system has generated numerous investigations of the quality of perinatal care (Clements et al., 2006, 2007; Declercq et al., 2007; Lazar et al., 2006; Shapiro-Mendoza et al., 2006; Tomashek et al., 2006).

Indiana: Child Health Improvement through Computer Automation System

The Child Health Improvement through Computer Automation (CHICA) system at Indiana Children's Health Services aims to strengthen parental involvement by asking parents about risks and concerns as part of a pediatric visit. Parental responses help ensure that physicians know about issues that need to be addressed and can shape the visit to make it more efficient.

CHICA is a computer-based decision support and EHR system for pediatric preventive care and disease management. Parents fill out a prescreening form in the waiting room that includes questions about risks, concerns, and reasons for the visit. The handwritten responses are then scanned and uploaded into the computer system, which generates customized items on a form used by the physician when he or she sees the patient. For example, if the parent has indicated that the child lives with a smoker, CHICA will prompt the pediatrician to discuss smoking cessation as well as the dangers of secondhand smoke (Downs et al., 2008). The information is tracked from clinic to clinic and from visit to visit.

Colorado: County Health Profiles

The Colorado Department of Health Care Policy and Financing (CDHCPF) has adopted the position that its role is to hold payers accountable for the health of the populations they serve (Wadhwa, 2010). To this end, CDHCPF uses a county health ranking model developed by the University of Wisconsin to examine the impact of policies and programs and population health factors on health outcomes. This model proposes that the physical and the social and economic environments contribute 50 percent to health outcomes, while factors within the health care system (clinical care and health behaviors) contribute the remaining 50 percent. The social and economic environment alone (rates of education, employment, income, family and social support, and community safety) is presumed to contribute 40 percent to population health outcomes. CDHCPF collects data from multiple state and federal sources and constructs health profiles for each county within the state. These county profiles organize health conditions and health care services into three categories: on the right track, needs improvement, and major challenges. This type of innovative practice requires expertise in working with multiple population health and administrative data sources, as well as statistical methods for comparing and analyzing data trends over time for selected populations.

Rhode Island: Asthma State Plan

One compelling example of a state-based partnership that uses data from multiple sources to address a chronic health problem is the Asthma State Plan adopted by the state of Rhode Island (RIACC, 2009). This plan is the result of a collaborative effort between the Rhode Island Department of Health and the Rhode Island Asthma Control Coalition, which consists of a variety of community health organizations. Recognizing that 11 percent of children in the state have asthma, the plan draws on an integrated chronic care health systems approach to effect change. This systems approach identifies 14 asthma-specific goals within five broad categories, which apply to both adults and children and include the following examples:

- Ensure that policies, programs, and systemwide changes are based on and evaluated using timely, comprehensive, and accurate asthma data.
- Decrease the disproportionate burden of asthma in racial and ethnic minority and low-income populations.
- Reduce exposure within schools to environmental asthma triggers, irritants, and asthmagens.

In developing a data system to implement various objectives under each goal, the Asthma State Plan does not seek to integrate multiple data sets, but rather relies on a strategy that designates an agency as the principal actor and specifies the data set that should be used to monitor progress toward achieving each objective. To reduce exposure within schools, for example, the Rhode Island databases used by the Department of Education provide the basis for monitoring the following key objective: "By 2014, increase the number of 'High Performance' schools that adopt construction, maintenance, and cleaning practices from 0 in 2008 to 20" (RIACC, 2009, p. 36).

Multiple state-level data sources are used to monitor performance, including the 2005 Rhode Island Behavioral Risk Factor Surveillance System (BRFSS), the 2008+ Rhode Island BRFSS Call-back Survey, and the Rhode Island Chronic Care Collaborative (RICCC) Asthma Database. The Rhode Island Asthma State Plan demonstrates that federal and state-based data systems can be used to support collective action and quality improvement efforts designed to address child health problems. Such efforts require dedicated financial and human resources, however, both to support the initial organizing, planning, and goal-setting efforts and to sustain the activities associated with data monitoring, analyses, and progress reports.

Philadelphia: Kids Integrated Data Set

The city of Philadelphia has established linkages among multiple data sets maintained by the departments of education, human services, law enforcement, and others. The Kids Integrated Data Set (KIDS) provides basic guidance for public officials in determining where resources can be matched with "hot spots" of vulnerable populations and neighborhoods. At present, however, health information cannot be linked effectively into the KIDS program because of legal and administrative restrictions that prevent "memorializing the link" between an individual child's health and educational records (Schwarz, 2010).

Austin, Texas: Children's Optimal Health

Based in Austin, Texas, Children's Optimal Health (COH) is aimed at improving children's health in the central Texas area through the use of geographic information system (GIS) mapping. The group is a nonprofit association consisting of approximately 50 members, including hospital systems, universities, businesses, and local agencies involved in health, education, and housing. COH does not aim to integrate separate data sources, but draws on a wide range of proprietary and public data sets that would otherwise never be shared. These data sets undergo a layering process that integrates the data without compromising the confidentiality of individual patients or the institutional data holders or violating legal restrictions such as those associated with the Health Insurance Portability and Accountability Act and the Family Educational Rights and Privacy Act. The layered data are fed into the GIS to form a succinct and powerful visualization—such as color-coded maps—of the community's health, which identifies social determinants (such as income or education levels) and highlights influential geographic factors (such as the location or clustering of specific businesses). These maps are then used by the participating groups within

COH to suggest steps for improvement and to formulate opportunities for collaborative policies (Sage et al., 2010).

In 2008, COH initiated a GIS mapping effort to address obesity trends among middle-school-aged children in Austin. First, the group sought data-sharing agreements from nearby hospital systems, federally qualified health centers, the city's housing authority, the Austin independent school district, organizations that offer services to youth and families, and a national health information exchange. The data sets produced from these agreements included data on students' body mass index, cardiovascular fitness, endurance, and flexibility, which could then be mapped to the locations of specific school districts. COH also collected police incident data that, once mapped, could account for less time spent outdoors because of a parent's or child's reduced sense of safety. A technical advisory committee ensured that all data were standardized and deidentified and offered initial interpretations of resulting maps. The final outcomes were presented at a community summit to engage the community in analyzing the findings and develop next steps (Sage et al., 2010).

SUMMARY

This chapter has provided an overview of child and adolescent health care quality measures, emerging opportunities to improve the development and use of measures, and unresolved difficulties that continue to challenge both the measurement of quality and the delivery of high-quality care for children and adolescents. A number of factors contribute to the current state of quality measurement. For example, the committee found that the motivations for creating and using quality measures for younger and older populations differ. One reason for this difference is the absence of private-sector incentives for the measurement and improvement of health care quality in younger populations. As a result, the state of health care quality measures for youth lags far behind that for adults. The absence of private-sector activity, coupled with the compelling need to improve health care quality and population health outcomes for children and adolescents, supports the need for a stronger public-sector presence in the design, collection, use, and reporting of such measures.

As described in this chapter, federal agencies have made some progress in addressing these shortcomings through the identification of an initial core set of standardized quality measures for children and adolescents. However, the exclusion of any measure for which validity, reliability, and feasibility have not been extensively documented has resulted in the neglect of measures for important areas of health for which evidence is limited (such as mental health, substance use, oral health, and relatively rare chronic conditions). Quality measures are especially important for the content of and follow-up on preventive and early intervention services for children and adolescents.

In addition, studies of vulnerable and marginalized populations of children and adolescents require greater attention to social and economic factors in assessing health care quality and health outcomes for children and adolescents. Some measures are available in these areas, but their implementation is limited in the absence of state and national data systems that support such measurement.

Although a number of measures of child and adolescent functional status exist, none have been accepted as "standard" measures. As noted in the previous chapter, there is no agreement on the appropriate domains for these measures, and little is known about the sensitivity of most such measures to medical care interventions.

This chapter has highlighted a number of emerging opportunities to improve the development and use of child and adolescent health care quality measures. For example, using a life-course approach to measurement provides a more comprehensive view of child and adolescent health care. A life-course perspective can inform understanding of the outcomes of preventive and early interventions, as well as the health consequences associated with early social environments. Incorporating this perspective will require longitudinal data sets that can follow population groups across episodes of care, as well as the management and measurement of care transitions across multiple settings and across time. Such transitions are especially salient for children and adolescents with special health care needs or chronic health conditions, as well as for the general population across specific life transitions, such as those from the prenatal stage to early childhood and from adolescence to young adulthood.

This chapter has provided examples of state and local efforts that encourage collaboration; foster the use of population health and administrative data sets among health care providers and their institutions and other service settings; support quality improvement practices; and inform coordinated interventions to prevent and mitigate health risk behaviors, as well as address the social and environmental contexts in which behaviors develop. These strategies can improve the timeliness of data collection and the transparency of data sources, with the ultimate goal of improving child and adolescent health care quality. However, taking these efforts to scale will require a full examination of Health Insurance Portability and Accountability Act regulations and state and local capacity to analyze, interpret, and report on data, among other issues.

Finally, additional work is needed to expand the existing collection of measures of child and adolescent health care quality. It will be necessary to underscore the need for broader availability of outcome measures across sectors; the collection and reporting of measures of social influences on health; and the creation of measures that can follow children and adolescents across different care settings, health plans, and multiple states over time. Clinical and comparative effectiveness research and the Centers of Excellence (U18) awards authorized by the CHIPRA legislation offer two important opportunities to build the evidence base for health care access and quality measures and to fill critical gaps, especially those gaps that address the specific characteristics and needs of younger populations. New initiatives associated with HIT and the creation of EHRs also offer substantial opportunities to foster the incorporation of children and adolescents into efforts to build the next generation of data sources and data collection methods. However, these efforts by themselves are unlikely to achieve this objective. Ultimately, greater alignment among federal agencies concerned with technology and quality measurement will be necessary.

6

Conclusions and Recommendations

The committee believes child and adolescent health is important in and of itself—as a measure of a society's values and capabilities—and as a direct determinant of subsequent productivity and later longevity. Timely, high-quality, readily accessible, and transparent information enables society to assess the impacts of programs and activities that may influence child and adolescent health. Such information enables society to compare the relative health of the nation's young people and the youth of other nations, as well as specific subgroups of American youth—defined by geography, race, socioeconomic status, or other characteristics—so we can make the policy and program changes that can achieve national health and health care goals. Similarly, measurement of the quality of children's health care enables society as a whole to understand the value of investments in health care services so as to make better decisions about these investments. Quality measures reveal which systems are functioning more or less effectively for which populations, again so we can improve the performance of those systems to achieve better short- and long-term outcomes, reduce suffering, advance safety, and achieve health equity.

Preceding chapters highlight the wealth of measures used to monitor the health status of children and adolescents and the quality of health care services they receive. Those chapters also point to the shortcomings and limitations of these measures and the challenges associated with integrating data sources and methods from diverse health and health care surveys and administrative records. While significant progress has been made, the nation has not yet balanced competing priorities and limited resources in developing measures that can support useful analyses of the extent to which children and adolescents in the United States are healthy or are receiving high-quality health care.

CONCLUSIONS

In reviewing the findings presented in the preceding chapters of this report, the committee formulated three sets of conclusions. The first set focuses on the nature, scope, and quality of *existing data sources* with information about child and adolescent health and health care quality. The second set involves conclusions about *gaps in measurement areas* that provide opportunities for improving future data collection, analysis, and reporting efforts broadly. These gaps focus in particular on the social and behavioral determinants of health and health care quality and the importance of incorporating a life-course perspective in existing data sets. The third set includes conclusions related to *gaps in methodological approaches* that would benefit from future attention. These three sets of conclusions provide the foundation for the recommendations that follow, which are framed by a stepwise approach to measuring health and health care quality for children and adolescents.

The Nature, Scope, and Quality of Existing Data Sources

- Multiple and independent federal and state data sources exist that include measures of the health and health care quality of children and adolescents.
- The fragmentation of existing data sources impedes access to and timely use of the information they collectively provide.
- Existing data sources have their individual strengths and limitations, but no single data set derived from these sources provides robust information about the health status or health care quality of the general population of children and adolescents.
- Lack of standardization in the measurement of disparities in health and health care quality limits the ability to identify, monitor, and address persistent health disparities among children and adolescents. The use of standardized definitions and measures for disparities is especially important as the nation moves toward greater reliance on computer-generated forms and other electronic data sources. Lessons learned from the use of standard formats for classification of race and ethnicity data, as well as for self-identification responses by informants (or parents), can inform the standardization process.
- Common definitions and consistent data collection methods would improve the standardization of common data elements (such as

insurance coverage) across multiple settings, such as health care, education, and human services, in federal and state data sets. Co-ordination among current national and state-level data collection efforts and the creation of common data elements could reduce duplication and maximize the effective use of resources.

Gaps in Measurement Areas

The conclusions in this area focus on the social and behavioral determinants of health and health care quality. Multiple longitudinal studies document the impact of physical and social environments (e.g., toxic exposures, safe neighborhoods, or crowded housing), behaviors (e.g., diet or the use of alcohol or drugs), and relationships (e.g., parent-child attachment) on the health status of children and adolescents and their use of health care services. Earlier IOM/NRC reports have documented the extent to which such information is lacking in existing federal health and health care data sets, and stressed that these contextual factors are key influences on the short- and long-term health outcomes of children and adolescents.

- Existing goal-setting efforts in the public and private sectors offer a foundation from which to develop national goals for children and adolescents in priority areas of health and health care quality.
- Quality measures for preventive services deserve particular attention for children and adolescents because most individuals in these age groups are generally healthy and because early interventions may prevent the onset of serious health disorders as the child or adolescent becomes an adult. Preventive measures could direct attention to both the content of screening procedures and the rate of use of follow-up services that were recommended in response to the identification of risk factors.
- Standardized measures of child health and the quality of relevant health care are important for all child health problems, but especially for preventable, ongoing, *or* serious health conditions. Moreover, the implications of the existence of a health condition may vary with the age of the child or adolescent. As noted in Chapter 4, child health problems include a large number of relatively rare conditions, such as sickle cell disease, which occurs only among certain racial and ethnic groups of children and adolescents. Many federal data sets do not have a sufficient number of children with these specific conditions to offer detailed analyses in the quality of care. In other cases, developmental conditions may be a source of concern within specific age groups. For example, an early sign of a health problem may be slower rates of physical growth, but later

implications may include poorer school achievement, perhaps due to repeated absences (Byrd and Weitzman, 1994; Weitzman et al., 1982), or behavioral issues that may further impede school success (Gortmaker et al., 1990). Special health conditions may vary in severity across different children and over time and have implications for adult health.

- Variations persist in data elements pertaining to race, ethnicity, income, wealth, and education. Core data elements for socioeconomic status need to be identified that can feasibly be collected in a standardized manner, while introducing a life-course approach that can be applied across multiple data sets, especially those that collect information about early stages of development.

- The health of other family members, especially parents and other caregivers, may directly affect the health of children and adolescents, as well as their access to and use of health care services. Family-focused measures (e.g., the health conditions affecting parents, their employment status, and family and household structure) are a new frontier for research in the development of measures. Understanding the relationship between parental and child health will involve new forms of data collection that can be used to analyze mother child and father child health patterns. The linkage between maternal and child health is one of the most important areas to explore. Family-focused measures will also improve understanding of parent-child relationships that influence the need for, access to, and use of health care services.

- With respect to social determinants of health, data are needed to determine those elements that offer timely potential for prediction of disparities. Key items for consideration are information on socioeconomic status, including family structure and family income in relation to family size; educational, literacy, and language proficiency levels of parents/guardians; neighborhood conditions (including rates of violence and mobility, school density and status, and environmental quality); and economic hardships, such as housing insecurity or homelessness and food insecurity/hunger.

- Race/ethnicity, socioeconomic status, primary language spoken at home, and parental English proficiency all affect disparities in health and health care and therefore are relevant topics for data collection for all children and adolescents. Determining the conditions under which racial and ethnic characteristics are an accurate proxy for social influences on health and health care quality is a significant challenge.

- Measures of health literacy are important for adults' ability to understand information that is relevant for children's healthy development and in ensuring adolescents' understanding of their own health status. These measures reside on the margins of health measures and deserve greater recognition in the identification of future research priorities and the testing of new measures in national surveys.

- Biological influences on the health of children and adolescents are an important focus for measures of health and health care quality; also important are measures of behaviors and levels of functioning. Functional status measures, for example, offer opportunities to describe health across multiple conditions, with direct implications for service needs, patterns of use, and care effectiveness. Measures focused on the needs of the "whole child," as opposed to individual clinical concerns, can address the distinct needs of children and adolescents, including their unique epidemiology, their dependent status, and their developmental stages. Functional status measures are one of the cornerstones recommended in *Children's Health, the Nation's Wealth* (IOM and NRC, 2004). Current child and adolescent health measures lack the capacity to capture important functional and developmental data; however, valid measures in these areas that have been tested across diverse populations do not yet exist. The inclusion of greater patient and family voice in the measurement of levels of functioning is an area that deserves particular attention.

- Measures of care transitions are important, especially for children with special health care needs. The creation and use of these measures would direct attention to episodes of care, as well as the design of consistent measures that can be used to follow children and adolescents over time across multiple care settings.

- New areas of focus entail place-based measurement, targeting selected geographic regions and population groups at the state, county, and even neighborhood levels. Place-based measurement for children's health and health care quality may be strengthened by efforts that draw explicitly on strategies described in the IOM report *Performance Measurement: Accelerating Improvement* (IOM, 2006b).

Methodological Areas That Deserve Attention

- Many data sources cannot be used to assess the status of specific groups of children and youth, particularly vulnerable populations who are at risk of poor health outcomes because of their health conditions or social circumstances. Implementing an integrated approach involves determining specific criteria for selecting reference groups, such as the following:

—age, gender, racial and ethnic characteristics, geographic location, and special health care needs;

—social and economic features, such as household income and parental educational levels;

—plan enrollment data at either a macro (i.e., public or private) or micro (i.e., Medicaid managed care or private point-of-service plan) level, length of plan enrollment, and eligibility criteria; and

—selected health conditions (such as asthma or mental health disorders) and parental health status.

- The selection of reference group criteria would benefit from interactions with state and local health officials, as well as those concerned with the health and health care quality of children and adolescents in their region, particularly underserved populations. The selection of criteria could also be guided by the perspectives of both consumers and users, who may regard the relevance and timeliness of the data as highly important, and those involved in data collection, who may be more concerned with validity, reliability, and accuracy.

- Greater transparency is necessary to expose the strengths and limitations of different surveys in tracking the status of key child and adolescent populations of interest; in identifying appropriate reference groups over time; and in implementing innovative measurement practices that can adapt to changing conditions, changing populations, and opportunities for health improvement. Such transparency is challenging, especially in circumstances where the data pool may be extremely small because of rare conditions, few providers or care settings, or stigma association with certain conditions. Experience with the creation and use of performance measures associated with the cystic fibrosis registry (Richesson et al., 2009), for example, illustrates how such transparency could be developed while protecting individual rights to privacy and confidentiality.

- Linking or aggregating databases (combining data derived from multiple jurisdictions, institutions, and population subgroups or from different time periods) would reduce variations among multiple data sources and decrease the burden of data collection on individual states, providers, health plans, and households.

—The time is ripe for developing collaborative efforts to improve the timeliness of data collection and the transparency of data sources in order to foster state and local efforts to improve health care quality. Such state and local efforts encourage collaboration; foster the use of population health and administrative data sets among health care providers and their institutions and other service settings; and support quality improvement practices.

—In some cases, data aggregation efforts have involved the creation of registries to pool data on immunization coverage, as well as data on selected rare health conditions (such as cystic fibrosis or childhood cancers) that involve complex health care services. Such registries can be extremely valuable in comparing health outcomes (such as mortality or hospitalization rates) among different providers and health care settings and identifying opportunities to introduce best practices that could improve health outcomes.

—Opportunities to create such registries may be available for other health conditions, such as sickle cell disease, HIV/AIDS, and mental health and behavioral disorders.

- While it is often difficult to connect data from the clinical records of children and adolescents enrolled in public health insurance plans to population health surveys and administrative data sets, such efforts will increase understanding of the social context and life-course influences that may affect children's health status and their access to and use and quality of health care services (IOM and NRC, 2004, p. 135). The legal challenges presented by laws such as the Health Insurance Portability and Accountability Act (HIPAA) and the Family Educational Rights and Privacy Act of 1974 (FERPA) deserve appropriate remedies, but they should not be viewed as insurmountable for efforts to link multiple data sets. Efforts to promote data sharing within individual states using, for example, the Medicaid databases and vital statistics records, deserve encouragement and support.

- Longitudinal data (with multiple observations for the same children/families over time) would enrich the quality of measures used in population health surveys and health care quality studies. Such data are critical to understanding the long-term implications of interventions and health status measures during prenatal development, infancy, childhood, and adolescence, and their relationship to adult health outcomes within a life-course framework (NRC, 1998, p. 1). Incorporation of a life-course perspective into health care quality measures for children and adolescents deserves serious consideration in the creation and design of a comprehensive measurement system. Despite the inevitable challenges for measurement, the life-course perspective is key, creative, underutilized, and promising. The emerging science of fetal and early childhood predictors of health outcomes lends particular importance to the need for longitudinal data sets. Incorporating this perspective could be achieved through longitudinal data sets that can follow population groups across multiple settings and across time to monitor the outcomes of preventive and early interventions, as well as the health consequences associated with early social environments.

- Electronic data capture and linkage would greatly enhance future measurement activity. Expanding data collection beyond geographic and claims information to capture state-level policy and community-level characteristics would enable analysis of the variability and impact of coverage, eligibility, and payment policies. Measurement efforts would be optimally useful if closely tied to current knowledge about specific functional health goals, meaningful use of health information technology, and established best practices for data extraction. Special attention will be needed to ensure that advances in electronic data capture adhere to existing privacy and confidentiality guidelines and laws. Ongoing attention will also be needed to resolve emerging issues related to privacy and confidentiality in future measurement efforts.
- While electronic health records have potential for significant retrieval of selected variables across multiple records, they do not necessarily offer conceptual or metric precision. The data are locked in a multitude of disparate systems designed for purposes other than analyses of health and health care quality.

A STEPWISE APPROACH TO MEASURING HEALTH AND HEALTH CARE QUALITY FOR CHILDREN AND ADOLESCENTS

The drivers for the creation and use of health and health care quality measures for younger populations are different from and lag far behind those for the development of quality measures for adult and elderly populations. The absence of strong private-sector incentives for the measurement of health care quality in younger populations, coupled with the compelling need to improve health care quality and population health outcomes for underserved children and adolescents, supports the need for a strong public presence in the design, collection, use, and reporting of such measures.

In reviewing early efforts and recent initiatives focused on improving health and health care quality measures for children and adolescents, the committee sought to build on the experience gained from earlier Institute of Medicine (IOM) health and health care quality studies (see Appendix C), legislative guidance, the Agency for Healthcare Research and Quality (AHRQ) core measures, efforts of the Centers for Medicaid and Medicare Services (CMS), and health care reform initiatives. Each of these efforts offers guidance for identifying important areas for measurement, but they have significant limitations. First, the variations among them impede consensus on the priorities for future quality measurement strategies. Second, areas that are important to the health and health care quality of children and adolescents continue to lack valid and reliable measures, as was noted earlier in the review of the core set of measures for children's health care quality recommended by the Secretary of Health and Human Services (HHS). Third, while many health care quality measures for children and adolescents (such as immunizations or safety procedures in administering medication) are comparable to those for the general adult population, others need to be adapted to the particular developmental needs of children and adolescents, which differ substantially from those of adults and may not be explicitly addressed in existing measures.

Federal agencies have made progress in addressing these shortcomings, such as the creation of an initial core group of standardized measures of quality of health care for children and adolescents. But the emphasis on using only valid, reliable, and feasible measures has resulted in neglecting the development of measures for important areas of health for which evidence is limited (such as mental health, substance use, oral health, and relatively rare chronic conditions), as well as for the content of and follow-up to preventive and early intervention services.

To address these shortcomings and limitations, the committee proposes a stepwise approach for improving measures of the health and health care quality of children and adolescents, based on the conclusions presented above. Strengthening the capacity of existing national and state-level data sets to provide routine guidance on areas of concern regarding the health and health care quality of children and adolescents could be achieved by improving the science as well as the use of measurement in five key areas that inform the steps in this approach. While the steps are proposed in a linear way, the committee recognizes that efforts may not adhere to this exact sequence, and back-and-forth movement may be necessary before the ultimate goal is achieved. The essential point is that each of the following steps is necessary in working toward a coherent system of measurement:

- **Step 1**—*Set shared health and health care quality goals for all children and adolescents in the United States*, especially those served by Medicaid and Children's Health Insurance Program (CHIP) health plans.
- **Step 2**—*Develop annual reports and standardized measures based on existing data sets of health and health care quality that can be collected and used to assess progress toward those goals.* This step focuses on achieving comparability across federal and state data sources, aligning the selection of measures with goals and priority

needs, removing measures that are no longer necessary, and targeting measures to provide more insight into the nature and severity
of health and health care disparities for underserved populations.

- Step 3—*Create new measures and data sources in priority areas*
  that can capture basic information about the behavioral and social
  conditions that exert profound influences on child and adolescent
  health and health care services.

- Step 4—*Improve methods for data collection, reporting, and analysis* in areas that are difficult to measure, linking existing data sets
  to make greater use of their contents and improving the timeliness
  of access to available data.

- Step 5—*Improve public and private capacities to use and report
  data*, drawing on existing data sources, as well as developing new
  federal–state and public–private partnerships to support special-
  population studies, the development and selection of measures, and
  the appropriate use of measures.

Figure 6-1 provides a graphic representation of the stepwise approach
to measuring health and health care quality for children and adolescents.
As depicted, the process is necessarily continuous and calls for evaluation of
the measurement system itself in terms of transparency, accessibility, timeliness, quality, and feasibility. The entire approach is supported by research
and evidence; survey, administrative, and medical records data; the health
information infrastructure; and stakeholders.

The committee's primary objective is to set in motion a process by
which progress that has been achieved in identifying key domains for
measuring the health of children and adolescents—by going beyond health
conditions to assess health functioning, health potential, and health influences—can be incorporated into existing and future efforts to measure the
quality of health care for these populations. The report *Children's Health,
the Nation's Wealth* (IOM and NRC, 2004, p. 1) demonstrates that some
valid and reliable measures already exist in each of these domains, and
many take a life-course perspective, derived primarily from population
health surveys. However, while rudimentary measures exist in some areas of
functioning and the social determinants of health, significant work needs to
be undertaken to develop consensus around the best available measures that
do not yet meet key thresholds of validity or reliability, but offer significant
promise in improving understanding of the social circumstances that influence children's health and health care quality.

In addition, extensive work has begun to take advantage of emerging technologies and other data collection methods that can support the
analysis of multiple variables from diverse data sources to provide more
timely and accessible information about the health and quality of health

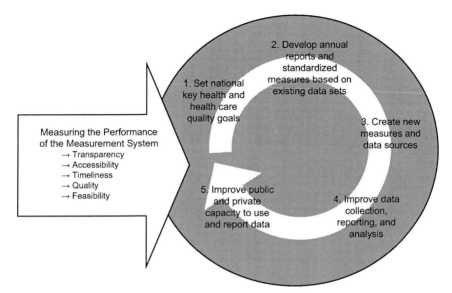

FIGURE 6-1 A stepwise approach to measuring health and health care quality for children and adolescents.

care for children and adolescents. Such efforts offer promise for informing the creation and selection of new measures, as well as the removal of comparatively inferior measures from administrative data sets as clinically rich electronic health records (EHRs) begin to emerge. Such electronic records hold the potential for identifying key relationships of interest that deserve consideration—such as those between health status and geographic location at different stages of development—provided such relationships can be established through the linkage of different data sources, the enhanced use of electronic data, or the development of new survey methods.

In the following sections, the committee offers recommendations for implementing each step of the proposed stepwise approach. In some areas, the committee offers specific guidance for implementing its recommendations, focusing in particular on those efforts that may be taken by the sponsors of this study, AHRQ and CMS. Box 6-1 provides a summary of key implementing actions for the committee's recommendations.

STEP 1: SET GOALS

Setting national and state-level goals for the health of children and adolescents would provide a structure within which to prioritize the next generation of health care quality measures, and would clarify the relative

BOX 6-1
Suggested Key Implementation Actions for the Committee's Recommendations

Secretary of Health and Human Services (HHS)

- Undertake a series of convening efforts designed to standardize definitions of race, ethnicity, special health care needs, and socioeconomic status in data sets pertaining to children and adolescents.
- Stimulate a series of research initiatives in diverse agencies to encourage the creation of valid and reliable indicators of the primary language spoken at home and parental English proficiency.
- Establish priority areas for future measures of health care disparities.

HHS Data Council

- Routinely convene experts in public health, health care quality, and data sources associated with public and private health plans to identify opportunities for coordinated and integrated measures of preventive services for children and adolescents.
- Coordinate with HHS agencies to validate functional and developmental measures that can apply to chronic health conditions for children and adolescents in existing data sets.
- Support efforts to identify and reconcile sources of variation among different child health surveys and to build consensus on the reference groups that merit consistent attention.

Federal Interagency Forum on Child and Family Statistics

- Undertake a series of convening efforts designed to standardize definitions of race, ethnicity, special health care needs, and socioeconomic status in data sets pertaining to children and adolescents.
- Work with other federal agencies (such as the Departments of Education and Justice) to identify opportunities to support state and local efforts that link health data for children and adolescents with school performance and community safety indicators.
- Work with other federal agencies to develop strategies for integrating multiple data sets into a comprehensive data system capable of monitoring influences on children's health outcomes.
- Work with other federal agencies to ensure that data on race/ethnicity, socioeconomic status, special health care needs, primary language spoken at home, and parental English proficiency are consistently collected in national and state surveys for all children and adolescents.

Agency for Healthcare Research and Quality (AHRQ) (in consultation with HHS)

- Identify priorities for future data aggregation efforts, and develop mechanisms to support these programs in public and private health care settings.

AHRQ and the Centers for Medicare and Medicaid Services (CMS)

- Assess current capacity to identify the social and economic status of children and adolescents in national and statewide data sources, and take steps to introduce associated measures where they are not available.
- Collaborate to support research and convening efforts focused on the development of measures that can be used to assess the content of basic preventive services associated with well-child visits, Early Periodic Screening, Diagnosis, and Treatment (EPSDT), and other preventive screens.
- Coordinate these efforts with evidence-based preventive services and programs for children and adolescents that are supported by other federal agencies.
- Conduct research on selected features of the families and neighborhoods of vulnerable populations of young people that exert significant influences on their health and health care quality.
- Introduce key measures for children and adolescents that capture such data as household income, levels of parental education, and family structure.
- Where feasible, introduce measures that can capture state-level policy and community characteristics.
- Develop guidelines to encourage greater transparency in monitoring the health outcomes (including mortality and morbidity rates) associated with the treatment of selected chronic conditions in different health settings and funded by different health plans.
- Convene a series of discussions with community leaders, educators, parents, and providers to explore approaches to linking diverse data sets through the use of unique identifiers while also protecting individual rights and respecting family privacy.
- Encourage collaboration with the National Health Information Network, the Key National Indicators Initiative, and related efforts to create community health maps and develop "smart targeting" techniques that focus on the status and particular needs of children enrolled in Medicaid and CHIP plans, as well as other vulnerable populations of children and adolescents.
- Convene state-based health plans to identify measures for key preventive health care strategies that could be incorporated into the core set of priority health care quality measures for children and adolescents.

roles of health care services and improvements in health care quality, as well as offer a basis for accountability, in achieving those goals. The goals could be derived as a set of critical objectives for children and adolescents from such sources as Healthy People 2010 and Healthy People 2020 for children and adolescents. They could also be reported as part of the annual national quality strategy and national prevention strategy reports prepared by the Secretary of HHS. In addition to specifying these goals, HHS agencies will need to establish lead agency roles in coordinating data linkage efforts. Questions to be resolved include the following:

- Should different agencies be responsible for health and health care data?
- Should health care services data be linked to efforts to improve quality and if so, at what level?
- Should different jurisdictions be encouraged or given incentives to coordinate and cooperate for efficiency in data coordination and linkage? How might this be achieved?

The answers to these questions will determine who has primary responsibility, and should be held accountable, for specific functions. Models to consider include designating a single agency with authority for coordinating multiple data sources, or, through interagency coordination efforts, building a robust data system with the capacity to collect information on important variables.

As discussed in Chapter 4, the committee built on earlier work that goes beyond the traditional focus on such indicators as morbidity, mortality, and chronic and acute conditions and identified seven priority areas to inform the setting of goals for health and health care quality for children and adolescents:

- childhood morbidity and mortality,
- chronic disease conditions,
- preventable common health conditions (especially mental and behavioral health and oral health),
- functional status,
- end-of-life conditions,
- health disparities, and
- social determinants of health.

These seven areas encompass the traditional measures of disease conditions, but also include new indicators of health and health care quality at the end of life and the social determinants of health. Pervading these seven areas is the need for a *life-course perspective* that can be used to examine how each area applies to different stages of development for infants, toddlers, children in middle childhood, and adolescents. As noted earlier, the recent IOM report, *Leading Health Indicators for Healthy People 2020*, stressed the importance of life-course approach and concluded that "the life course approach provides a useful framework for viewing health determinants and their relative importance at different stages of life, and for guiding the development of targeted health policies, programs, and actions to improve health" (IOM, 2011b). This current committee reaffirms the importance of setting national goals within a life-course perspective to focus attention on the need to develop positive indicators of health and well-being for different age groups and encourage the development of conditions and services that support such positive outcomes.

Frieden (2010) and others have identified an array of strategies that contribute to improving health outcomes: individual counseling and education, clinical interventions, long-lasting protective interventions (such as immunizations), changes in the environmental context for individual decision making (such as the use of protective equipment), and strategies addressing socioeconomic factors that influence health status (such as reducing poverty or increasing educational achievement). For specific populations—for example, those with life-threatening conditions such as cystic fibrosis or cancer—high-quality clinical care is a direct determinant of health; for more general populations, the latter strategies, such as public health or legal interventions that reduce exposure to tobacco or improve social and economic well-being, may be stronger influences on health outcomes.

Recommendation 1: The Secretary of Health and Human Services (HHS) should convene an interagency group to establish national health and health care quality goals for children and adolescents within a life-course framework.

The absence of a specified set of national goals that can guide measurement of the health and health care quality of children and adolescents and inform the health care quality improvement activities of multiple agencies creates a situation in which multiple measures exist without a clear sense of importance, priority, or connectedness. Federal and state agencies need to achieve consensus on a set of goals that captures the areas most important to monitor and measure, regardless of the quality of data sources and methods currently available to support the assessment of performance in achieving those goals. Existing measures can then be mapped against the goals to highlight areas in which measures are already available and identify areas that are important to monitor but lack valid and reliable measures.

HHS agencies can then assess the degree to which their grant-making priorities and research initiatives align with the established health and health care quality goals for children and adolescents.

The above seven priority areas often overlap and cannot be considered in isolation; however, each presents unique measurement challenges and opportunities that merit separate consideration. Most of the existing health and health care quality measures for children and adolescents are focused on the first two areas and draw extensively on administrative data sets. However, important initiatives have emerged within a few data sources that provide opportunities to build new measures in the remaining five areas. These initiatives warrant increased support because of their capacity to inform the next generation of health care quality measures, as well as the emerging health information technology infrastructure. Population health data sources, in particular, offer valuable resources to support new health care quality measures that go beyond traditional measures associated with treatment for acute and chronic disease.

In addition to support for these initiatives, extensive collaboration will be required among multiple agencies and sectors, as well as other key stakeholders and consumers of the data, to develop the next generation of measures, especially in areas that involve disparities, social and behavioral determinants of health, and a life-course perspective. Interagency working groups and public–private collaborations will need to be formed and charged to develop action steps with defined timelines. Agency leaders will need to be designated to assume responsibility and accountability for developing measures and data sets that can address these gaps in a timely way.

Multiple public- and private-sector efforts are already under way to identify priority health and health care quality goals for children and adolescents, such as indicators included in Healthy People 2010 and 2020 (HHS, 2000a), the annual child well-being reports prepared by the Interagency Forum on Child and Family Statistics (FIFCFS, 2009), the Kids Count activities supported by the Annie E. Casey Foundation (Mather and Adams, 2006), and the annual Child Well-Being Index supported by the Foundation for Child Development (Land and FCD, 2010). These efforts draw on multiple data sources of varying quality and focus on different areas of interest. A national goal-setting effort for child and adolescent health and health care priorities could draw attention to those areas in which advances in the quality of health care services can contribute to improvements in health outcomes. This effort could also focus attention on opportunities for advances in public health or social policy to make important contributions.

STEP 2: DEVELOP ANNUAL REPORTS AND STANDARDIZED MEASURES BASED ON EXISTING DATA SETS

The goal-setting effort of Step 1 would highlight areas in which measurement of the quality of child and adolescent health and health care services is strong, as well as areas in which valid and reliable measures do not yet exist, areas that are difficult to measure, and populations that are difficult to reach. Step 2 focuses attention on the need to develop annual reports and standardized measures in the seven priority areas based on existing data sets, building on the multiple efforts of professional, public, and private-sector organizations.

While a large number of measures exist, efforts to monitor and improve the health and health care quality of children and adolescents are hampered by the absence of routine annual reports that focus on child and adolescent health and health care quality, as well as variations in both the measures themselves and the underlying data sources that support them. In the latter area, the committee has identified two issues of particular concern: (1) the absence of consistent measurement of disparities in health and health care quality to support the development of targeted interventions at the national and state levels, and (2) the retention of unnecessary or obsolete measures resulting from the adoption of standardized core measure sets over time, which can be addressed through a periodic review process.

Existing Opportunities to Include Children and Adolescents in Annual HHS Reports

The Secretary of HHS is already required to produce annual reports on health care quality and disparities (HHS, 2010a, 2010b), as well as annual reports on national prevention initiatives (HHS, 2011b; NPC, 2010). These reports provide valuable opportunities to include specific attention to children and adolescents and to draw attention to the ways in which their needs may different from those of older populations.

Standardized Measurement of Disparities in Health and Health Care

The changing demography of America's youth increases the importance of recognizing and addressing pervasive disparities and inequities in child and adolescent health and health care. As with the measurement of health and health care quality, the measurement of disparities involves multiple dimensions and criteria. Though many studies measure disparities in terms of racial or ethnic differences, disparities also involve issues of gender, household income, educational status of the child or parent, insurance type, and medical practice setting (see Chapter 2).

Individual states are inconsistent in the way they classify race and ethnicity data in the Medicaid Statistics Information System (MSIS) (see Chapter 5). These inconsistencies highlight the importance of technical and methodological approaches that can reduce variation while allowing for individual choice. This issue is not unique to health and health care quality data for children and adolescents. Federal and state statistical systems would benefit from opportunities to exchange insight and experience in developing effective solutions. This is a recurrent theme throughout this report, as reflected in the committee's recommendations and the suggested key implementation actions outlined below and summarized in Box 6-1.

The composition of population groups that are represented in existing data sets, as well as the methodological limitations of the survey measures and administrative data themselves, deserve significant attention. One study of Consumer Assessment of Healthcare Providers and Systems (CAHPS)-like questions about patient experiences of care, for example, has called attention to variations in the applicability of the survey items to people with different cultural or other social traits (Morales et al., 2001). The absence of language diversity and the lack of rigorous methodological work on the cross-cultural validity of multiple survey measures are notable shortcomings in existing health care quality data sets. These shortcomings are especially evident in evaluating the patient-centeredness component of care, when parents are asked to assess their child's general status, their satisfaction with the services their child has received, and/or the extent to which their child's health needs have been adequately addressed.

Assessment of children's and adolescents' health will benefit from efforts to (1) adopt standardized definitions and measures of these characteristics, (2) routinely include socioeconomic information (minimally household income as an increment of the federal poverty level and educational attainment of parents), and (3) introduce data on language proficiency in existing data collection on the health and health care quality of children and adolescents. All these actions will be increasingly important in response to the growing poverty rates and increasing racial and ethnic heterogeneity of younger populations.

As noted earlier in this report, compared with U.S. adults, U.S. children and adolescents are disproportionately of nonwhite race/ethnicity, a fact of particular significance because poor and minority children have greater special health care needs than their nonpoor and white counterparts (Flores, 2010). Children and adolescents in these groups also are more frequently insured through public health plans. For example, more than 50 percent of African American and 48 percent of Latino children have public insurance such as Medicaid or CHIP (DeNavas-Walt et al., 2010). Thus the development of health indicators that can provide a basis for considering the health status of these groups in relationship to the general population of children and adolescents is a particularly urgent need.

Recommendation 2a: The Secretary of HHS should include specific measures of the health and health care quality of children and adolescents in annual reports to Congress as part of the Secretary's national quality and prevention strategy initiatives.

Recommendation 2b: These measures should include standardized definitions of race/ethnicity, socioeconomic status, and special health care needs, with the goal of identifying and eliminating disparities in health and health care quality within a life-course framework. Identifying and reducing disparities in health and health care will require collecting data on race/ethnicity, socioeconomic status, special health care needs, primary language spoken at home, and parental English proficiency for all children and adolescents.

Disparities in health and health care can be assessed by collecting data on race/ethnicity, socioeconomic status, special health care needs, primary language spoken at home, and parental English proficiency for all children and adolescents. Specific actions that could be taken to implement this recommendation include the following:

- All HHS agencies, especially AHRQ and CMS, could assess their current capacity to identify the social and economic status of children and adolescents in national and statewide data sources and take steps to introduce associated measures where they are not available.
- The Federal Interagency Forum on Child and Family Statistics could undertake a series of convening efforts to standardize definitions of race, ethnicity, special health care needs, and socioeconomic status in data sets pertaining to children and adolescents.
- The Federal Interagency Forum on Child and Family Statistics could work with other federal agencies to ensure that data on race/ethnicity, socioeconomic status, special health care needs, primary language spoken at home, and parental English proficiency are consistently collected in national and state surveys for all children and adolescents.
- The Secretary of HHS could stimulate a series of research initiatives within diverse agencies to encourage the creation of valid and reliable measures of the primary language spoken at home and parental English proficiency.

- The Secretary of HHS could establish priority areas for future measures of health care disparities, including disparities of health care access and utilization. Suggested areas include
  —prenatal care and neonatal development (i.e., prematurity and birth weight),
  —early childhood preventive care services and school readiness,
  —transitions from adolescence to young adulthood,
  —children with special health care needs (e.g., Down syndrome, cystic fibrosis),
  —oral health,
  —mental and behavioral health (including substance abuse), and
  —health care access and utilization.

A Periodic Review Process

As national health and health care quality goals change over time, certain measures or data sources may become obsolete or unnecessary, new data sources and measurement methods may emerge, and gaps may develop in areas that are important to monitor but difficult to measure. A process needs to be in place for conducting routine reviews of the recommended core set of standardized measures to identify those that are no longer appropriate for monitoring, those that support timely and reliable assessments of health and health care quality, and gaps that could benefit from investments in research to stimulate measurement in areas that are difficult to assess or for populations that are difficult to reach.

Standardization can produce measures with the potential to aid in robust comparative assessments across jurisdictions and time periods, but it often comes at a cost if lessons learned through the application of such measures are not shared with those involved in the development and selection of measures (McDonald, 2008). Standardization may result in the adoption of suboptimal measures at any given time based on the data sources available and the status of measure development. A periodic review process can help ensure that standardization does not result in the entrenchment of suboptimal measures (i.e., those that do not respond to changes in clinical evidence, understanding of the determinants of health, or measurement science). A periodic review process should include assessing each measure from the standardized core set to determine whether there is new evidence or information about the characteristics of the measure, its underlying data sources, or its application context (McDonald, 2008; Pancholi and Geppert, 2008), as well as to consider how it could incorporate features of new similar measures. The results of this assessment would provide a basis to revise, replace, or retire measures when justified. The evidence base for measures and associated data elements applicable to children and adolescents is limited compared with that for the adult population (McDonald, 2009). As a result, new information is likely to emerge rapidly, making a continual learning environment for measures for children and adolescents even more important.

The committee tried to avoid wherever possible major new demands for state-level data collection beyond current capacities without identifying resources to support such efforts. In some cases, many states are already collecting, analyzing, and reporting important child health data, as noted in prior chapters. Strengthening these efforts while providing additional funding to those states without these capacities can make the improvement of national child and adolescent health data more feasible. States often are required to report important data in such areas as health events and service provision as a condition for receipt of federal funding. In such cases, standardization in data collection efforts (through the creation of common data elements) and in the format for reporting may be a feasible route to the goal of improving the quality of national statistics on child health and health care. In other cases, new surveys may be needed to complement existing efforts. Ultimately, the national goal should be focused on developing useful measures of health and health care quality that address the priorities and needs of the users of the data.

The periodic review process provides an opportunity to address effective and valid data collection approaches and to ensure that respondents (especially parents and adolescents) are clear about the meaning and intent of the questions being asked. This is an important concern as parents may feel they need to put the best face on their children's health status. In the case of adolescents, many parents may honestly not know about all the sources of health care that their children have accessed. Important validation efforts are therefore needed as new concepts in such areas as care coordination, prevention, and medical homes assume a larger role in health care delivery.

Recommendation 3: The Secretary of HHS should develop a strategy for continuous improvement of the system for collecting, analyzing, and reporting health and health care quality measures for children and adolescents. This strategy should include periodic review of those measures that are used, recommended, or required by the federal government.

The AHRQ work on quality indicators initiated under the Evidence-based Practice Center Program is one example of this type of process that already exists at the federal level and could potentially be replicated for any standardized measures or measure sets. The development and maintenance of the AHRQ quality indicators are grounded in the methods of evidence-based medicine, applied to measurement. Initially, AHRQ and Healthcare Cost and Utilization Project (HCUP) partners requested an evidence project to refine the original HCUP quality indicators. The motivation for this refinement was to meet the needs of those who were collecting the data and were working within their states to supply hospitals, legislators, policy makers, and the public at large with meaningful information based on the routinely collected administrative data sets available at the time.

As the program evolved, AHRQ initiated a support contract to ensure ongoing refinement of the indicators, including retirement of measures. Thus the guiding philosophy of the program is continuous quality improvement based on user experience and changes in medical evidence. In addition, the program includes expansions within domains and data sets initially covered, as well as expansions to new domains without ties to any particular data set to reflect new priorities in health care. Throughout the process, AHRQ and the quality indicator team have continued to innovate to expand measurement methods, always evaluating measures from initial assessment to implementation, followed by feedback and support throughout their life in the field. Documentation of the revision, replacement/expansion, and retirement of measures is available on a website (AHRQ, 2008) so that users of the measures have standard specifications but know that annual updates will reflect any new information.

STEP 3: CREATE NEW MEASURES AND DATA SOURCES IN PRIORITY AREAS

As noted above, most of the current health and health care quality measures for children and adolescents are focused on significant causes of mortality and morbidity and chronic health conditions (Beal et al., 2004). Among the seven priority areas, preventive services and the social determinants of health—using a life-course perspective—deserve particular emphasis in the development of measures of the health and quality of health care for children and adolescents.

Measures Addressing Preventive Services

The core set of measures for children's health care quality recommended by the Secretary of HHS includes a strong emphasis on preventive services, but it lacks a similar emphasis in important areas that are particularly relevant for children and adolescents, such as oral health and mental and behavioral disorders. For example, dental caries are the leading cause of infectious disease among children and adolescents (HHS, 2000b). Likewise, in any given year, the percentage of young people with mental, emotional, or behavioral disorders is estimated to be between 14 and 20 percent (IOM, 2009c). Such disorders can include early drug or alcohol use or antisocial or aggressive behavior and violence that frequently emerge during childhood and adolescence. These disorders are included in selected data sources, but they frequently are omitted from national surveys. In addition, many children and adolescents in troubled circumstances (such as child welfare systems or juvenile detention centers) are not included in routine survey samples, and their family history or residential placements are not included in administrative records.

> **Recommendation 4: The Secretary of HHS should develop new measures of health and health care quality focused on preventive services with a life-course perspective. These measures should focus on common health conditions among children and adolescents, especially in the areas of oral health and mental and behavioral health, including substance abuse.**

The new National Prevention Strategy mandated in the Affordable Care Act offers an opportunity to improve the quality of data sources with respect to the measurement of preventive services for children and adolescents. This effort would benefit from collaboration among multiple HHS agencies:

- AHRQ and CMS could provide collaborative support for research and convening efforts focused on the development of measures that can be used to assess the content of basic preventive services associated with well-child visits, early periodic screening, diagnosis, and treatment (EPSDT), and other preventive screens.
- AHRQ and CMS could coordinate these efforts with evidence-based preventive services and programs for children and adolescents that are supported by other federal agencies (such as the Healthy Start program supported by the Health Resources and Services Administration [HRSA] and selected public health screening efforts for sexually transmitted infections, underage drinking, and substance use).
- The HHS Data Council could routinely convene experts in public health, health care quality, and data sources associated with public and private health plans to identify opportunities for coordinated and integrated measures of preventive services for children and adolescents.
- AHRQ and CMS should convene state-based health plans to identify measures for key preventive health care strategies that could be incorporated into the core set of priority health care quality measures for children and adolescents.

- While the creation of consistent measures that can be used to assess health care quality for diverse populations deserves substantial attention, additional effort is necessary to develop a system that can foster the implementation and use of such measures. Recent legislative initiatives such as the Affordable Care Act and other federal efforts to support the development of health information technology offer substantial opportunities to foster the inclusion of children and adolescents in these efforts to build the next generation of data sources and data collection methods.

- Some aspects of these changes will likely support implementation of the approach proposed in this report aimed at improving quality measurement and outcomes for children. For example, increased emphasis on payment for outcomes and other value-based payment strategies will necessitate an increased investment in data collection and analysis, as well as the development of new quality metrics that correspond to the new service delivery structures, especially those that focus on preventive interventions for children and adolescents. Other aspects of these changes may impede progress toward the approach proposed by the committee. For example, increased use of bundled payments may reduce the amount or quality of administrative data available to measure care content and processes. These cross-currents reinforce the importance of measuring quality and outcomes for children for private payers, in addition to Medicaid and CHIP, and including measures at multiple levels of the health care system (e.g., the physician, plan, and accountable care organization [ACO] levels).

Measures Addressing Social and Behavioral Determinants of Health Using a Life-Course Perspective

While the need for improved measures of health care disparities and preventive services has already attracted attention, few data sources currently provide opportunities to incorporate new measures in such areas as the social and behavioral determinants of health or incorporate a life-course approach to measuring health functioning and health potential. Measures in these areas would facilitate important analyses and reporting on child and adolescent health and health care quality, and deserve special consideration given the dependent status of children and adolescents and the growing numbers who live in poor and low-income families. In generating the necessary measures and data sources in these areas, extensive collaboration among multiple public and private stakeholders will be necessary.

Recommendation 5: The Secretary of HHS should support interagency collaboration within HHS to develop measures, data sources, and reporting focused on relationships between the social determinants of health and the health and health care quality of children and adolescents.

Recommendation 6: The Secretary of HHS should encourage interagency collaboration within HHS to introduce a life-course perspective that strengthens the capacity of existing data sources to measure health conditions, levels of functioning, and health influences (including access to and quality of care) for children and adolescents.

Specific actions that could be taken to implement these recommendations include the following:

- The HHS Data Council could support efforts to identify and reconcile sources of variation among different child health surveys and to build consensus on the reference age, racial/ethnic, and socioeconomic groups that merit consistent attention.
- The HHS Data Council could coordinate with HHS agencies to validate functional and developmental measures that can apply to chronic health conditions for children and adolescents in existing data sets. This effort would involve testing similar measures of functional status across different health conditions and populations to establish thresholds and categories and to highlight key dimensions of functional status, including calibration of parental/youth reporting and intervention strategies. Such efforts might also include measures of family care and intergenerational care in existing survey efforts.
- AHRQ and CMS could collaborate with other HHS agencies (particularly HRSA and the Centers for Disease Control and Prevention [CDC]) to conduct research on selected features of the families and neighborhoods of vulnerable populations of young people that exert significant influences on their health and health care quality (such as family structure, rates of mobility, and violence).
- AHRQ and CMS could adopt key measures for children and adolescents that capture data in such areas as household income, levels of parental education, and family structure. Such measures already exist, for example, in population health databases such as the NSCH and NS-CSHCN, but have yet to be introduced in health care quality data sources.

- The effort to introduce social determinants into new and existing data sets in other federal agencies will require
  —identifying key aspects of socioeconomic status to be incorporated into data collection efforts,
  —prioritizing other factors as standard elements in data collection efforts, and
  —prioritizing the data sources to be modified to include these elements.
- Where feasible, AHRQ and CMS should introduce measures that can capture state-level policy and community characteristics. Such data will enable analysis of the variability and impact of coverage, eligibility, and payment policies, which may vary across multiple jurisdictions. This effort would benefit from additional investments in research design and survey instruments. Child and adolescent health status and health care quality may be directly influenced by the capacity of the health care resources within communities. Eligibility for and use of available services may also be affected by state and national criteria and regulations and their implementation.
- The Federal Interagency Forum on Child and Family Statistics could develop coordinated strategies for sharing results from longitudinal studies of children and adolescents with those who design and analyze population health and administrative data sets for these populations. The gaps between these separate efforts prevent the discovery of key data elements or relationships emerging from longitudinal studies that could strengthen the quality of data sources that rely on other methods. Longitudinal data focus attention on the sequence of conditions, experiences, and resources that influence child health outcomes. Infant mortality rates in certain regions, for example, may result not from the scarcity or low quality of neonatal facilities but from the absence of high-quality prenatal care for pregnant women, especially those who have difficulty navigating health care services because of limited English proficiency, changes in employment or family structure, or low health literacy. Placing more emphasis on achieving high-quality care in neonatal facilities may have a limited pay-off when the real problem resides in behavioral, educational, and social factors, such as legal restrictions on public health care services for undocumented immigrants.
- The HHS Secretary could stimulate the development of registries and other data aggregation strategies for rare but chronic conditions that affect many children and adolescents (such as cystic fibrosis and sickle cell disease). Such strategies will provide a basis for analyzing practices and disparities in hospital and ambulatory care settings and identifying opportunities for quality improvement.

Recommendation 7: The Secretary of HHS should place priority on interactions between HHS agencies and other federal agencies to strengthen the capacity to link data sources in areas related to behavioral health and the social determinants of health and health care quality.

In addition to the internal interagency collaboration with the U.S. Department of Health (as suggested in Recommendation 5), opportunities exist to foster integration of federal data sets that could link health and health care quality data to other child and adolescent outcomes, in areas such as education, employment, and public safety. These collaborative efforts would require interactions between HHS agencies and other federal departments. Specific actions that could be taken to implement this recommendation include the following:

- The HHS Data Council could work with other federal agencies (such as the Departments of Education and Justice) to identify opportunities to support state and local efforts that link health data for children and adolescents with school performance and community safety indicators, with special consideration of the challenges created by HIPAA and FERPA regulations.
- The Federal Interagency Forum on Child and Family Statistics could work with other federal agencies to develop strategies for integrating multiple data sets into a comprehensive data system capable of monitoring influences on children's health outcomes, including
  —environmental indicators that inform analyses of interactions between health influences and child health conditions;
  —geographic indicators that facilitate comparisons of health and nonhealth factors linked across population health survey(s), claims data, administrative records, EHRs, and other data sources; and
  —encouragement for the inclusion of innovative measures in current population health surveys, such as diet, nutrition, and media exposure for children and adolescents, as well as other measures that respond to changing technologies and emerging health concerns.

STEP 4: IMPROVE DATA COLLECTION, REPORTING, AND ANALYSIS

The Importance of Data Aggregation and Transparency

Several strategies can be used to improve data sources and methods for data collection, reporting, and analysis: (1) data aggregation strategies, including the use of registries and data linkage opportunities; (2) the development of mechanisms to foster greater transparency of performance indicators; (3) the use of unique identifiers that allow analysts to link data on the same child from different administrative data sets to obtain a more robust profile of the characteristics of the child and his or her social context and health and educational outcomes (for an in-depth analysis of unique identifiers, see IOM, 2010b); and (4) greater use of longitudinal studies, which follow the same cohort of children over time to monitor their health conditions and the health care services they receive.

The importance of longitudinal measurement has been cited in multiple other studies (see, for example, the IOM report on performance measurement, IOM, 2006b, pp. 119–120). Longitudinal measurement fosters child-centered analysis, breaking down the divisions among data created by the different silos of the health care system and other service settings that engage the child and his or her family. Longitudinal measures are especially useful in monitoring care transitions, from hospital to ambulatory care, from primary care to other service settings, and from pediatric care to adult care settings (the times when breakdowns and errors in care are most likely to occur) (Coleman and Berenson, 2004). Longitudinal studies also enable assessment of whether the child's or adolescent's needs have been identified and met within an appropriate care setting. In addition, longitudinal measurement is necessary to determine both the short- and long-term outcomes of care, identifying intervening factors that may enhance or impede the effects of a high-quality health care system.

Creating opportunities to link data across multiple health care settings, as well as connecting health and health care data to education and human service data sources, will improve timeliness and foster greater transparency as to the multiple factors that affect the well-being of children and adolescents. Such efforts will require both methodological and technical advances and the resolution of concerns related to privacy and data sharing. Timely and transparent data sets can also help in explaining to participants the rationale for data collection efforts, including their purpose and the means by which the data will be used to assist their own and other children and adolescents nationwide. This understanding is key to ensuring that all segments of the population, including marginalized groups, will be fully represented in survey and administrative data sources. Patient advocacy and other community-based organizations can play an outreach role in the community so that underrepresented populations will not interpret participation negatively.

Enhancing Timeliness: Moving Health and Health Care Quality Data into the Digital Age

The rationale for timeliness is obvious—information that lags or is collected only infrequently is of little value in informing program and policy decisions. Similarly, decision making is impaired by poor-quality data that reflect the health or quality of health care services for children and adolescents neither truthfully nor precisely. Transparency is necessary if the data are to be believable; otherwise, the data will not lead to action. Accessibility is critical as well if the data are to inform public discourse and lead to prompt action.

Linking data across multiple health care settings, as well as linking administrative records to education and human service data systems, will improve timeliness and foster greater transparency as to the multiple factors that affect the health and health care quality of children and adolescents.

> **Recommendation 8: The Secretary of HHS should identify significant opportunities to link data across health care, education, and human service settings, with the goal of improving timeliness and fostering greater transparency as to the multiple factors that affect the health of children and adolescents and the quality of services (including health care, educational, and social services) aimed at addressing those factors.**

> **Recommendation 9: The Secretary of HHS should promote policy, research, and convening efforts that can facilitate linkages among digital data sets while also resolving legal and ethical concerns about privacy and data sharing.**

Specific actions to be considered in implementing these recommendations include the following:

- The HHS Data Council, in consultation with various other HHS agencies, such as AHRQ, HRSA, CDC, and the National Center for Health Statistics (NCHS), could identify priorities for future data aggregation efforts and develop mechanisms to support these programs in public and private health care settings.
- AHRQ and CMS, in consultation with other HHS agencies, could develop guidelines to encourage greater transparency in monitoring the health outcomes (including mortality and morbidity rates)

associated with the treatment of selected chronic conditions in different health settings and funded by different health plans.

- CMS could expand and improve access to Medicaid data for quality measurement in child and adolescent health, including improving states' access to encounter data (e.g., from the MSIS), resolving anomalies in state-level claims and enrollment records, and encouraging states to link to other databases (e.g., the National Vital Statistics System [NVSS]).

- Use of a unique identifier would facilitate aggregation of data and longitudinal studies, especially for children who are served in multiple public and private settings. Establishment of a system of unique identifiers would require cooperation across multiple institutions and providers of care. When a unique identifier is not available, statistical methods can be used for matching across data sets, but problems of duplication and undercoverage make this approach challenging. CMS has already developed unique identifiers for health records that are collected as part of the MSIS (see Chapter 5). The state-assigned identifier can be used consistently to identify a given individual across different years and different enrollment periods, making it possible to track Medicaid beneficiaries over time within the state. At present, however, it is not possible to track children and adolescents who move to different state jurisdictions. The MSIS has not been widely used for national reporting under CHIPRA, but HHS is now in the early stages of collecting and analyzing annual MSIS data within 6 months of state submission.

- AHRQ and CMS could develop a series of demonstration experiments involving the use of unique identifiers to foster life-course analyses and to strengthen the capacity to link records across multiple health care settings, as well as to link health data with sources of education and community safety data. Such experiments should build on innovative local and regional models that are already employing unique identifiers in data warehouses, such as the Kids Integrated Data Set (KIDS) initiative in Philadelphia and the Multi-State Foster Care Data Archive administered by the Chapin Hall Center for Children.

- AHRQ and CMS could convene a series of discussions with community leaders, educators, parents, and providers to explore solutions for linking diverse data sets through the use of unique identifiers while also protecting individual rights and respecting family privacy.

- AHRQ and CMS could encourage collaboration with the National Health Information Network, the Key National Indicators Initiative, and related efforts to create community health maps and develop "smart targeting" techniques (seeking niche populations based on predetermined criteria) that focus on the status and particular needs of children enrolled in Medicaid and CHIP plans, as well as other vulnerable populations of children and adolescents.

STEP 5: IMPROVE PUBLIC AND PRIVATE CAPACITIES TO USE AND REPORT DATA

The conclusions presented earlier in this chapter emerged from the committee's review of research studies on the measurement of health, health care quality, and health disparities for children and adolescents. These studies consistently demonstrate that improving measurement in these areas requires building capacities to use and report data at the federal and state levels. The emerging health information technology infrastructure offers an opportunity to emphasize the distinct needs of children and adolescents and to link those needs to family data in health information exchanges, for example, as well as to supplement traditional electronic information with data from other sources (including parents). These linked data sets could track children across public and private data sources, as well as link with public health data through birth certificates and newborn screening data sets.

Simply building more capacity will not suffice, however. It will also be important to develop an integrated approach that can aggregate and combine measures of the health status of children and adolescents (drawn from population health surveys) with measures of health care quality for those services that are actually used by children, adolescents, and their families. Additionally, measures are needed with which to compare the quality and utilization of services with the types and severity of children's health needs due to chronic health disorders or risk factors that make them vulnerable to adverse health outcomes.

Efforts to build federal, state, and even local capacity for place-based measures can resolve some of the current difficulties of integrating health measures, measures of social context and other health influences, and health care quality measures focused on services within the health care setting. Such efforts will require innovative approaches to compiling and extracting data from existing surveys and databases. They will also require a conceptual framework that can prioritize and operationalize key measures of social context and health influences, as well as criteria that can be used to designate the appropriate reference groups of common interest. Some states are prepared to serve as laboratories for the creation of new measures for difficult-to-measure indicators or difficult-to-reach populations, and they would benefit from the development of incentives that would encourage voluntary compliance now.

At the same time, improving federal and state data collection capacity will not be sufficient to ensure that the data will lead to better child and adolescent health outcomes. Collaboration needs to be strengthened between those who collect the data and those who are expected to use the data to shape current and future interventions in health care and other service-based or community settings. Fostering this collaboration involves investing in the capacity of communities, states, providers, consumers, and others to use the data effectively to drive decision making in light of limited resources, as well as to monitor changes given the introduction of new policies or investments over time. Capacity for the use of data on health and health care quality also involves understanding the importance of tailoring interventions to the needs of different racial/ethnic, geographic, and other segments of the population and tracking longitudinally how disparities respond to changes in health care resources, processes, and policies.

> **Recommendation 10: The Secretary of HHS should establish a timetable for all states to report on a core set of standardized measures that can be used in the health information technology infrastructure to assess health and health care quality for children and adolescents. Congress and HHS should formulate alternative strategies (through incentive awards, demonstration grants, and technical assistance, for example) that would enable states to develop the necessary data sources and analyses to meet such requirements.**

Progress has occurred within various data collection efforts on forming collaborations with the states and public–private partnerships that can foster the creation and use of health and health care quality measures addressing the particular needs of children and adolescents. However, much remains to be done, and federal leadership can provide guidance to establish policy regarding standard and minimum data elements, to create forums for consensus building, and to sponsor research in areas where new measures or existing measures could be tested with diverse reference groups. The report *Children's Health, the Nation's Wealth* (IOM and NRC, 2004) emphasizes the need for federal leadership in taking responsibility for measuring and monitoring the health of children and adolescents. That report also calls for the creation of a specific unit within HHS to address "development, coordination, standardization, and validation of data across the multiple HHS data collection agencies, to support state-level use of data, and to facilitate coordination across federal departments" (IOM and NRC, 2004, p. 6). To date, the problems associated with multiple data collection efforts across multiple federal agencies persist. While the creation of a high-level unit with responsibility and resources for tracking health data on children and adolescents across multiple agencies remains elusive, some steps could be taken now to undertake the policy actions, convening efforts, and research initiatives described above.

Building capacity at the national, state, and local levels is critical to ensure the use of available indicators and performance measures.

- AHRQ could foster such capacity building by funding demonstration grants for the development and testing of national data linkage models incorporating content and communication standards that facilitate the aggregation of state- and agency-specific health and health care quality measures for children and adolescents. Ideally, these projects would assess the value of these linkages, the timeliness of data access, the usefulness of existing data sources, and opportunities to streamline redundant data collection efforts.
- State-level data are needed to monitor performance, accountability, and improvements in the health status and quality of care of children and adolescents. While states are routinely burdened with data collection requirements for numerous federal programs, they frequently lack the capacity to conduct their own analyses of state-level data sources. Some states have initiated innovative practices aimed at moving beyond traditional data silos, as described in Chapter 5.
- Also of value would be local-area studies addressing specific communities with unmet needs, particularly those that cut across state jurisdictions or that require analysis of selected demographic groups (such as children whose primary language at home is not English). Such studies would focus attention on selected reference groups that require more intensive and coordinated strategies because of their high rates of mobility, frequent turnover with multiple health plans, and high risk of poor health conditions. Data linkage and data "layering" strategies, such as those that have been demonstrated in Austin and Philadelphia (as described in Chapter 5), deserve further consideration and support as well.

FINAL OBSERVATIONS

The direction of policy and resources toward improving the health and health care quality of children and adolescents in recent years is an encouraging sign that the distinct needs of these populations are being recognized. Such efforts could build on the experience and expertise associated with measures of health and health care quality for adults, but they also need to recognize the unique needs of children and adolescents. Opportunities are available now to apply the conclusions and recommendations set forth in this chapter to enhance the measures used in population health surveys and administrative data sources. Recognizing that individuals and organizations may disagree about the best means of achieving the essential intent of a particular recommendation, the committee proposes a national dialogue on the characteristics and key features of the recommendations themselves before the course by which they might be incorporated into public policy or private practice is charted.

Implementation of the recommendations presented in this chapter call for strong national and state-based leadership, as well as modest additional resources to go beyond traditional boundaries and incorporate data elements that can deepen our understanding of the complex interactions among health, health care quality, and the social determinants of health for children and adolescents. Innovations in electronic technologies and data gathering methods offer opportunities to create new measures that can inform our understanding of important health disparities, preventable health conditions, the social determinants of health, and a life-course approach to the assessment of health and health care quality for America's children and adolescents.

References

AAP (American Academy of Pediatrics). 2002. The medical home. *Pediatrics* 110(1):184.

Abma, J. C., G. M. Martinez, W. D. Mosher, and B. S. Dawson. 2004. Teenagers in the United States: Sexual activity, contraceptive use, and childbearing, 2002. *Vital Health Statistics* 23(24):1-48.

ACF (Administration for Children and Families). 2010. Trends in foster care and adoption: FY 2002-FY 2008. In *Source: AFCARS data, U.S. Children's Bureau, Administration for Children, Youth and Families*. Rockville, MD: HHS.

Adams, S. H., P. W. Newacheck, M. J. Park, C. D. Brindis, and C. E. Irwin, Jr. 2007. Health insurance across vulnerable ages: Patterns and disparities from adolescence to the early 30s. *Pediatrics* 119(5):e1033-e1039.

AHIP and RWJF (America's Health Insurance Plans and The Robert Wood Johnson Foundation). 2006. *Collection and use of race and ethnicity data for quality improvement: 2006 AHIP-RWJF Survey of Health Insurance Plans* (issue brief). Washington, DC: AHIP.

AHRQ (Agency for Healthcare Research and Quality). 2003. *Care of children and adolescents in U.S. hospitals*. AHRQ Publication No. 04-0004. Rockville, MD: HHS.

AHRQ. 2008. *AHRQ quality indicators*. http://qualityindicators.ahrq.gov/ (accessed December 3, 2010).

AHRQ. 2010a. *Data & surveys*. http://www.ahrq.gov/data/ (accessed November 19, 2010).

AHRQ. 2010b. *Medical Expenditure Panel Survey*. http://www.meps.ahrq.gov/mepsweb/ (accessed November 19, 2010).

AHRQ. 2010c. *Background report for the request for public comment on initial, recommended core set of children's healthcare quality measures for voluntary use by Medicaid and CHIP programs*. http://www.ahrq.gov/chipra/corebackground/corebacktab.htm (accessed November 16, 2010).

AHRQ. 2010d. *CHIPRA Pediatric Healthcare Quality Measures Program Centers of Excellence (U18)*. http://grants.nih.gov/grants/guide/rfa-files/RFA-HS-11-001.html (accessed November 16, 2010).

AHRQ. 2010e. *First meeting of the Subcommittee on Quality Measures for Children in Medicaid and Children's Health Insurance Programs: Transcript of Barbara Dailey.* http://ahrq.hhs.gov/chipra/chipra/snac072209/sesstranscra.htm (accessed October 15, 2010).

AHRQ. 2010f. *Initial core set of children's healthcare quality measures.* http://www.ahrq.gov/chipra/listtable.htm (accessed November 16, 2010).

AHRQ. 2010g. *Lessons learned from the process used to identify an initial core quality measure set for children's health care in Medicaid and CHIP: A report from the Subcommittee on Children's Healthcare Quality Measures for Medicaid and CHIP Programs (SNAC).* http://www.ahrq.gov/chipra/lessons.htm (accessed November 16, 2010).

AHRQ. 2010h. *Request for public comment on initial, recommended core set of children's healthcare quality measures for voluntary use by Medicaid and CHIP programs background report.* http://www.ahrq.gov/chipra/corebackground/corebackgrnd.pdf (accessed November 16, 2010).

AHRQ. 2011. *Health literacy interventions and outcomes: An update of the literacy and health outcomes systematic review of the literature.* Rockville, MD: HHS.

Akinbami, L. J. 2006. *The state of childhood asthma, United States, 1980-2005.* Hyattsville, MD: NCHS.

Akinbami, L. J., and K. C. Schoendorf. 2002. Trends in childhood asthma: Prevalence, health care utilization, and mortality. *Pediatrics* 110(2):315-322.

Alessandrini, E. A., K. N. Shaw, W. B. Bilker, D. F. Schwarz, and L. M. Bell. 2001. Effects of Medicaid managed care on quality: Childhood immunizations. *Pediatrics* 107(6): 1335-1342.

Alexander, B. T. 2006. Fetal programming of hypertension. *American Journal of Physiology. Regulatory, Integrative and Comparative Physiology* 290(1):R1-R10.

Altman, B., E. Rasch, and J. Madans. 2006. Disability measurement matrix: A tool for the coordination of measurement purpose and instrument development. In *International views on disability measures: Moving toward comparative measurement (Research in social science and disability, volume 4)*, edited by B. Altman and S. Barnartt. Amsterdam, Netherlands: Emerald Group Publishing Limited. Pp. 263-284.

Anda, R. F., D. W. Brown, S. R. Dube, J. D. Bremner, V. J. Felitti, and W. H. Giles. 2008. Adverse childhood experiences and chronic obstructive pulmonary disease in adults. *American Journal of Preventive Medicine* 34(5):396-403.

Anderson, L. M., S. C. Scrimshaw, M. T. Fullilove, and J. E. Fielding. 2003. The Community Guide's model for linking the social environment to health. *American Journal of Preventive Medicine* 24(Suppl. 3):12-20.

Anderson, R. N., A. M. Miniño, D. L. Hoyert, and H. M. Rosenberg. 2001. *Comparability of cause of death between ICD–9 and ICD–10: Preliminary estimates.* Hyattsville, MD: NCHS.

Andresen, E. M., T. K. Catlin, K. W. Wyrwich, and J. Jackson-Thompson. 2003. Retest reliability of surveillance questions on health related quality of life. *Journal of Epidemiology and Community Health* 57(5):339-343.

Arnett, J. J. 2000. Emerging adulthood: A theory of development from the late teens through the twenties. *American Psychologist* 55(5):469-480.

Arnett, J. J. 2004. *Emerging adulthood: The winding road from the late teens through the twenties.* New York: Oxford University Press.

Arnett, J. J. 2006. Emerging adulthood: Understanding the new way of coming of age. In *Emerging adults in America: Coming of age in the 21st century*, edited by J. Arnett and J. Tanner. Washington, DC: American Psychological Association. Pp. 3-18.

Averett, S. L., D. I. Rees, and L. M. Argys. 2002. The impact of government policies and neighborhood characteristics on teenage sexual activity and contraceptive use. *American Journal of Public Health* 92(11):1773-1778.

Baker, D. W., R. M. Parker, M. V. Williams, W. C. Coates, and K. Pitkin. 1996. Use and effectiveness of interpreters in an emergency department. *Journal of the American Medical Association* 275(10):783-788.

Barker, D. J. P. 2002. Fetal programming of coronary heart disease. *Trends in Endocrinology and Metabolism* 13(9):364-368.

Baydar, N. 1995. Consequences for children of their birth planning status. *Family Planning Perspectives* 27(6):228-234.

Bayley, N. 1993. *Bayley scales of infant development* (2nd ed.). San Antonio, TX; Toronto: Psychological Corporation.

Beal, A., J. Co, D. Dougherty, T. Jorsling, J. Kam, J. Perrin, and H. Palmer. 2004. Quality measures for children's health care. *Pediatrics* 113(1):199-209.

Ben-Shlomo, Y., and D. Kuh. 2002. A life course approach to chronic disease epidemiology: Conceptual models, empirical challenges and interdisciplinary perspectives. *International Journal of Epidemiology* 31(2):285-293.

Berdahl, T., P. L. Owens, D. Dougherty, M. C. McCormick, Y. Pylypchuk, and L. A. Simpson. 2010. Annual report on health care for children and youth in the United States: Racial/ethnic and socioeconomic disparities in children's health care quality. *Academic Pediatrics* 10(2):95-118.

Bernard, S. J., L. J. Paulozzi, and D. L. J. Wallace. 2007. Fatal injuries among children by race and ethnicity—United States, 1999-2002. *MMWR Surveillance Summaries* 56(5):1-16.

Bethell, C. D. 2010 (unpublished). *Presentation on NQF Child Stream: Key concepts and population-based health and quality of care summary.* Washington, DC: National Quality Forum.

Bethell, C., C. Peck, and E. Schor. 2001. Assessing health system provision of well-child care: The Promoting Healthy Development Survey. *Pediatrics* 107(5):1084-1094.

Bethell, C. D., D. Read, R. E. Stein, S. J. Blumberg, N. Wells, and P. W. Newacheck. 2002. Identifying children with special health care needs: Development and evaluation of a short screening instrument. *Ambulatory Pediatrics* 2(1):38-48.

Bethell, C., C. Reuland, and B. Latzke. 2007. *The Promoting Healthy Development Survey (PHDS)-PLUS: Implementation guidelines for Medicaid and other settings, February 7.* New York: The Commonwealth Fund.

Bethell, C., and P. Newacheck. 2010 (unpublished). Overview and potential relevance of three MCHB lead national surveys to deliberations of the IOM Committee on Pediatric Health and Health Care Measures (NSCH, NS-CSHCN, NSECH). Prepared for the IOM Committee on Pediatric Health and Health Care Quality Measures.

Bickman, L., J. Samson, and C. Lapare. in press. *Improving the quality of mental health services through CHIPRA: You can't get there from here.*

Bilheimer, L. 2010. *Community health data initiative & health indicators warehouse.* http://www.ncvhs.hhs.gov/100617p1.pdf (accessed February 16, 2011).

Black, R., S. Morris, and J. Bryce. 2003. Where and why are 10 million children dying every year? *Lancet* 361(9376):2226-2234.

Blewett, L., and M. Davern. 2006. Meeting the need for state-level estimates of health insurance coverage: Use of state and federal survey data. *Health Services Research* 41(3 Pt. 1):946-975.

Bloom, B., R. Cohen, and G. Freeman. 2010. Summary health statistics for U.S. children: National Health Interview Survey, 2009. *Vital and Health Statistics* 10(247).

Blumberg, S. J., and J. V. Luke. 2007. Coverage bias in traditional telephone surveys of low-income and young adults. *Public Opinion Quarterly* 71(5):734-749.

Blumberg, S. J., L. Olson, M. Frankel, L. Osborn, C. Becker, K. Srinath, and P. Giambo. 2003. *Design and operation of the National Survey of Children with Special Health Care Needs, 2001.* Hyattsville, MD: NCHS.

Blumberg, S. J., J. V. Luke, and M. L. Cynamon. 2006. Telephone coverage and health survey estimates: Evaluating the need for concern about wireless substitution. *American Journal of Public Health* 96(5):926-931.

Blumenshine, P., S. Egerter, C. J. Barclay, C. Cubbin, and P. A. Braveman. 2010. Socioeconomic disparities in adverse birth outcomes: A systematic review. *American Journal of Preventive Medicine* 39(3):263-272.

Booske, B., and UWPHI. 2010. *County health rankings: Our approach.* http://www.county-healthrankings.org/our-approach (accessed October 27, 2010).

Borse, N. N., J. Gilchrist, A. M. Dellinger, R. A. Rudd, M. Ballesteros, and D. A. Sleet. 2008. *Childhood injury report: Patterns of unintentional injuries among 0-19 year olds in the United States, 2000-2006.* Atlanta, GA: National Center for Injury Prevention and Control, CDC.

Braveman, P. A. 2006. Health disparities and health equity: Concepts and measurement. *Annual Review of Public Health* 27(1):167-194.

Braveman, P. A., and C. Barclay. 2009. Health disparities beginning in childhood: A life-course perspective. *Pediatrics* 124(Suppl. 3):S163-S175.

Braveman, P. A., S. A. Egerter, C. Cubbin, and K. S. Marchi. 2004. An approach to studying social disparities in health and health care. *American Journal of Public Health* 94(12):2139-2148.

Braveman, P. A., C. Cubbin, S. Egerter, S. Chideya, K. S. Marchi, M. Metzler, and S. Posner. 2005. Socioeconomic status in health research. *Journal of the American Medical Association* 294(22):2879-2888.

Braveman, P. A., C. Cubbin, S. Egerter, D. R. Williams, and E. Pamuk. 2010. Socioeconomic disparities in health in the United States: What the patterns tell us. *American Journal of Public Health* 100(Suppl. 1):S186-S196.

Braveman, P. A., S. A. Egerter, and R. E. Mockenhaupt. 2011. Broadening the focus: The need to address the social determinants of health. *American Journal of Preventive Medicine* 40(Suppl. 1):S4-S18.

Brick, J. M., P. D. Brick, S. Dipko, S. Presser, C. Tucker, and Y. Yuan. 2007. Cell phone survey feasibility in the U.S.: Sampling and calling cell numbers versus landline numbers. *Public Opinion Quarterly* 71(1):23-39.

Brousseau, D. C., R. G. Hoffmann, J. Yauck, A. B. Nattinger, and G. Flores. 2005. Disparities for Latino children in the timely receipt of medical care. *Ambulatory Pediatrics* 5(6):319-325.

Brown, D. W., R. F. Anda, V. J. Felitti, V. J. Edwards, A. M. Malarcher, J. B. Croft, and W. H. Giles. 2010. Adverse childhood experiences are associated with the risk of lung cancer: A prospective cohort study. *BMC Public Health* 10:20.

Burbano O'Leary, S. C., S. Federico, and L. C. Hampers. 2003. The truth about language barriers: One residency programs experience. *Pediatrics* 111(5):e569-e573.

BUSPH (Boston University School of Public Health). 2010. *Pregnancy to Early Life Longitudinal Linkage (PELL).* https://sph.bu.edu/index.php/menu-id-452.html?task=view (accessed December 3, 2010).

Byrd, R. S., and M. L. Weitzman. 1994. Predictors of early grade retention among children in the United States. *Pediatrics* 93(3):481-487.

Cagney, K. A., C. R. Browning, and D. M. Wallace. 2007. The Latino paradox in neighborhood context: The case of asthma and other respiratory conditions. *American Journal of Public Health* 97(5):919-925.

CAHMI (Child and Adolescent Health Measurement Initiative). 2006. *National Survey of Children with Special Health Care Needs.* http://cshcndata.org/Content/Default.aspx (accessed July 1, 2010).

CAHMI. 2010. *Child and Adolescent Health Measurement Initiative (CAHMI): Young Adult Health Care Survey (YAHCS)*. http://www.ahrq.gov/chtoolbx/measure7.htm (accessed February 22, 2011).

Call, K., M. Davern, and L. Blewett. 2007. Estimates of health insurance coverage: Comparing state surveys with the current population survey. *Health Affairs* 26(1):269-278.

Callahan, S. T., and W. O. Cooper. 2004. Gender and uninsurance among young adults in the United States. *Pediatrics* 113(2):291-297.

Callahan, S. T., R. F. Winitzer, and P. Keenan. 2001. Transition from pediatric to adult-oriented health care: A challenge for patients with chronic disease. *Current Opinion in Pediatrics* 13(4):310-316.

Cassedy, A., G. Fairbrother, and P. W. Newacheck. 2008. The impact of insurance instability on children's access, utilization, and satisfaction with health care. *Ambulatory Pediatrics* 8(5):321-328.

CBO (Congressional Budget Office). 2003. *How many people lack health insurance and for how long?* Washington, DC: U.S. Government Printing Office.

CDC (Centers for Disease Control and Prevention). 1991. Consensus set of health status indicators for the general assessment of community health status—United States. *MMWR: Morbidity & Mortality Weekly Report* 40(27):449-451.

CDC. 1999. Achievements in public health, 1900-1999 impact of vaccines universally recommended for children—United States, 1990-1998. *MMWR: Morbidity & Mortality Weekly Report* 48(12):243-248.

CDC. 2006. *CDC injury fact book*. Atlanta, GA: CDC.

CDC. 2008. Youth risk behavior surveillance—United States, 2007. *MMWR Surveillance Summary* 57(SS-4).

CDC. 2009. *Detailed PRAMS methodology*. http://www.cdc.gov/prams/methodology.htm (accessed November 30, 2010).

CDC. 2010a. *ACE Study participant demographics*. http://www.cdc.gov/ace/demographics.htm (accessed December 2, 2010).

CDC. 2010b. *Adverse Childhood Experiences (ACE) Study: About the study*. http://www.cdc.gov/ace/about.htm (accessed December 1, 2010).

CDC. 2010c. *Adverse Childhood Experiences (ACE) Study: Future directions*. http://www.cdc.gov/ace/future.htm (accessed December 2, 2010).

CDC. 2010d. *Pregnancy Risk Assessment Monitoring System (PRAMS): Participating PRAMS states*. http://www.cdc.gov/prams/states.htm (accessed October 27, 2010).

CDC. 2011. CDC health disparities and inequalities report—United States, 2011. *Morbidity and Mortality Weekly Report* 60(Suppl):3-9.

CDCHU (Center on the Developing Child at Harvard University). 2010. *The foundations of lifelong health are built in early childhood*. Boston, MA: Harvard University.

CFAR (Center for Functional Assessment Research). 1993. Guide for the uniform data set for medical rehabilitation for children (WeeFIM). In *Uniform data system for medical rehabilitation*. Buffalo, NY: State University of New York at Buffalo.

Chuang, Y. C., C. Cubbin, D. Ahn, and M. A. Winkleby. 2005. Effects of neighbourhood socioeconomic status and convenience store concentration on individual level smoking. *Journal of Epidemiology and Community Health* 59(7):568-573.

Clements, K. M., W. D. Barfield, M. Kotelchuck, K. G. Lee, and N. Wilber. 2006. Birth characteristics associated with early intervention referral, evaluation for eligibility, and program eligibility in the first year of life. *Maternal Child Health Journal* 10(5):433-441.

Clements, K. M., W. D. Barfield, M. F. Ayadi, and N. Wilber. 2007. Preterm birth-associated cost of early intervention services: An analysis by gestational age. *Pediatrics* 119(4):e866-e874.

CMS (Centers for Medicare & Medicaid Services). 2010. Initial core set of children's health-care quality measures for voluntary use by Medicaid and CHIP programs (CMS–2474–NC). *Federal Register* 74(248):68846-68849.

Cohen, A. L., F. Rivara, E. K. Marcuse, H. McPhillips, and R. Davis. 2005. Are language barriers associated with serious medical events in hospitalized pediatric patients? *Pediatrics* 116(3):575-579.

Cohen, S. 2004. *Integrated survey designs: A framework for nonresponse bias reduction through the linkage of surveys, administrative and secondary data.* Working Paper No. 04001. Rockville, MD: AHRQ.

Coleman, E. A., and R. A. Berenson. 2004. Lost in transition: Challenges and opportunities for improving the quality of transitional care. *Annals of Internal Medicine* 141(7):533-536.

Corso, P. S., V. J. Edwards, X. Fang, and J. A. Mercy. 2008. Health-related quality of life among adults who experienced maltreatment during childhood. *American Journal of Public Health* 98(6):1094-1100.

Costello, E., A. Angold, B. Burns, D. Stangl, D. Tweed, A. Erkanli, and C. Worthman. 1996. The Great Smoky Mountains Study of Youth: Goals, design, methods, and the prevalence of DSM-III-R disorders. *Archives of General Psychiatry* 53(12):1129-1136.

CQAIMH (Center for Quality Assessment and Improvement in Mental Health). 2010. *The national inventory of mental health quality measures.* http://www.cqaimh.org/NIMHQM.htm (accessed March 15, 2010).

Crane, J. A. 1997. Patient comprehension of doctor-patient communication on discharge from the emergency department. *Journal of Emergency Medicine* 15(1):1-7.

Cutler, D., and G. Miller. 2004. *The role of public health improvements in health advances: The 20th century United States.* Boston, MA: NBER.

CWLA (Child Welfare League of America). 2010. *The nation's children.* Arlington, VA: Special tabulation of the Adoption and Foster Care Analysis Reporting System (AFCARS) by National Data Archive for Child Abuse and Neglect (NDACAN) and CWLA.

Danseco, E., T. Miller, and R. Spicer. 2000. Incidence and costs of 1987-1994 childhood injuries: Demographic breakdowns. *Pediatrics* 105(2):E27.

Davern, M., J. Klerman, J. Ziegenfuss, V. Lynch, and G. Greenberg. 2009. A partially corrected estimate of Medicaid enrollment and uninsurance: Results from an imputational model developed off linked survey and administrative data. *Journal of Economic and Social Measurement* 34(4):219-240.

Declercq, E., M. Barger, H. J. Cabral, S. R. Evans, M. Kotelchuck, C. Simon, J. Weiss, and L. J. Heffner. 2007. Maternal outcomes associated with planned primary cesarean births compared with planned vaginal births. *Obstetrics & Gynecology* 109(3):669-677.

DeNavas-Walt, C., B. D. Proctor, and J. C. Smith. 2009. Income, poverty, and health insurance coverage in the United States: 2008. In *Current population reports: Consumer income, P60-235*, edited by U.S. Census Bureau. Washington, DC: U.S. Government Printing Office.

DeNavas-Walt, C., B. D. Proctor, and J. C. Smith. 2010. *Income, poverty, and health insurance coverage in the United States.* Washington, DC: U.S. Government Printing Office.

Denny, J. C., A. Spickard, K. B. Johnson, N. B. Peterson, J. F. Peterson, and R. A. Miller. 2009. Evaluation of a method to identify and categorize section headers in clinical documents. *Journal of the American Medical Informatics Association* 16(6):806-815.

DesRoches, C. M., E. G. Campbell, S. R. Rao, K. Donelan, T. G. Ferris, A. Jha, R. Kaushal, D. E. Levy, S. Rosenbaum, A. E. Shields, and D. Blumenthal. 2008. Electronic health records in ambulatory care—a national survey of physicians. *New England Journal of Medicine* 359(1):50-60.

Dietrich, T., C. Culler, R. I. Garcia, and M. M. Henshaw. 2008. Racial and ethnic disparities in children's oral health: The National Survey of Children's Health. *Journal of the American Dental Association* 139(11):1507-1517.

Dietz, W. H. 1994. Critical periods in childhood for the development of obesity. *American Journal of Clinical Nutrition* 59(5):955-959.

Diez Roux, A. V., and C. Mair. 2010. Neighborhoods and health. *Annals of the New York Academy of Sciences* 1186(1):125-145.

Divi, C., R. G. Koss, S. P. Schmaltz, and J. M. Loeb. 2007. Language proficiency and adverse events in US hospitals: A pilot study. *International Journal for Quality in Health Care* 19(2):60-67.

Doan, S., L. Bastarache, S. Klimkowski, J. C. Denny, and H. Xu. 2010. Integrating existing natural language processing tools for medication extraction from discharge summaries. *Journal of the American Medical Informatics Association* 17(5):528-531.

Donabedian, A. 1988. The quality of care: How can it be assessed? *Journal of the American Medical Association* 260(12):1743-1748.

Dong, M., W. H. Giles, V. J. Felitti, S. R. Dube, J. E. Williams, D. P. Chapman, and R. F. Anda. 2004. Insights into causal pathways for ischemic heart disease: Adverse Childhood Experiences Study. *Circulation* 110(13):1761-1766.

Dougherty, D., and L. A. Simpson. 2004. Measuring the quality of children's health care: A prerequisite to action. *Pediatrics* 113(1):185-198.

Downs, S. M., V. Zhu, V. Anand, P. G. Biondich, and A. E. Carroll. 2008. The CHICA smoking cessation system. *AMIA Annual Symposium Proceedings* 166-170.

Doyle, L. W., and P. J. Anderson. 2010. Adult outcome of extremely preterm infants. *Pediatrics* 126(2):342-351.

Drolet, B. C., and K. B. Johnson. 2008. Categorizing the world of registries. *Journal of Biomedical Informatics* 41(6):1009-1020.

Dube, S. R., R. F. Anda, V. J. Felitti, D. P. Chapman, D. F. Williamson, and W. H. Giles. 2001. Childhood abuse, household dysfunction, and the risk of attempted suicide throughout the life span: Findings from the Adverse Childhood Experiences Study. *Journal of the American Medical Association* 286(24):3089-3096.

Dye, B., S. Tan, V. Smith, B. Lewis, L. Barker, G. Thornton-Evans, P. I. Eke, E. D. Beltrá n-Aguilar, A. M. Horowitz, and C.-H. Li. 2007. *Trends in oral health status: United States, 1988-1994 and 1999-2004.* Hyattsville, MD: NCHS.

Edwards, V. J., R. F. Anda, V. J. Felitti, and S. R. Dube. 2004. *Adverse childhood experiences and health-related quality of life as an adult.* In *Health consequences of abuse in the family: A clinical guide for evidence-based practice,* edited by K. A. Kendall-Tackett. Washington, DC: American Psychological Association.

Eisen, M. 1980. *Conceptualization and measurement of health for children in the health insurance study.* Santa Monica, CA: The Rand Corporation.

Elixhauser, A. 2008. *Hospital stays for children 2006.* HCUP statistical brief #56. Rockville, MD: AHRQ.

Evensen, K. A. I., S. Steinshamn, A. E. Tjønna, T. Stølen, M. A. Høydal, U. Wisløff, A.-M. Brubakk, and T. Vik. 2009. Effects of preterm birth and fetal growth retardation on cardiovascular risk factors in young adulthood. *Early Human Development* 85(4):239-245.

Fairbrother, G., R. Sebastien, J. McAuliffe, and L. Simpson. 2010 (unpublished). *Monitoring changes in health care for children and families.* Child Policy Research Center.

Felitti, V. J., R. F. Anda, D. Nordenberg, D. F. Williamson, A. M. Spitz, V. Edwards, M. P. Koss, and J. S. Marks. 1998. Relationship of childhood abuse and household dysfunction to many of the leading causes of death in adults. The Adverse Childhood Experiences (ACE) Study. *American Journal of Preventive Medicine* 14(4):245-258.

Femina, D. D., C. A. Yeager, and D. O. Lewis. 1990. Child abuse: Adolescent records vs. adult recall. *Child Abuse & Neglect* 14(2):227-231.

Ferris, T. G., D. Dougherty, D. Blumenthal, and J. M. Perrin. 2001. A report card on quality improvement for children's health care. *Pediatrics* 107(1):143-155.

Feudtner, C., R. M. Hays, G. Haynes, J. R. Geyer, J. M. Neff, and T. D. Koepsell. 2001. Deaths attributed to pediatric complex chronic conditions: National trends and implications for supportive care services. *Pediatrics* 107(6):e99.

Feudtner, C., K. R. Hexem, M. Shabbout, J. A. Feinstein, J. Sochalski, and J. H. Silber. 2009. Prediction of pediatric death in the year after hospitalization: A population-level retrospective cohort study. *Journal of Palliative Medicine* 12(2):160-169.

Fielding, J., S. Teutsch, and L. Breslow. 2010. A framework for public health in the United States. *Public Health Reviews* 32(1):174-189.

FIFCFS (Federal Interagency Forum on Child and Family Statistics). 2009. *America's children: Key national indicators of well-being, 2009.* Washington, DC: U.S. Government Printing Office.

FIFCFS. 2010. *America's children in brief: Key national indicators of well-being.* Washington, DC: U.S. Government Printing Office.

Fine, A., and M. Kotelchuck. 2010. *Rethinking MCH: The life course model as an organizing framework concept paper.* Rockville, MD: HHS.

Fiser, D. H., N. Long, P. K. Roberson, G. Hefley, K. Zolten, and M. Brodie-Fowler. 2000a. Relationship of pediatric overall performance category and pediatric cerebral performance category scores at pediatric intensive care unit discharge with outcome measures collected at hospital discharge and 1- and 6-month follow-up assessments. *Critical Care Medicine* 28(7):2616-2620.

Fiser, D. H., J. M. Tilford, and P. K. Roberson. 2000b. Relationship of illness severity and length of stay to functional outcomes in the pediatric intensive care unit: A multi-institutional study. *Critical Care Medicine* 28(4):1173-1179.

Flores, G. 2005. The impact of medical interpreter services on the quality of health care: A systematic review. *Medical Care Research and Review* 62(3):255-299.

Flores, G. 2009. *Achieving optimal health and healthcare for all children: How we can eliminate racial and ethnic disparities in children's health and healthcare.* Washington, DC: First Focus.

Flores, G. 2010. Racial and ethnic disparities in the health and health care of children. *Pediatrics* 125(4):e979-e1020.

Flores, G., and S. C. Tomany-Korman. 2008. The language spoken at home and disparities in medical and dental health, access to care, and use of services in US children. *Pediatrics* 121(6):e1703-e1714.

Flores, G., M. Abreu, I. Schwartz, and M. Hill. 2000. The importance of language and culture in pediatric care: Case studies from the Latino community. *The Journal of Pediatrics* 137(6):842-848.

Flores, G., M. Abreu, and S. C. Tomany-Korman. 2005a. Limited English proficiency, primary language at home, and disparities in children's health care: How language barriers are measured matters. *Public Health Report* 120(4):418-430.

Flores, G., L. Olson, and S. C. Tomany-Korman. 2005b. Racial and ethnic disparities in early childhood health and health care. *Pediatrics* 115(2):e183-e193.

Forrest, C. B., L. Simpson, and C. Clancy. 1997. Child health services research: Challenges and opportunities. *Journal of the American Medical Association* 277(22):1787-1793.

Frawley, W. J., P. Shapiro, and C. J. Matheus. 1992. Knowledge discovery in databases—an overview. *AI Magazine* 13:57-70.

Freed, G. L., S. J. Clark, D. E. Pathman, and R. Schectman. 1999. Influences on the receipt of well-child visits in the first two years of life. *Pediatrics* 103(4):864-869.

Frieden, T. R. 2010. A framework for public health action: The health impact pyramid. *American Journal of Public Health* 100(4):590-595.

Gaillard, D., P. Passilly-Degrace, and P. Besnard. 2008. Molecular mechanisms of fat preference and overeating. *Annals of the New York Academy of Sciences* 1141:163-175.

GAO (General Accounting Office). 1997. *Health insurance: Coverage leads to increased health care access for children.* Washington, DC: U.S. Government Printing Office.

Garasky, S., S. D. Stewart, C. Gundersen, B. J. Lohman, and J. C. Eisenmann. 2009. Family stressors and child obesity. *Social Science Research* 38(4):755-766.

Gardner, H. G. 2007. Office-based counseling for unintentional injury prevention. *Pediatrics* 119(1):202-206.

Gardner, W., K. J. Kelleher, K. Pajer, and J. V. Campo. 2004. Follow-up care of children identified with ADHD by primary care clinicians: A prospective cohort study. *The Journal of Pediatrics* 145(6):767-771.

Giles-Corti, B., and R. J. Donovan. 2002. The relative influence of individual, social and physical environment determinants of physical activity. *Social Science and Medicine* 54(12):1793-1812.

Gillman, M. W. 2005. Developmental origins of health and disease. *New England Journal of Medicine* 353(17):1848-1850.

Godfrey, K. M., and D. J. Barker. 2001. Fetal programming and adult health. *Public Health Nutrition* 4(2b):611-624.

Goodwin, P. Y., W. D. Mosher, and A. Chandra. 2010. *Marriage and cohabitation in the United States: A statistical portrait based on Cycle 6 (2002) of the National Survey of Family Growth.* Hyattsville, MD: NCHS.

Gortmaker, S. L., D. K. Walker, M. Weitzman, and A. M. Sobol. 1990. Chronic conditions, socioeconomic risks, and behavioral problems in children and adolescents. *Pediatrics* 85(3):267-276.

Grossman, D. C., J. W. Krieger, J. R. Sugarman, and R. A. Forquera. 1994. Health status of urban American Indians and Alaska natives: A population-based study. *Journal of the American Medical Association* 271(11):845-850.

Guagliardo, M. F., S. J. Teach, Z. J. Huang, J. M. Chamberlain, and J. G. Joseph. 2003. Racial and ethnic disparities in pediatric appendicitis rupture rate. *Academic Emergency Medicine* 10(11):1218-1227.

Gundersen, C., B. J. Lohman, S. Garasky, S. Stewart, and J. Eisenmann. 2008. Food security, maternal stressors, and overweight among low-income US children: Results from the National Health and Nutrition Examination Survey (1999-2002). *Pediatrics* 122(3).

Guo, S. S., and W. C. Chumlea. 1999. Tracking of body mass index in children in relation to overweight in adulthood. *The American Journal of Clinical Nutrition* 70(1 Part 2):145S-148S.

Guyer, B., M. A. Freedman, D. M. Strobino, and E. J. Sondik. 2000. Annual summary of vital statistics: Trends in the health of Americans during the 20th century. *Pediatrics* 106(6):1307-1317.

Guyer, B., S. Ma, H. Grason, K. Frick, D. Perry, A. Sharkey, and J. McIntosh. 2009. Early childhood health promotion and its life course health consequences. *Academic Pediatrics* 9(3):142-149, e141-e171.

Hack, M. 2009. Adult outcomes of preterm children. *Journal of Developmental & Behavioral Pediatrics* 30(5):460-470.

Hack, M., D. J. Flannery, M. Schluchter, L. Cartar, E. Borawski, and N. Klein. 2002. Outcomes in young adulthood for very-low-birth-weight infants. *New England Journal of Medicine* 346(3):149-157.

Haggerty, R. J., K. J. Roghmann, and I. B. Pless. 1993. *Child health and the community.* New Brunswick, NJ: Transaction Publishers.

Halfon, N., and M. Hochstein. 2002. Life course health development: An integrated framework for developing health, policy, and research. *Milbank Quarterly* 80(3):433-479, iii.

Halfon, N., M. Schuster, W. Valentine, and E. McGlynn. 1998. Improving the quality of healthcare for children: Implementing the results of the AHSR research agenda conference. *Health Services Research* 33(4):955-976.

Halfon, N., L. Olson, M. Inkelas, R. Mistry, H. Sareen, L. Lange, M. Hochstein, and J. Wright. 2002. Summary statistics from the National Survey of Early Childhood Health, 2000 National Center for Health Statistics. *Vital Health Statistics* 15(3).

Hartman, M., A. Catlin, D. Lassman, J. Cylus, and S. Heffler. 2008. U.S. health spending by age, selected years through 2004. *Health Affairs* 27(1):w1-w12.

Hasnain-Wynia, R., D. Pierce, and M. Pittman. 2004. *Who, when, and how the current state of race, ethnicity, and primary language data collection in hospitals.* New York: The Commonwealth Fund.

Hawkins, A. O., V. S. Kantayya, and C. Sharkey-Asner. 2010. Health literacy: A potential barrier in caring for underserved populations. *Disease-a-Month* 56(12):734-740.

HCUP (Healthcare Cost and Utilization Project). 2006. *The KIDS' inpatient database.* http://www.hcup-us.ahrq.gov/kidoverview.jsp (accessed November 19, 2010).

Hennessey, C., D. Moriarty, M. Zack, P. Scherr, and R. Brackbill. 1994. Measuring health-related quality of life for public health surveillance. *Public Health Reports* 109:665-672.

Heron, M. 2010. Deaths: Leading causes for 2006. *National Vital Statistics Reports* 58(14).

Heron, M., P. D. Sutton, J. Xu, S. J. Ventura, D. M. Strobino, and B. Guyer. 2010. Annual summary of vital statistics: 2007. *Pediatrics* 125(1):4-15.

HHS (U.S. Department of Health and Human Services). 2000a. *Healthy people 2010: Understanding and improving health* (2nd ed.). Washington, DC: HHS.

HHS. 2000b. *Oral health in America: A Report of the Surgeon General.* Rockville, MD: National Institute of Dental and Craniofacial Research, NIH.

HHS. 2003. *Directory of health and human services data resources.* http://aspe.hhs.gov/datacncl/DataDir/index.shtml (accessed November 19, 2010).

HHS. 2006. *Children and secondhand smoke exposure. Excerpts from the health consequences of involuntary exposure to tobacco smoke: A report of the Surgeon General.* Atlanta, GA: HHS.

HHS. 2008. *The National Survey of Children with Special Health Care Needs Chartbook 2005-2006.* Edited by HRSA and MCHB. Rockville, MD: HHS.

HHS. 2009. Medicaid and CHIP programs; initial core set of children's healthcare quality measures for voluntary use by Medicaid and CHIP programs. *Federal Register* 74(248):68846-68849.

HHS. 2010a. *Establishing a holistic framework to reduce inequities in HIV, viral hepatitis, STDs, and tuberculosis in the United States.* Atlanta, GA: CDC.

HHS. 2010b. *Foundation health measures.* http://www.healthypeople.gov/2020/about/tracking.aspx (accessed January 24, 2011).

HHS. 2010c. *Annual report on the quality of care for children in Medicaid and CHIP.* https://www.cms.gov/MedicaidCHIPQualPrac/Downloads/secrep.pdf (accessed November 15, 2010).

HHS. 2010d. *National Health Care Quality Strategy Plan.* http://www.hhs.gov/news/reports/quality/nationalhealthcarequalitystrategy.pdf (accessed November 15, 2010).

HHS. 2011a. *Understanding health information privacy.* http://www.hhs.gov/ocr/privacy/hipaa/understanding/index.html (accessed February 7, 2011).

HHS. 2011b. *Building healthier communities by investing in prevention.* http://www.healthcare.gov/news/factsheets/prevention02092011b.html (accessed February 25, 2011).

HHS, HRSA, and MCHB (U.S. Department of Health and Human Services, Health Resources and Services Administration, and Maternal and Child Health Bureau). 2009. *Child health USA 2008-2009.* Rockville, MD: HHS.

Hogan, D., and M. Msall. 2008. *Key indicators of child and youth well-being: Completing the picture,* edited by B. V. Brown. New York: Lawrence Erlbaum Associates.

Hoilette, L. K., S. J. Clark, A. Gebremariam, and M. M. Davis. 2009. Usual source of care and unmet need among vulnerable children: 1998-2006. *Pediatrics* 123(2):e214-e219.

Homer, C. J., L. C. Kleinman, and D. A. Goldman. 1998. Improving the quality of care for children in health systems. *Health Services Research* 33(4 Pt. 2):1091-1109.

Horn, I., and A. Beal. 2004. Child health disparities: Framing a research agenda. *Ambulatory Pediatrics* 4(4):269-275.

How, S. K. H., A. K. Fryer, D. McCarthy, C. Schoen, and E. L. Schor. 2011. *Securing a healthy future: The Commonwealth Fund State Scorecard on Child Health System Performance, 2011.* New York: The Commonwealth Fund.

Hoyert, D. L., and J. A. Martin. 2002. Vital statistics as a data source. *Seminars in Perinatology* 26(1):12-16.

Hu, D. J., and R. M. Covell. 1986. Health care usage by Hispanic outpatients as function of primary language. *The Western Journal of Medicine* 144(4):490-493.

Iglehart, J. K. 2007. The battle over SCHIP. *New England Journal of Medicine* 357(10):957-960.

IOM (Institute of Medicine). 1988. *The future of public health.* Washington, DC: National Academy Press.

IOM. 1991. *Disability in America: Toward a national agenda for prevention.* Washington, DC: National Academy Press.

IOM. 1993. *Access to health care in America.* Washington, DC: National Academy Press.

IOM. 1995. *The best intentions: Unintended pregnancy and the well-being of children and families.* Washington, DC: National Academy Press.

IOM. 1999. *To err is human: Building a safer health system.* Washington, DC: National Academy Press.

IOM. 2001a. *Crossing the quality chasm: A new health system for the 21st century.* Washington, DC: National Academy Press.

IOM. 2001b. *Envisioning the National Healthcare Quality Report.* Washington, DC: National Academy Press.

IOM. 2003a. *Unequal treatment: Confronting racial and ethnic disparities in health care.* Washington, DC: The National Academies Press.

IOM. 2003b. *When children die: Improving palliative and end-of-life care for children and their families.* Washington, DC: The National Academies Press.

IOM. 2005. *Preventing childhood obesity: Health in the balance.* Washington, DC: The National Academies Press.

IOM. 2006a. *Preterm birth: Causes, consequences, and prevention.* Washington, DC: The National Academies Press.

IOM. 2006b. *Performance measurement: Accelerating improvement.* Washington, DC: The National Academies Press.

IOM. 2006c. Rewarding provider performance: Aligning incentives in Medicare. In *Pathways to quality health care.* Washington, DC: The National Academies Press.

IOM. 2006d. Medicare's Quality Improvement Organization Program: Maximizing potential. In *Pathways to quality health care.* Washington, DC: The National Academies Press.

IOM. 2007. *The future of disability in America.* Washington, DC: The National Academies Press.

IOM. 2009a. *America's uninsured crisis: Consequences for health and health care.* Washington, DC: The National Academies Press.

IOM. 2009b. *Beyond the HIPAA privacy rule: Enhancing privacy, improving health through research.* Washington, DC: The National Academies Press.

IOM. 2009c. *Preventing mental, emotional, and behavioral disorders among young people: Progress and possibilities.* Washington, DC: The National Academies Press.

IOM. 2009d. *Race, ethnicity, and language data: Standardization for health care quality improvement.* Washington, DC: The National Academies Press.

IOM. 2010a. *Future directions for the national healthcare quality and disparities reports.* Washington, DC: The National Academies Press.

IOM. 2010b. *Clinical data as the basic staple of health learning: Creating and protecting a public good: Workshop summary.* Washington, DC: The National Academies Press.

IOM. 2011a. *For the public's health: The role of measurement in action and accountability.* Washington, DC: The National Academies Press.

IOM. 2011b. *Leading health indicators for Healthy People 2020: Letter report.* Washington, DC: National Academies Press.

IOM and NRC (Institute of Medicine and National Research Council). 2004. *Children's health, the nation's wealth: Assessing and improving child health.* Washington, DC: The National Academies Press.

IOM and NRC. 2009a. *Adolescent health services: Missing opportunities.* Washington, DC: The National Academies Press.

IOM and NRC. 2009b. *Weight gain during pregnancy: Reexamining the guidelines.* Washington, DC: The National Academies Press.

James, S., S. J. Charlemagne, A. B. Gilman, Q. Alemi, R. L. Smith, P. R. Tharayil, and K. Freeman. 2010. Post-discharge services and psychiatric rehospitalization among children and youth. *Administration and Policy in Mental Health* 37(5):433-445.

Johnson, K. B., C. S. Gadd, D. Aronsky, K. Yang, L. Tang, V. Estrin, J. K. King, and M. Frisse. 2008. The MidSouth eHealth Alliance: Use and impact in the first year. *AMIA Annual Symposium Proceedings* 333-337.

Johnson, R. C., and R. F. Schoeni. 2007. *The influence of early-life events on human capital, health status, and labor market outcomes over the life course, Working Paper Series, Institute for Research on Labor and Employment, UC Berkeley.* Berkeley, CA: Goldman School of Public Policy University of California Berkeley.

Jones, B. H. 2004. Safety and stability for foster children: A developmental perspective. *From the Future of Children, A publication of the David and Lucile Packard Foundation* 14(1):16.

Jordan, J. E., R. H. Osborne, and R. Buchbinder. 2010. Critical appraisal of health literacy indices revealed variable underlying constructs, narrow content and psychometric weaknesses. *Journal of Clinical Epidemiology* 64(4):366-379.

Joyce, T. J., R. Kaestner, and S. Korenman. 2000. The effect of pregnancy intention on child development. *Demography* 37(1):83-84.

Kataoka, S., L. Zhang, and K. Wells. 2002. Unmet need for mental health care among U.S. children: Variation by ethnicity and insurance status. *American Journal of Psychiatry* 159(9):1548-1555.

Kavanagh, P. L., W. G. Adams, and C. J. Wang. 2009. Quality indicators and quality assessment in child health. *Archives of Disease in Childhood* 94(6):458-463.

Kawachi, I., and L. Berkman. 2003. *Neighborhoods and health.* New York: Oxford University Press.

Kaye, N., J. May, and M. Abrams. 2006. *State policy options to improve delivery of child development services: Strategies from the eight ABCD states.* New York: The Commonwealth Fund.

Kenney, G., J. Holahan, and L. Nichols. 2006. Toward a more reliable federal survey for tracking health insurance coverage and access. *Health Services Research* 41(3 Pt. 1):918-945.

KFF (Kaiser Family Foundation). 2008. *Data source: Estimated number of children enrolled in CHIP with family income at or below 200% Federal Poverty Level (FPL), FY2008.* http://www.statehealthfacts.org/savemap.jsp?cat=4&ind=658 (accessed November 29, 2010).

Kirby, D. 2007. *Emerging answers 2007: Research findings on programs to reduce teen pregnancy and sexually transmitted diseases.* Washington, DC: The National Campaign to Prevent Teen Pregnancy.

Kirkman-Liff, B., and D. Mondragon. 1991. Language of interview: Relevance for research of southwest Hispanics. *American Journal of Public Health* 81(11):1399-1404.

Kitsantas, P., L. R. Pawloski, and K. F. Gaffney. 2010. Maternal prepregnancy body mass index in relation to Hispanic preschooler overweight/obesity. *European Journal of Pediatrics* 169(11):1361-1368.

Klein, R. J., and S. A. Hawk. 1992. *Health status indicators: Definitions and national data.* Rockville, MD: HHS, CDC, Public Health Services, and NCHS.

Klerman, J., M. Davern, K. Call, V. Lynch, and J. Ringel. 2009. Understanding the current population survey's insurance estimates and the Medicaid "undercount." *Health Affairs* 28(6):w991-w1001.

Kogan, M. D., G. R. Alexander, B. W. Jack, and M. C. Allen. 1998. The association between adequacy of prenatal care utilization and subsequent pediatric care utilization in the United States. *Pediatrics* 102(1):25-30.

Koh, H. K. 2010. A 2020 vision for healthy people. *New England Journal of Medicine* 362(18):1653-1656.

Kuh, D., and Y. Ben-Shlomo. 1997. *A life course approach to chronic disease epidemiology.* Oxford: Oxford Medical Publications.

Kuhlthau, K. A., A. C. Beal, T. G. Ferris, and J. M. Perrin. 2002. Comparing a diagnosis list with a survey method to identify children with chronic conditions in an urban health center. *Ambulatory Pediatrics* 2(1):58-62.

Kulich, M., M. Rosenfeld, C. H. Goss, and R. Wilmott. 2003. Improved survival among young patients with cystic fibrosis. *The Journal of Pediatrics* 142(6):631-636.

Kutner, M., E. Greenberg, Y. Jin, and C. Paulsen. 2006. *The health literacy of America's adults: Results from the 2003 National Assessment of Adult Literacy* (NCES 2006–483). Washington, DC: National Center for Education Statistics.

Lalonde, M. 1981. *A new perspective on the health of Canadians: A working document.* Ottowa, Canada: Ministry of Supply and Services.

Land, K. C., and FCD (Foundation for Child Development). 2010. *Child and Youth Well-being Index (CWI).* New York: FCD.

Landon, B. E., E. C. Schneider, S. L. Normand, S. H. Scholle, L. G. Pawlson, and A. M. Epstein. 2007. Quality of care in Medicaid managed care and commercial health plans. *Journal of the American Medical Association* 298(14):1674-1681.

Landraf, J. L., L. Abetz, and J. E. Ware. 1996. *The Child Health Questionnaire User's Manual.* Boston, MA: The Health Institute, New England Medical Center.

Laraia, B. A., A. M. Siega-Riz, J. S. Kaufman, and S. J. Jones. 2004. Proximity of supermarkets is positively associated with diet quality index for pregnancy. *Preventive Medicine* 39(5):869-875.

Larson, N. I., M. T. Story, and M. C. Nelson. 2009. Neighborhood environments. Disparities in access to healthy foods in the U.S. *American Journal of Preventive Medicine* 36(1):74-81.e10.

Lazar, J., M. Kotelchuck, A. Nannini, and M. Barger. 2006. Identifying multiple gestation groups using state-level birth and fetal death certificate data. *Maternal Child Health Journal* 10(3):225-228.

Leatherman, S., and D. McCarthy. 1999. Public disclosure of health care performance reports: Experience, evidence and issues for policy. *International Journal for Quality in Health Care* 11(2):93-98.

Leatherman, S., and D. McCarthy. 2004. *Quality of health care for children and adolescents: A chartbook.* http://www.commonwealthfund.org/usr_doc/leatherman_pedchartbook_700.pdf (accessed November 16, 2010).

Lee, N. E., A. K. De, and P. A. Simon. 2006. School-based physical fitness testing identifies large disparities in childhood overweight in Los Angeles. *Journal of the American Dietetic Association* 106(1):118-121.

Lepkowski, J., W. Mosher, K. Davis, R. Groves, and V. H. J. 2010. *The 2006-2010 National Survey of Family Growth: Sample design and analysis of a continuous survey.* Hyattsville, MD: NCHS.

The Lewin Group. 2000 (unpublished). *Commissioned planning material for National Children's Study.* Hyattsville, MD: NCHS.

Lindberg, L. D., and M. Orr. 2011. Neighborhood-level influences on young men's sexual and reproductive health behaviors. *American Journal of Public Health* 101(2):271-274.

Linet, M. S., L. A. Ries, M. A. Smith, R. E. Tarone, and S. S. Devesa. 1999. Cancer surveillance series: Recent trends in childhood cancer incidence and mortality in the United States. *Journal of the National Cancer Institute* 91(12):1051-1058.

Little, R. J. A. 1982. Direct standardization: A tool for teaching linear models for unbalanced data. *The American Statistician* 36(1):38-43.

Lohman, B. J., S. Stewart, C. Gundersen, S. Garasky, and J. C. Eisenmann. 2009. Adolescent overweight and obesity: Links to food insecurity and individual, maternal, and family stressors. *Journal of Adolescent Health* 45(3):230-237.

Lotstein, D. S., M. McPherson, B. Strickland, and P. W. Newacheck. 2005. Transition planning for youth with special health care needs: Results from the National Survey of Children with Special Health Care Needs. *Pediatrics* 115(6):1562-1568.

Ludwig, D. S., and J. Currie. 2010. The association between pregnancy weight gain and birthweight: A within-family comparison. *The Lancet* 376(9745):984-990.

MacTaggart, P. 2010 (unpublished). *Overview of development & use of quality measures for children.* George Washington University Medical Center.

Mangione-Smith, R., A. H. DeCristofaro, C. M. Setodji, J. Keesey, D. J. Klein, J. L. Adams, M. A. Schuster, and E. A. McGlynn. 2007. The quality of ambulatory care delivered to children in the United States. *New England Journal of Medicine* 357(15):1515-1523.

Mannino, D. M., M. Siegel, C. Husten, D. Rose, and R. Etzel. 1996. Environmental tobacco smoke exposure and health effects in children: Results from the 1991 National Health Interview Survey. *Tobacco Control* 5(1):13-18.

Marmot, M. G., and R. G. Wilkinson. 1999. *Social determinants of health.* Oxford: Oxford University Press.

Marmot, S., S. Friel, R. Bell, T. A. Houweling, and S. Taylor. 2008. Closing the gap in a generation: Health equity through action on the social determinants of health. *The Lancet* 372(9650):1661-1669.

Marquis, M. S., and S. H. Long. 2002. The role of public insurance and the public delivery system in improving birth outcomes for low-income pregnant women. *Medical Care* 40(11):1048-1059.

Martinez, G., A. Chandra, J. Abma, J. Jones, and W. D. Mosher. 2006. *Fertility, contraception, and fatherhood: Data on men and women from Cycle 6 (2002) of the National Survey of Family Growth.* Hyattsville, MD: NCHS.

Martinez, G., J. Abma, and C. Copen. 2010. *Educating teenagers about sex in the United States.* Hyattsville, MD: NCHS.

Mather, M., and D. Adams. 2006. *A KIDS COUNT/PRB: Report on Census 2000: The risk of negative child outcomes in low-income families.* Baltimore, MD: Ann E. Casey Foundation.

Mattingly, M., and M. Stransky. 2010. Young child poverty in 2009: Rural poverty rate jumps to nearly 29 percent in second year of recession. *Carsey Institute Issue Brief* (17).

McCormick, M. C., J. S. Litt, V. C. Smith, and J. A. F. Zupancic. 2011. Prematurity: An overview and public health implications. *Annual Review of Public Health* 32(1).

McDonald, K. M. 2008. *Future validation and improvement of the AHRQ QI.* http://quality indicators.ahrq.gov/downloads/usermeeting2008/McDonald_Future%20Validation.ppt (accessed December 3, 2010).

McDonald, K. M. 2009. Approach to improving quality: The role of quality measurement and a case study of the Agency for Healthcare Research and Quality Pediatric Quality Indicators. *Pediatric Clinics of North America* 56(4):815-829.

McGlynn, E. A., C. L. Damberg, E. A. Kerr, and M. A. Schuster. 2000. *Quality of care for children and adolescents: A review of selected clinical conditions and quality indicators.* Santa Monica, CA: Rand.

MCHB (Maternal and Child Health Bureau). 2010. *Title V Information System.* https://perf data.hrsa.gov/MCHB/TVISReports/default.aspx (accessed February 22, 2011).

McPherson, M., P. Arango, H. Fox, C. Lauver, M. McManus, P. W. Newacheck, J. M. Perrin, J. P. Shonkoff, and B. Strickland. 1998. A new definition of children with special health care needs. *Pediatrics* 102(1):137-139.

Meier, A. M. 2007. Adolescent first sex and subsequent mental health. *American Journal of Sociology* 112(6):37.

Mejia, G. C., J. A. Weintraub, N. F. Cheng, W. Grossman, P. Z. Han, K. R. Phipps, and S. A. Gansky. 2010. Language and literacy relate to lack of children's dental sealant use. *Community Dentistry and Oral Epidemiology* [Epub ahead of print].

Merikangas, K. R., J.-P. He, M. Burstein, S. A. Swanson, S. Avenevoli, L. Cui, C. Benjet, K. Georgiades, and J. Swendsen. 2010a. Lifetime prevalence of mental disorders in U.S. adolescents: Results from the National Comorbidity Survey Replication–Adolescent Supplement (NCS-A). *Journal of the American Academy of Child and Adolescent Psychiatry* 49(10):980-989.

Merikangas, K. R., J.-P. He, D. Brody, P. W. Fisher, K. Bourdon, and D. S. Koretz. 2010b. Prevalence and treatment of mental disorders among US children in the 2001-2004 NHANES. *Pediatrics* 125(1):75-81.

Merrick, N. J., R. Houchens, S. Tillisch, B. Berlow, and C. Landon. 2001. Quality of hospital care of children with asthma: Medicaid versus privately insured patients. *Journal of Health Care for the Poor and Underserved* 12(2):192-207.

Miller, E., J. Y. Lee, D. A. DeWalt, and W. F. Vann, Jr. 2010. Impact of caregiver literacy on children's oral health outcomes. *Pediatrics* 126(1):107-114.

Miller, W., P. Simon, and S. Maleque. 2009. *Beyond health care: New directions to a healthier America.* Washington, DC: The Robert Wood Johnson Foundation Commission to Build a Healthier America.

Miller, W. D., C. E. Pollack, and D. R. Williams. 2011. Healthy homes and communities: Putting the pieces together. *American Journal of Preventive Medicine* 40(Suppl. 1):S48-S57.

Morales, L. S., M. N. Elliott, R. Weech-Maldonado, K. L. Spritzer, and R. D. Hays. 2001. Differences in CAHPS® adult survey reports and ratings by race and ethnicity: An analysis of the National CAHPS® Benchmarking Data 1.0. *Health Services Research* 36(3):595-617.

Morland, K., S. Wing, and A. D. Roux. 2002. The contextual effect of the local food environment on residents' diets: The Atherosclerosis Risk in Communities Study. *American Journal of Public Health* 92(11):1761-1767.

Moster, D., R. T. Lie, and T. Markestad. 2008. Long-term medical and social consequences of preterm birth. *New England Journal of Medicine* 359(3):262-273.

Mulye, T. P., M. J. Park, C. D. Nelson, S. H. Adams, C. E. Irwin Jr., and C. D. Brindis. 2009. Trends in adolescent and young adult health in the United States. *Journal of Adolescent Health* 45(1):8-24.

NCHS (National Center for Health Statistics). 1973. *Examination and health history findings among children and youths, 6-17 years, United States.* DHEW Publication No. (HRA) 74-1611, ser. 11, No. 129. Hyattsville, MD: U.S. Government Printing Office.

NCHS. 2004. *Health, United States: With chartbook on trends in the health of Americans.* Hyattsville, MD: HHS.

NCHS. 2009a. *About the State and Local Area Integrated Telephone Survey.* http://www.cdc. gov/nchs/slaits/about_slaits.htm (accessed November 19, 2010).

NCHS. 2009b. *Health, United States, 2009: With special feature on medical technology.* Hyattsville, MD: U.S. Government Printing Office.

NCHS. 2009c. *National Survey of Children's Health.* http://www.cdc.gov/nchs/slaits/nsch.htm (accessed November 19, 2010).

NCHS. 2010a. *National Health and Nutrition Examination Survey 2007-2008 Overview.* Hyattsville, MD: CDC.

NCHS. 2010b. *Report of the SLAITS and NIS Review Panel to the NCHS Board of Scientific Counselors (BSC).* http://www.cdc.gov/nchs/data/bsc/bsc_slaits_final_report.htm (accessed April 16, 2010).

NCHS. 2011a. *Health Data Interactive.* http://www.cdc.gov/nchs/hdi.htm (accessed January 24, 2011).

NCHS. 2011b. *National Health Interview Survey.* http://www.cdc.gov/nchs/nhis.htm (accessed February 1, 2011).

NCHS. 2011c. *National Immunization Survey.* http://www.cdc.gov/nchs/nis.htm (accessed February 1, 2011).

NCHS and CDC. 2006. *NHANES analytic and reporting guidelines.* Hyattsville, MD: HHS.

NCQA (National Committee for Quality Assurance). 2009. *Medicaid managed care benchmarking project final report.* Washington, DC: NCQA.

NCQA. 2010. *HEDIS & quality measurement.* http://www.ncqa.org/tabid/59/Default.aspx (accessed January 24, 2011).

NCVHS (National Committee on Vital and Health Statistics). 2010. *Toward enhanced information capacities for health: An NCVHS concept paper.* Washington, DC: HHS.

Nersesian, W. S. 1988. Infant mortality in socially vulnerable populations. *Annual Review of Public Health* 9:361-377.

Neumark-Sztainer, D., M. Story, P. J. Hannan, and J. Croll. 2002. Overweight status and eating patterns among adolescents: Where do youths stand in comparison with the Healthy People 2010 objectives? *American Journal of Public Health* 92(5):844-851.

Newacheck, P. W., and S. E. Kim. 2005. A national profile of health care utilization and expenditures for children with special health care needs. *Archives of Pediatrics and Adolescent Medicine* 159(1):10-17.

Newacheck, P. W., D. C. Hughes, and J. J. Stoddard. 1996. Children's access to primary care: Differences by race, income, and insurance status. *Pediatrics* 97(1):26-32.

Newacheck, P. W., J. Stoddard, D. Hughes, and M. Pearl. 1998a. Health insurance and access to primary care for children. *New England Journal of Medicine* 338(8):513-519.

Newacheck, P., B. Strickland, J. Shonkoff, J. Perrin, M. McPherson, M. McManus, C. Lauver, H. Fox, and P. Arango. 1998b. An epidemiologic profile of children with special health care needs. *Pediatrics* 102(1 Pt. 1):117-123.

NICHD (National Institute for Child Health and Development). 2007. *Add Health Study.* http://www.nichd.nih.gov/health/topics/add_health_study.cfm (accessed March 31, 2011).

NIH (National Institutes of Health). 2010a. *Health Services Research Information Central (HSRIC).* http://www.nlm.nih.gov/hsrinfo/datasites.html (accessed November 19, 2010).

NIH. 2010b. *Death among children and adolescents.* http://www.nlm.nih.gov/medlineplus/ency/article/001915.htm (accessed November 30, 2010).

NIH. 2010c. *NIH's National Children's Study begins recruiting at 30 locations.* http://www.nih.gov/news/health/sep2010/nichd-22.htm (accessed November 30, 2010).

NPC (National Prevention Council). 2010. *2010 Annual Status Report: National Prevention, Health Promotion and Public Health Council.* Washington, DC: NPC.

NQF (National Quality Forum). 2011. *Child health quality measures.* http://www.qualityforum.org/Projects/c-d/Child_Health_Quality_Measures_2010/Child_Health_Quality_Measures_2010.aspx (accessed February 16, 2011).

NRC (National Research Council). 1998. Longitudinal surveys of children. In *The Compass Series.* Washington, DC: National Academy Press.

NRC. 2000. *From neurons to neighborhoods: The science of early child development.* Washington, DC: National Academy Press.

NRC. 2007. *Engaging privacy and information technology in a digital age.* Washington, DC: The National Academies Press.

NRC. 2010. *Databases for estimating health insurance coverage for children: A workshop summary.* Washington, DC: The National Academies Press.

NRC and IOM. 1995. *Integrating federal statistics on children: Report of a workshop.* Washington, DC: National Academy Press.

NRC and IOM. 2008. *National children's study research plan: A review.* Washington, DC: The National Academies Press.

NSCAW Research Group (National Survey of Child and Adolescent Well-Being Research Group). 2002. Methodological lessons from the National Survey of Child and Adolescent Well-Being: The first three years of the USA's first national probability study of children and families investigated for abuse and neglect. *Children and Youth Services Review* 25(6/7):513-541.

Nutbeam, D. 2000. Health literacy as a public health goal: A challenge for contemporary health education and communication strategies into the 21st century. *Health Promotion International* 15(3):259-267.

OECD (Organisation for Economic Co-operation and Development). 2010a. *OECD health data 2010: How does the US compare?* Paris, France: OECD Health Division.

OECD. 2010b. "Infant mortality," *OECD factbook 2010: Economic, environmental and social statistics.* Paris: OECD Publishing.

Ogden, C. L., M. D. Carroll, L. R. Curtin, M. M. Lamb, and K. M. Flegal. 2010. Prevalence of high body mass index in US children and adolescents, 2007-2008. *Journal of the American Medical Association* 303(3):242-249.

OJJDP (Office of Juvenile Justice and Delinquency Prevention). 2008. *How OJJDP is serving children, families, and communities.* http://www.ncjrs.gov/pdffiles1/ojjdp/225036.pdf (accessed November 16, 2010).

Olson, L. M., S. F. Tang, and P. W. Newacheck. 2005. Children in the United States with discontinuous health insurance coverage. *New England Journal of Medicine* 353(4):382-391.

Orszag, P. 2007. Letter to Max Baucus, Chairman, Committee on Finance, United States Senate, July 24, Washington, DC.

Otto, R., J. Greenstein, M. Johnson, and R. Friedman. 1992. Prevalence of mental disorders among youth in the juvenile justice system. In *Responding to the mental health needs among youth in the juvenile justice system,* edited by J. J. Cocozza. Seattle, WA: National Coalition for the Mentally Ill in the Criminal Justice System. Pp. 7-48.

Owen, C. G., R. M. Martin, P. H. Whincup, G. Davey-Smith, M. W. Gillman, and D. G. Cook. 2005a. The effect of breastfeeding on mean body mass index throughout life: A quantitative review of published and unpublished observational evidence. *American Journal of Clinical Nutrition* 82(6):1298-1307.

Owen, C. G., R. M. Martin, P. H. Whincup, G. D. Smith, and D. G. Cook. 2005b. Effect of infant feeding on the risk of obesity across the life course: A quantitative review of published evidence. *Pediatrics* 115(5):1367-1377.

Owens, P. L., J. Thompson, A. Elixhauser, and K. Ryan. 2003. *Care of children and adolescents in U.S. hospitals.* Rockville, MD: AHRQ.

PAC (President's Advisory Commission on Consumer Protection and Quality in the Health Care Industry). 1998. *Quality first: Better health care for all Americans—final report to the President of the United States.* Washington, DC: U.S. Government Printing Office.

Pachter, L. M., and C. García Coll. 2009. Racism and child health: A review of the literature and future directions. *Journal of Developmental and Behavioral Pediatrics* 30(3):255-263.

Palfrey, J. 2006. Child health in America: Making a differnce through advocacy. Baltimore, MD: The Johns Hopkins University Press.

Pancholi, M., and J. Geppert. 2008. *AHRQ quality indicators 101: Background and introduction to the AHRQ QIs.* http://qualityindicators.ahrq.gov/downloads/Webinar2008/917webinarslides.ppt (accessed December 3, 2010).

Parsons, T. J., C. Power, S. Logan, and C. D. Summerbell. 1999. Childhood predictors of adult obesity: A systematic review. *International Journal of Obesity and Related Metabolic Disorders* 23(Suppl. 8):S1-S107.

Pati, S., Z. Mohamad, A. Cnaan, J. Kavanagh, and J. A. Shea. 2010. Influence of maternal health literacy on child participation in social welfare programs: The Philadelphia experience. *American Journal of Public Health* 100(9):1662-1665.

Pearlin, L. I., S. Schieman, E. M. Fazio, and S. C. Meersman. 2005. Stress, health, and the life course: Some conceptual perspectives. *Journal of Health and Social Behavior* 46(2):205-219.

Perrin, J. M, S. R. Bloom, and S. L. Gortmaker. 2007. The increase of chronic childhood conditions in the U.S. *Journal of the American Medical Association* 297(24):2755-2759.

Peterson, C. L., and R. Burton. 2007. *The U.S. health care spending: Comparison with other OECD countries* (RL 34175). http://digitalcommons.ilr.cornell.edu/key_workplace/311/ (accessed May 3, 2010).

PHS (Public Health Service). 1980. *Promoting health/preventing disease: Objectives for the nation.* Rockville, MD: HHS.

Pickett, K. E., and M. Pearl. 2001. Multilevel analyses of neighbourhood socioeconomic context and health outcomes: A critical review. *Journal of Epidemiology and Community Health* 55(2):111-122.

Pollack, C. E., S. Chideya, C. Cubbin, B. Williams, M. Dekker, and P. Braveman. 2007. Should health studies measure wealth? A systematic review. *American Journal of Preventive Medicine* 33(3):250-264.

Pollack, M. M., R. Holubkov, P. Glass, J. M. Dean, K. L. Meert, J. Zimmerman, K. J. S. Anand, J. Carcillo, C. J. L. Newth, R. Harrison, D. F. Willson, C. Nicholson, and Eunice Kennedy Shriver National Institute. 2009. Functional Status Scale: New pediatric outcome measure. *Pediatrics* 124(1):E18-E28.

Reidpath, D. D., and P. Allotey. 2003. Infant mortality rate as an indicator of population health. *Journal of Epidemiology and Community Health* 57(5):344-346.

RIACC (Rhode Island Asthma Control Coalition). 2009. *Reducing the burden of asthma in Rhode Island: Asthma State Plan 2009-2014.* Providence, RI: Department of Health.

Richardson, L. P., D. DiGiuseppe, M. Garrison, and D. A. Christakis. 2003. Depression in Medicaid-covered youth: Differences by race and ethnicity. *Archives of Pediatrics & Adolescent Medicine* 157(10):984-989.

Richesson, R. L., H. S. Lee, D. Cuthbertson, J. Lloyd, K. Young, and J. P. Krischer. 2009. An automated communication system in a contact registry for persons with rare diseases: Scalable tools for identifying and recruiting clinical research participants. *Contemporary Clinical Trials* 30(1):55-62.

Roberts, D. H., G. S. Gilmartin, N. Neeman, J. E. Schulze, S. Cannistraro, L. H. Ngo, M. D. Aronson, and J. W. Weiss. 2009. Design and measurement of quality improvement indicators in ambulatory pulmonary care. *Chest* 136(4):1134-1140.

Rodriguez, M. A., M. A. Winkleby, D. Ahn, J. Sundquist, and H. C. Kraemer. 2002. Identification of population subgroups of children and adolescents with high asthma prevalence: Findings from the Third National Health and Nutrition Examination Survey. *Archives of Pediatrics & Adolescent Medicine* 156(3):269-275.

Roesler, J., and M. Ostercamp. 2000. Pediatric firearm injury in Minnesota, 1998. Fatal and nonfatal firearm injuries among Minnesota youth. *Minnesota Medicine* 83(9):57-60.

Roghmann, K., and I. Pless. 1993. Acute illness. In *Child health and the community*, 2nd ed., edited by R. Haggerty, K. Roghmann, and I. Pless. New Brunswick, NJ: Transaction Publishers.

Romano, P. S. 2000. Should health plan quality measures be adjusted for case mix? *Medical Care* 38(10):977-980.

Sable, M. R., and A. A. Herman. 1997. The relationship between prenatal health behavior advice and low birth weight. *Public Health Reports* 112(4):332-339.

Sage, W. M., M. Balthazar, S. Kelder, S. Millea, S. Pont, and M. Rao. 2010. Mapping data shape community responses to childhood obesity. *Health Affairs* 29(3):498-502.

SAMHSA (Substance Abuse and Mental Health Services Administration). 2007. *Results from the 2006 National Survey on Drug Use and Health: National findings*. Rockville, MD: HHS.

Sandler, A. D., D. Brazdziunas, W. C. Cooley, L. González De Pijem, D. Hirsch, T. A. Kastner, M. E. Kummer, R. D. Quint, E. S. Ruppert, W. C. Anderson, B. Crider, P. Burgan, C. Garner, M. McPherson, L. Michaud, M. Yeargin-Allsopp, J. D. Cartwright, C. P. Johnson, and K. Smith. 2001. Developmental surveillance and screening of infants and young children. *Pediatrics* 108(1):192-196.

Satcher, D. 2000. Eliminating racial and ethnic disparities in health: The role of the ten leading health indicators. *Journal of the National Medical Association* 92(7):315-318.

Satel, S., and J. Klick. 2006. *The health disparities myth diagnosing the treatment gap*. http://www.aei.org/docLib/20060201_SatelKlickPR_g.pdf (accessed November 16, 2010).

Savitz, D. A., and R. B. Ness. 2010. Saving the National Children's Study. *Epidemiology* 21(5):598-601.

Scal, P., T. Evans, S. Blozis, N. Okinow, and R. Blum. 1999. Trends in transition from pediatric to adult health care services for young adults with chronic conditions. *Journal of Adolescent Health* 24(4):259-264.

Scanlon, M. C., J. M. Harris, 2nd, F. Levy, and A. Sedman. 2008. Evaluation of the Agency for Healthcare Research and Quality pediatric quality indicators. *Pediatrics* 121(6):e1723-e1731.

Schoendorf, K. C., and A. M. Branum. 2006. The use of United States vital statistics in perinatal and obstetric research. *American Journal of Obstetrics and Gynecology* 194(4):911-915.

Schoenman, J. A., J. P. Sutton, A. Kintala, D. Love, and R. Maw. 2005. *The value of hospital discharge databases*. Final report submitted to the AHRQ under contract number 282-98-0024. Rockville, MD: AHRQ.

Scholle, S. H., S. L. Sampsel, N. E. Davis, and E. L. Schor. 2009. *Quality of child health care: Expanding the scope and flexibility of measurement approaches*. New York: The Commonwealth Fund.

Schuster, M. A., T. Franke, and C. B. Pham. 2002. Smoking patterns of household members and visitors in homes with children in the United States. *Archives of Pediatrics & Adolescent Medicine* 156(11):1094-1100.

Schuster, M. A., E. A. McGlynn, and R. H. Brook. 2005. How good is the quality of health care in the United States? *Milbank Quarterly* 83(4):843-895.

Schwarz, D. 2010 (unpublished). *Workshop on pediatric health and health care quality measurement and information needs*. Philadelphia, PA.

Selling, K. E., J. Carstensen, O. Finnstrom, A. Josefsson, and G. Sydsjo. 2008. Hospitalizations in adolescence and early adulthood among Swedish men and women born preterm or small for gestational age. *Epidemiology* 19(1):63-70.

Serdula, M., D. Ivery, R. Coates, D. Freedman, D. Williamson, and T. Byers. 1993. Do obese children become obese adults? A review of the literature. *Preventive Medicine* 22(2):167-177.

SHADAC and RWJF (State Health Access Data Assistance Center and The Robert Wood Johnson Foundation). 2009. *Comparing federal government surveys that count uninsured people in America*. Princeton, NJ: RWJF.

Shapiro-Mendoza, C. K., K. M. Tomashek, M. Kotelchuck, W. Barfield, J. Weiss, and S. Evans. 2006. Risk factors for neonatal morbidity and mortality among "healthy," late preterm newborns. *Seminars in Perinatology* 30(2):54-60.

Shi, L., and G. D. Stevens. 2005. Disparities in access to care and satisfaction among U.S. children: The roles of race/ethnicity and poverty status. *Public Health Report* 120(4): 431-441.

Shin, Hyon, and Robert Kominski. 2010. *Language use in the United States: 2007*. In American Community Survey Reports, ACS-12. Washington, DC: U.S. Census Bureau.

Shone, L. P., A. W. Dick, C. Brach, K. S. Kimminau, B. J. LaClair, E. A. Shenkman, J. F. Col, V. A. Schaffer, F. Mulvihill, P. G. Szilagyi, J. D. Klein, K. VanLandeghem, and J. Bronstein. 2003. The role of race and ethnicity in the State Children's Health Insurance Program (SCHIP) in four states: Are there baseline disparities, and what do they mean for SCHIP? *Pediatrics* 112(6 Pt. 2):e521.

Shone, L. P., A. W. Dick, J. D. Klein, J. Zwanziger, and P. G. Szilagyi. 2005. Reduction in racial and ethnic disparities after enrollment in the State Children's Health Insurance Program. *Pediatrics* 115(6):e697-e705.

Shonkoff, J., W. Boyce, and B. McEwen. 2009. Neuroscience, molecular biology, and the childhood roots of health disparities: Building a new framework for health promotion and disease prevention. *Journal of the American Medical Association* 301(21):2252-2259.

Shufelt, J. L., and J. J. Cocozza. 2006. *Youth with mental health disorders in the juvenile justice system: Results from a multi-state prevalence study*. New York: National Center for Mental Health and Juvenile Justice.

Singh, G. K., and M. D. Kogan. 2007. Widening socioeconomic disparities in US childhood mortality, 1969-2000. *American Journal of Public Health* 97(9):1658-1665.

Singh, G. K., and S. M. Yu. 1996. US childhood mortality, 1950 through 1993: Trends and socioeconomic diffferentials. *American Journal of Health* 86(4):505-512.

Smith, V., J. Edwards, E. Reagan, and D. Roberts. 2009. *Medicaid and CHIP strategies for improving child health*. New York: The Commonwealth Fund.

Sondik, E. J., D. T. Huang, R. J. Klein, and D. Satcher. 2010. Progress toward the Healthy People 2010 goals and objectives. *Annual Review of Public Health* 31(1):271-281.

Sparrow, S. S., D. A. Balla, and D. V. Cicchetti. 2006. *Vineland-II: Teacher rating form manual; Vineland adaptive behavior scales; A revision of the Vineland social maturity scale by E. A. Doll* (2nd ed.). Minneapolis, MN: Pearson Assessments.

Stagner, M. W., and J. M. Zweigl. 2007. *Indicators of youth health and well-being: Taking the long view*, edited by B. V. Brown. New York: Lawrence Erlbaum Associates.

Starfield, B. 2004. U.S. child health: What's amiss, and what should be done about it? *Health Affairs* 23(5):165-170.

Starfield, B., M. Bergner, M. Ensminger, A. Riley, S. Ryan, B. Green, P. McGauhey, A. Skinner, and S. Kim. 1993. Adolescent health status measurement: Development of the child health and illness profile. *Pediatrics* 91(2):430-435.

Starmer, J., and D. Giuse. 2008. A Real-time ventilator management dashboard: Toward hardwiring compliance with evidence-based guidelines. *AMIA Annual Symposium Proceedings* 702-706.

Starmer, J., and L. R. Waitman. 2006. Orders and evidence-based order sets—Vanderbilt's experience with CPOE ordering patterns between 2000 and 2005. *AMIA Annual Symposium Proceedings* 1108.

Stein, R. E. K., and D. J. Jessop. 1990. Functional Status II(R): A measure of child health status. *Medical Care* 28(11):1041-1055.

Stein, R. E. K., E. C. Perrin, I. B. Pless, S. L. Gortmaker, J. M. Perrin, D. K. Walker, and M. Weitzman. 1987. Severity of illness: Concepts and measurements. *The Lancet* 330(8574):1506-1509.

Stephenson, J. 2000. Palliative and hospice care needed for children with life-threatening conditions. *Journal of the American Medical Association* 284(19):2437-2438.

Story, M., K. M. Kaphingst, R. Robinson-O'Brien, and K. Glanz. 2008. Creating healthy food and eating environments: Policy and environmental approaches. *Annual Review of Public Health* 29:253-272.

Swallen, K. C., E. N. Reither, S. A. Haas, and A. M. Meier. 2005. Overweight, obesity, and health-related quality of life among adolescents: The National Longitudinal Study of Adolescent Health. *Pediatrics* 115(2):340-347.

Swamy, G. K., T. Østbye, and R. Skjærven. 2008. Association of preterm birth with long-term survival, reproduction, and next-generation preterm birth. *Journal of the American Medical Association* 299(12):1429-1436.

Sturm, R., J. S. Ringel, and T. Andreyeva. 2003. Geographic disparities in children's mental health care. *Pediatrics* 112(4):e308.

Szilagyi, P. G., and E. L. Schor. 1998. The health of children. *Health Services Research* 33(4 Pt. 2):1001-1039.

Tang, S. F., L. M. Olson, and B. K. Yudkowsky. 2003. Uninsured children: How we count matters. *Pediatrics* 112(2):e168-e173.

Thompson, J. W., K. W. Ryan, S. D. Pinidiya, and J. E. Bost. 2003. Quality of care for children in commercial and Medicaid managed care. *Journal of the American Medical Association* 290(11):1486-1493.

Tomashek, K. M., C. K. Shapiro-Mendoza, J. Weiss, M. Kotelchuck, W. Barfield, S. Evans, A. Naninni, and E. Declercq. 2006. Early discharge among late preterm and term newborns and risk of neonatal morbidity. *Seminars in Perinatology* 30(2):61-68.

Udry, J. R., P. S. Bearman, and K. M. Harris. 2009. *The National Longitudinal Study of Adolescent Health: Research Design.* http://www.cpc.unc.edu/projects/addhealth/design (accessed December 1, 2010).

UNICEF (United Nations Children's Fund). 2007. *Child poverty in perspective: An overview of child well-being in rich countries.* New York: UNICEF.

Urban Institute and Kaiser Commission. 2010. *Medicaid enrollees and expenditures by enrollment group, 2007.* http://facts.kff.org/chart.aspx?ch=465 (accessed November 29, 2010).

U.S. Congress (106th). 1999. *Healthcare Research and Quality Act of 1999*. Washington, DC: Government Printing Office.

U.S. Congress (111th). 2009. *State Child Well-Being Research Act of 2009*. Washington, DC: Government Printing Office.

U.S. Preventive Services Task Force. 2009. Screening and treatment for major depressive disorder in children and adolescents: U.S. Preventive Services Task Force recommendation statement. *Pediatrics* 123:1223-1228.

Van Berkestijn, L., M. Kastein, A. Lodder, R. De Melker, and M.-L. Bartelink. 1999. How do we compare with our colleagues? Quality of general practitioner performance in consultations for non-acute abdominal complaints. *International Journal for Quality in Health Care* 11(6):475-486.

Van Cleave, J., S. Gortmaker, and J. Perrin. 2010. Dynamics of obesity and chronic health conditions among children and youth. *Journal of the American Medical Association* 303(7):623-630.

Van der Lee, J., L. Mokkink, M. Grootenhuis, H. Heymans, and M. Offringa. 2007. Definitions and measurement of chronic health conditions in childhood: A systematic review. *Journal of the American Medical Association* 297(24):2741-2751.

van Dyck, P. C., M. McPherson, B. B. Strickland, K. Nesseler, S. J. Blumberg, M. L. Cynamon, and P. W. Newacheck. 2002. The National Survey of Children with Special Health Care Needs. *Ambulatory Pediatrics* 2(1):29-37.

Ventura, S. J., J. C. Abma, and W. D. Mosher. 2009. Estimated pregnancy rates for the United States, 1990–2005: An update. *National Vital Statistics Reports* 58(4).

Vest, J. 2009. Health information exchange and healthcare utilization. *Journal of Medical Systems* 33(3):223-231.

Villegas, Andrew. 2011. *Medicaid Coverage Explained 2009*. Available from http://www.npr.org/templates/story/story.php?storyId=113339184 (accessed March 14, 2011).

Wadhwa, S. 2010. *Measuring children's health and health care*. Presentation to Committee on Pediatric Health and Health Care Quality Measures, March 23, 2010, Washington, DC. http://iom.edu/~/media/Files/Activity%20Files/Quality/PediatricQualityMeasures/Sandeep%20Wadhwa_3_23_10.ashx (accessed December 2, 2010).

Wasserman, G., S. Ko, and L. McReynolds. 2004. *Assessing the mental health status of youth in juvenile justice settings, Juvenile Justice Bulletin*. Washington, DC: U.S. Department of Justice, Office of Justice Programs, Office of Juvenile Justice and Delinquency Prevention.

Weinburg, D. 2003. *Using the Survey of Income and Program Participation for Policy Analysis* (paper no. 240). Washington, DC: U.S. Census Bureau.

Weiss, B. D., and R. Palmer. 2004. Relationship between health care costs and very low literacy skills in a medically needy and indigent medicaid population. *The Journal of the American Board of Family Practice* 17(1):44-47.

Weitzman, M., L. V. Klerman, G. Lamb, J. Menary, and J. J. Alpert. 1982. School absence: A problem for the pediatrician. *Pediatrics* 69(6):739-746.

White, P. H. 2002. Access to health care: Health insurance considerations for young adults with special health care needs/disabilities. *Pediatrics* 110(6 Pt. 2):1328-1335.

WHO (World Health Organization). 1948. Preamble to the Constitution of the World Health Organization as adopted by the International Health Conference, New York, 19-22 June, 1946; signed on 22 July 1946 by the representatives of 61 States (and entered into force on 7 April 1948). *Official Records of the World Health Organization* (2):100.

WHO. 2008. *Closing the gap in a generation: Health equity through action on the social determinants of health. Final report of the Commission on Social Determinants of Health.* Geneva, Switzerland: WHO.

WHO. 2010. *International Classification of Functioning, Disability and Health (ICF)*. http://www.who.int/classifications/icf/en/ (accessed November 16, 2010).

Williams, L. M. 1995. Recovered memories of abuse in women with documented child sexual victimization histories. *Journal of Traumatic Stress* 8(4):649-673.

Williams, D. R., and M. Sternthal. 2010. Understanding racial-ethnic disparities in health. *Journal of Health and Social Behavior* 51(Suppl. 1):S15-S27.

Williams, D. R., M. Sternthal, and R. J. Wright. 2009. Social determinants: Taking the social context of asthma seriously. *Pediatrics* 123(Suppl. 3):S174-S184.

Wise, P. H. 2009. Confronting social disparities in child health: A critical appraisal of life-course science and research. *Pediatrics* 124(Suppl. 3):S203-S211.

Wood, D. L., C. Corey, H. E. Freeman, and M. F. Shapiro. 1992. Are poor families satisfied with the medical care their children receive? *Pediatrics* 90(1):66-70.

Xu, J., K. D. Kochanek, S. L. Murphy, and B. Tejada-Vera. 2010. Deaths: Final data for 2007. *National Vital Statistics Reports* 58(19).

Zaslavsky, A. M. 2001. Statistical issues in reporting quality data: Small samples and casemix variation. *International Journal for Quality in Health Care* 13(6):481-488.

Zaydfudim, V., L. A. Dossett, J. M. Starmer, P. G. Arbogast, I. D. Feurer, W. A. Ray, A. K. May, and C. W. Pinson. 2009. Implementation of a real-time compliance dashboard to help reduce SICU ventilator-associated pneumonia with the ventilator bundle. *Archives of Surgery* 144(7):656-662.

Zito, J., A. Derivan, C. Kratochvil, D. Safer, J. Fegert, and L. Greenhill. 2008. Off-label psychopharmacologic prescribing for children: History supports close clinical monitoring. *Child and Adolescent Psychiatry and Mental Health* 2(1):24.

A

List of Acronyms

AAP	American Academy of Pediatrics
ABCD	Assuring Better Child Health and Development
ACA	Patient Protection and Affordable Care Act
ACE	Adverse Childhood Experiences Study
ACO	accountable care organization
ACS	American Community Survey
ADD	attention-deficit disorder
Add Health	National Longitudinal Study of Adolescent Health
ADHD	attention-deficit/hyperactivity disorder
ADL	activities of daily life
AHRQ	Agency for Healthcare Research and Quality
AMA-PPMC	American Medical Association-Physician Practice Management Company
ARRA	American Recovery and Reinvestment Act
ASQ	Ages and Stages Questionnaires
BINS	Bayley Infant Neurodevelopmental Screens
BMI	body mass index
BRFSS	Behavioral Risk Factor Surveillance Survey
CAHMI	Child and Adolescent Health Measurement Initiative
CAHPS	Consumer Assessment of Healthcare Providers and Systems
CBO	Congressional Budget Office
CCS	Clinical Classification System

CCU	critical care unit
CDC	Centers for Disease Control and Prevention
CDHCPF	Colorado Department of Health Care Policy and Financing
CHICA	Child Health Improvement through Computer Automation
CHIP	Children's Health Insurance Program
CHIPRA	Children's Health Insurance Program Reauthorization Act
CHP	Center for Health Policy
CMS	Centers for Medicare and Medicaid Services
COH	Children's Optimal Health
CPI	Consumer Price Index
CPS	Current Population Survey
CSHCN	Children with special health care needs
CWI	Child Well-Being Index
DRC	Data Resource Center for Child and Adolescent Health
DX	diagnosis
EBP	evidence-based practice
ECLS-B	Early Childhood Longitudinal Study-Birth Cohort
ECLS-K	Early Childhood Longitudinal Study-Kindergarten Class
ED	emergency department
EDC	Education Development Center
E-HIE	electronic health information exchange
EHR	electronic health record
EPA	Environmental Protection Agency
EPC	Evidence-based Practice Center
EPSDT	Early and periodic screening, diagnosis and treatment
ETS	Educational Testing Service
FAcct	Foundation for Accountability
FERPA	Family Educational Rights and Privacy Act of 1974
FIFCFS	Federal Interagency Forum on Child and Family Statistics
FPL	federal poverty level
GIS	geographic information system
GSMS	Great Smoky Mountains Study
HCUP	Healthcare Cost and Utilization Project
HEDIS	Healthcare Effectiveness Data and Information Set
HHS	U.S. Department of Health and Human Services

HIPAA	Health Insurance Portability and Accountability Act
HIT	Health information technology
HITECH	Health Information Technology for Economic and Clinical Health
HRSA	Health Resources and Services Administration
ICD-9	*International Classification of Diseases*, Ninth Revision
ICD-10	*International Classification of Diseases*, Tenth Revision
ICF	*International Classification of Functioning*
ICU	intensive care unit
IHS	Indian Health Service
IOM	Institute of Medicine
IQI	Inpatient Quality Indicator
IT	information technology
KID	Kids' Inpatient Database
KIDS	Kids Integrated Data Set
MACPAC	Medicaid and CHIP Payment and Access Commission
MCH	maternal and child health
MCHB	Maternal and Child Health Bureau
MCO	managed care organization
MEPS	Medical Expenditure Panel Survey
MMIS	Medicaid Management Information System
MOU	Memorandum of Understanding
MSIS	Medicaid Statistical Information System
MST	multisystemic therapy
NAMCS	National Ambulatory Medical Care Survey
NCES	National Center for Education Statistics
NCHHSTP	National Center for HIV/AIDS, Viral Hepatitis, STD, and TB Prevention (Centers for Disease Control)
NCHS	National Center for Health Statistics
NCQA	National Committee for Quality Assurance
NCS	National Children's Study
NDACAN	National Data Archive on Child Abuse and Neglect
NDI	National Death Index
NEDS	Nationwide Emergency Department Sample
NHAMC	National Hospital Ambulatory Medical Care Survey
NHANES	National Health and Nutrition Examination Survey
NHCS	National Health Care Survey
NHDS	National Hospital Discharge Survey
NHES	National Household Education Surveys

NHHCS	National Home and Hospice Care Survey
NHIS	National Health Interview Survey
NICHQ	National Initiative for Children's Healthcare Quality
NICHSR	National Information Center on Health Services Research and Health Care Technology
NICU	neonatal intensive care unit
NIH	National Institutes of Health
NIMH	National Institute of Mental Health
NIS	National Immunization Survey
NIS	Nationwide Inpatient Sample
NORC	National Opinion Research Center
NQF	National Quality Forum
NRC	National Research Council
NS-CSHCN	National Survey of Children with Special Health Care Needs
NSAF	National Survey of American Families
NSCAW	National Survey of Child and Adolescent Well-being
NSCH	National Survey of Children's Health
NSECH	National Survey of Early Childhood Health
NSFG	National Survey of Family Growth
NVSS	National Vital Statistics System
ODD	oppositional defiant disorder
OMB	Office of Management and Budget
PCOR	Primary Care and Outcomes Research
PCP	primary care provider
PDI	Pediatric Quality Indicator
Pedi-QS	Pediatric Data Quality System Collaborative Measure Workgroup
PEDS	Parents' Evaluations of Developmental Status
PELL	Pregnancy to Early Life Longitudinal
PHDS	Promoting Healthy Development Survey
PHR	personal health record
PQI	Prevention Quality Indicator
PQRI	Physician Quality Reporting Initiative
PRAMS	Pregnancy Risk Assessment and Monitoring System
PROMIS	Patient-Reported Outcomes Measurement Information System
PSI	Patient Safety Indicator
PSID	Panel Survey of Income Dynamics
PSQIA	Patient Safety and Quality Improvement Act of 2005

QISMC	Quality Improvement System for Managed Care
QSDE	Qualified State-Designated Entity
QUAL	Quality

RIACC	Rhode Island Asthma Control Coalition
RICCC	Rhode Island Chronic Care Collaborative
RWJF	Robert Wood Johnson Foundation

SASD	State Ambulatory Surgery Databases
SCHIP	State Children's Health Insurance Program (now CHIP)
SED	severe emotional distress
SEDD	State Emergency Department Databases
SEER	Surveillance, Epidemiology, and End Results
SID	State Inpatient Databases
SIDS	sudden infant death syndrome
SIPP	Survey of Income and Program Participation
SLAITS	State and Local Area Integrated Telephone Survey
SNAC	AHRQ Subcommittee on Quality Measures for Children in Medicaid and Children's Health Insurance Programs
SNOMED	Systematized Nomenclature of Medicine
SSI	Supplemental Security Income
STD	sexually transmitted disease
STI	sexually transmitted infection

TB	tuberculosis

UCLA	University of California, Los Angeles
UCSF	University of California, San Francisco

WHO	World Health Organization
WIC	Supplemental Nutrition Program for Women, Infants, and Children
WISQARS™	Web-based Injury Statistics Query and Reporting System
WPPSI	Wechsler Preschool and Primary Scale of Intelligence

YAHCS	Young Adult Health Care Survey
YRBS	Youth Risk Behavior Survey

B

Workshop Agenda and Participants

**Workshop on Pediatric Health and Health Care Quality
Measurement and Information Needs**

Agenda

March 23, 2010

WORKSHOP GOALS:
- To highlight unmet measurement and information needs from a broad group of data users
- To gather information to support the development of a framework, a subset of measures, and a data system for child health and health care quality measures
- To illustrate innovative and exemplary data collection efforts to support the development of a framework for a comprehensive data support system

WORKSHOP ORGANIZATION:
The workshop will be comprised of four sessions featuring speaker presentations followed by panel discussions (15 minutes per speaker presentation; 30 minutes for each panel discussion).

The panels are organized to hear the perspectives of four major stakeholder groups:

PANEL 1:	Patients and Parents
PANEL 2:	Providers
PANEL 3:	Payers
PANEL 4:	Policy makers

PROGRAM:

8:40A   Welcome Remarks
                        Gordon H. DeFriese, Ph.D., Committee Chair

8:55A – 9:40A   **Panel 1: Patients and Parents**
                        Moderator: **Maxine Hayes, M.D., M.P.H.,** State
                        Health Officer, State of Washington, Department of
                        Health, *Committee Member*

                        Nora Wells, M.Ed., Director of Research Activities,
                        Family Voices
                        Darcy Gruttadaro, J.D., Director of the Child and
                        Adolescent Action Center, National Alliance on
                        Mental Illness
                        Judith Thierry, D.O., M.P.H., Maternal and
                        Child Health Coordinator, Office of Clinical and
                        Preventive Services, Indian Health Service,
                        U.S. Department of Health and Human Services

9:40A – 10:10A   **Panel 1 Discussion**

10:30A – 11:15A   **Panel 2: Providers**
                        Moderator: **Glenn Flores, M.D.,** Judith and
                        Charles Ginsburg Chair in Pediatrics, Department
                        of Pediatrics, University of Texas Southwestern
                        Medical Center at Dallas, *Committee Member*

                        Linda Juszczak, D.N.Sc., M.P.H., M.S., C.P.N.P.,
                        Executive Director, National Association of School-
                        Based Health Care
                        Ed Schor, M.D., Vice President, State High
                        Performance Health Systems Program, The
                        Commonwealth Fund
                        Xavier Sevilla, M.D., Chief of Pediatrics, Manatee
                        County Rural Health Services, Inc., Whole
                        Child Pediatrics, and Chair, American Academy
                        of Pediatrics Steering Committee on Quality
                        Improvement and Management

11:15A – 11:45A   **Panel 2 Discussion**

11:45A – 12:30P   **Panel 3: Payers**
Moderator: **Alan Weil, J.D., M.P.P.,** Executive
Director, National Academy for State Health Policy,
Committee Member

Russell Frank, M.S., CHIP Director, Vermont
Department of Health
Foster Gesten, M.D., Medical Director, Office
of Health Insurance Programs, New York State
Department of Health
Sandeep Wadhwa, M.D., M.B.A., Medicaid
Director and Chief Medical Officer, Colorado
Department of Health Care Policy and Financing

12:30P – 1:00P   **Panel 3 Discussion**

2:00P – 2:45P   **Panel 4: Policy makers**
Moderator: **Claire Brindis, Dr.P.H.,** Executive
Director, Philip R. Lee Institute for Health Policy
Studies and for the National Adolescent Health
Information and Innovation Center, University of
California, San Francisco, *Committee Member*

Richard G. Kronick, Ph.D., Deputy Assistant
Secretary for Health Policy, U.S. Department of
Health and Human Services
Don Schwarz, M.D., M.P.H., Deputy Mayor and
Health Commissioner, City of Philadelphia
Joe Thompson, M.D., M.P.H., Surgeon General,
Office of the Surgeon General, State of Arkansas

2:45P – 3:15P   **Panel 4 Discussion**

3:15P – 3:50P   Public Comments

3:50P – 4:00P   Closing Remarks and Adjournment
Gordon H. DeFriese, Ph.D., Committee Chair

PARTICIPANT LIST

Committee Members:

Gordon H. DeFriese, Ph.D. (*Chair*), Cecil G. Sheps Center for Health Service Research, University of North Carolina at Chapel Hill

Paula A. Braveman, M.D., M.P.H., Center on Social Disparities in Health, University of California, San Francisco

Claire D. Brindis, Dr.P.H., Philip R. Lee Institute for Health Policy Studies, University of California, San Francisco

Barbara J. Burns, Ph.D., Department of Psychiatry and Behavioral Sciences, Duke University School of Medicine

Glenn Flores, M.D., Department of Pediatrics, University of Texas Southwestern Medical Center at Dallas

Gary L. Freed, M.D., M.P.H., Department of Pediatrics, University of Michigan Health Systems

Deborah A. Gross, D.N.Sc., Department of Acute and Chronic Care, Johns Hopkins School of Nursing

Maxine Hayes, M.D., M.P.H., State of Washington, Department of Health

Charles J. Homer, M.D., M.P.H., National Initiative for Children's Healthcare Quality

Kevin B. Johnson, M.D., M.S., Department of Biomedical Informatics and Department of Pediatrics, Vanderbilt University School of Medicine

Genevieve Kenney, Ph.D., The Urban Institute

Marie C. McCormick, M.D., Sc.D., Department of Society, Human Development and Health, School of Public Health, Harvard University

Kathryn M. McDonald, M.M./M.B.A., Center for Primary Care and Outcomes Research, Stanford University School of Medicine

Michael J. O'Grady, Ph.D., Health Policy and Evaluation Department, National Opinion Research Corporation at the University of Chicago

Alan R. Weil, J.D., M.P.P., National Academy for State Health Policy

Alan M. Zaslavsky, Ph.D., Department of Health Care Policy, Harvard Medical School

Workshop Presenters:

Russell Frank, M.S., Vermont Department of Health

Foster Gesten, M.D., Office of Health Insurance Programs, New York State Department of Health

Darcy Gruttadaro, J.D., Child and Adolescent Action Center, National Alliance for the Mentally Ill

Linda Juszczak, D.N.Sc., M.S., M.P.H., National Assembly on School-Based Health Care

Richard G. Kronick, Ph.D., Office of Health Policy, HHS Office of the Assistant Secretary for Planning and Evaluation

Edward L. Schor, M.D., The Commonwealth Fund

Donald F. Schwarz, M.D., M.P.H., City of Philadelphia

Xavier Sevilla, M.D., Manatee County Rural Health Services Inc., Whole Child Pediatrics

Judith Thierry, D.O., M.P.H., F.A.A.P., Maternal and Child Health, HHS Indian Health Service

Joseph W. Thompson, M.D., M.P.H., Center for Health Improvement, State of Arkansas

Sandeep Wadhwa, M.D., M.B.A., Colorado Department of Health Care Policy and Financing

Nora Wells, M.S.Ed., Family Voices

National Academies Staff:

Rosemary Chalk, Study Director

Patti Simon, Program Officer

Pamella Atayi, Senior Program Assistant

Chelsea Bodnar, Christine Mirzayan Science and Technology Policy Fellow

Wendy Keenan, Program Associate

Julienne Palbusa, Research Assistant

Registered Attendees:

Jennifer Burks, Health Resources and Services Administration

Tim S. Bushfield, U.S. Government Accountability Office

Barbara A. Dailey, Centers for Medicare and Medicaid Services

Maushami DeSoto, Agency for Healthcare Research and Quality

Denise Dougherty, Agency for Healthcare Research and Quality

Elaine Duffee, Engelberg Center for Health Care Reform

Sarah Edwards, The National Academies, Christine Mirzayan Science and Technology Policy Fellow

Michael Ellwood, National Association of Children's Hospitals and Related Institutions

Gerry Fairbrother, Cincinnati Children's Hospital Medical Center

Richard Fenton, National Association of State Medicaid Directors

Patricia Franklin, National Association of Pediatric Nurse Practitioners

Rita Munley Gallagher, American Nurses Association
Mengfei Huang, The National Academies, Christine Mirzayan Science
    and Technology Policy Fellow
David Keller, HHS Office of the Assistant Secretary for Planning and
    Evaluation
Kristina Krasnov, The National Academies, Christine Mirzayan Science
    and Technology Policy Fellow
Marcia Lillie-Blanton, The George Washington University
Hannah S. Locke, U.S. Government Accountability Office
Susan L. Lukacs, Centers for Disease Control and Prevention
Patricia MacTaggart, The George Washington University
Nick Manetto, B&D Consulting
Jessica L. McAuliffe, Cincinnati Children's Hospital Medical Center
Poornima Nayak, American Public Human Services Association
Sarah Hudson Scholle, National Committee for Quality Assurance
Ellen Schwalenstocker, National Association of Children's Hospitals and
    Related Institutions
Katie Sellers, Association of State and Territorial Health Officials
Alan E. Simon, Centers for Disease Control and Prevention
Jan Strozer, National Assembly on School-Based Health Care
Caroline Taplin, HHS Office of the Assistant Secretary for Planning and
    Evaluation
Tatiana Zenzano, HHS Office of Public Health and Science

C

Private-Sector Initiatives to Advance Health Care Quality and the Development of Quality Measures

This appendix reviews a number of private-sector initiatives to advance health care quality and the development of quality measures, catalyzed by the Institute of Medicine's (IOM) seminal series of reports on quality of care.

THE IOM QUALITY SERIES

The first wave of the quality movement was shaped by a number of forces—pressure to control health care spending, a demand for greater accountability in health care, urgent calls for improved patient safety, and an overall push for better national health outcomes. In 1990, the IOM provided what has become an enduring and widely used definition of quality of care: "Quality of care is the degree to which health services for individuals and populations increase the likelihood of desired health outcomes and are consistent with current professional knowledge."

In the years that followed, a series of landmark reports, legislation, and innovations shaped the field of quality improvement. Two such reports, *To Err Is Human: Building a Safer Health System* (IOM, 1999) and *Crossing the Quality Chasm: A New Health System for the 21st Century* (IOM, 2001), described serious quality gaps in health care and envisioned a new health system to bridge the quality chasm, respectively. They built on experience with quality measurement and quality improvement in other industries, such as transportation safety, and embraced the classical Donabedian framework (Donabedian, 1988) of structure, process, and outcomes. The reports laid out six specific aims for health care quality improvement:

safety, timeliness, effectiveness, efficiency, equity, and patient-centeredness. *Crossing the Quality Chasm* emphasized the shift in health care from acute to chronic care, noting that "chronic conditions are now the leading cause of illness, disability, and death; they affect almost half the population and account for the majority of health care expenditures" (IOM, 2001).

A later series of IOM reports (IOM, 2006a, 2006b, 2006c) proposed a rigorous, systematic, and quantifiable approach for using the above six aims to promote quality measurement in the health care system. These studies offered strategies for evaluating the performance of managed care organizations, health plans or programs, and hospitals, as well as individual practitioners, and made suggestions for how these measures could be used to induce changes in practice through financial rewards or penalties. Some progress has been made—primarily in the area of patient safety among adults (Leape and Berwick, 2005)—but nearly a decade later, significant gaps in quality persist.

Several IOM reports have reviewed an array of public- and private-sector initiatives aimed at improving health care quality (IOM, 2006a, 2006b, 2006c). These studies have focused primarily on the quality of adult health care. They reflect a bias toward the need for quality measures that can help improve the management of complex, chronic conditions, as well as health care services that are commonly associated with hospitalization or require intensive procedures or interactions with multiple health care providers.

The initial IOM health care quality framework was augmented by a later approach that called attention to adapting quality measures to a patient-centered focus, emphasizing the stages of an individual's health status: preventive services ("staying healthy"), acute treatment ("getting better"), chronic conditions ("living with illness"), and end-of-life care.

DEVELOPMENT OF INITIAL QUALITY MEASURES FOR CHILDREN AND ADOLESCENTS

Concern about the quality of care, particularly chronic care, gave rise to efforts to assess the effectiveness of care for the chronically ill. The National Quality Forum (NQF) is a private-sector standards-setting organization whose efforts center on the evaluation and endorsement of standardized performance measures. Since its establishment in 1999, NQF has endorsed more than 500 measures covering all aspects of care (i.e., ambulatory, hospital and facility, and palliative care). However, measures relevant to or developed specifically for children and adolescents failed to receive early attention. This was the result of NQF's initial focus on high-need and high-cost conditions (largely in response to its private health plan funders' priorities). This approach inevitably created a focus on adults, since this population has the highest prevalence of chronic conditions.

NQF held its first meeting specifically on measures for children in 2004. This gathering led to the identification of several priority areas in which measures existed, but few measures were endorsed since no consensus regarding their validity and reliability and the feasibility of their use had been established (Simpson et al., 2007). After the 2004 meeting, it would be several years before NQF would once again be able to focus specifically on children and adolescents. Despite these limitations, NQF has endorsed numerous quality measures either specifically for or inclusive of children and adolescents. In addition, at least some of the measures aimed at adults might be relevant to children, adolescents, or young adults with some modification (Simpson and Fairbrother, 2010).

In 2009, the Department of Health and Human Services expanded the scope of the contract with NQF to include a focus on Medicaid and the State Children's Health Insurance Program (SCHIP), thus supporting NQF's efforts to enhance the number and scope of endorsed measures relevant to children and adolescents and to better incorporate the needs of young people into the ongoing priorities.

EXPANSION OF MEASURE DEVELOPMENT AND QUALITY IMPROVEMENT

In the mid-1990s, the National Committee for Quality Assurance (NCQA) convened a pediatric measurement advisory panel to expand the scope of measures relevant to children in the Healthcare Effectiveness Data and Information Set (HEDIS©), which at the time was quite limited (Forrest et al., 1997). In addition, the Child and Adolescent Health Measurement Initiative (CAHMI) was launched at the Foundation for Accountability (FAcct) to bring a focus on consumer-driven measures as a key component of quality measurement. Together, these two organizations developed a set of priorities for measure development that helped shape the next decade's work on quality measurement. At the same time, the National Initiative for Children's Healthcare Quality (NICHQ) was established in 1999 to complement measure development with quality improvement activities. And the 1999 reauthorization of the Agency for Healthcare Research and Quality (AHRQ) included children as one of the named priority populations.

The ensuing years saw slow but steady progress in the number of measures available for assessing the quality of care for children (Beal et al., 2004; Dougherty and Simpson, 2004; Kavanagh et al., 2009; Miller et al., 2005; Schwalenstocker et al., 2008). For example, the Joint Commission on Accreditation of Healthcare Organizations worked with the Pediatric Data Quality System Collaborative Measure Workgroup (Pedi-QS) to develop indicators for reviewing the delivery of inpatient asthma care and care provided in the pediatric intensive care unit (Scanlon et al., 2007;

Schwalenstocker et al., 2008). With funding from the Centers for Medicare and Medicaid Services (CMS), the RAND Corporation developed a set of more than 400 outpatient indicators for children and adolescents and used them to assess the quality of care in landmark studies on quality of care for adults (McGlynn et al., 2003) and for children and adolescents (Mangione-Smith et al., 2007). Yet issues related to the feasibility and cost of large-scale abstraction from medical records inhibit the use of these indicators.

At a 2010 conference convened by NICHQ and NQF to promote alignment with national priorities and child health measures, stakeholders identified key drivers, or essential levers, that together are necessary and sufficient to achieve progress toward quality improvement goals: payment reform, public reporting, professional development, performance measurement, research and knowledge dissemination, and system capacity (Homer et al., 2010). Stakeholders believed that, in addition to the presence of appropriate measures, these drivers were likely to be powerful levers for change in child and adolescent health.

Numerous privately funded entities are engaged in developing measures for assessing the quality of health care for children and adolescents (NCQA, RAND, NICHQ, CAHMI, the American Medical Association-Physician Practice Management Company [AMA-PPMC], the Joint Commission). Although a process exists for reviewing and endorsing measures (NQF), disconnects persist between the *availability* of such measures and their *use*. First the Children's Health Insurance Program Reauthorization Act (CHIPRA), then the Affordable Care Act (ACA), changed the landscape. A mandate and an urgency now exist, especially around measures focused on accountability and value in service delivery. More attention needs to be given to medical records data as a source for quality measurement. For example, many HEDIS measures (implemented by State Medicaid and CHIP programs) are hybrid measures that require both administrative claims data and data from medical records abstraction to score. Moreover, the clinical detail found in medical records is especially important in developing prevention measures (e.g., content of well-child visits). However, the primary focus of this study (based on the committee's scope of work, as described in Chapter 1) was to consider the major national population-based reporting systems sponsored by the federal government. Thus, the committee acknowledges the value of medical records abstraction and recognizes the current constraints in making medical records data more widely available for quality measurement purposes without making specific recommendations on the future use of these data.

REFERENCES

Beal, A., J. Co, D. Dougherty, T. Jorsling, J. Kam, J. Perrin, and H. Palmer. 2004. Quality measures for children's health care. *Pediatrics* 113(1):199-209.

Donabedian, A. 1988. The quality of care: How can it be assessed? *Journal of the American Medical Association* 260(12):1743-1748.

Dougherty, D., and L. A. Simpson. 2004. Measuring the quality of children's health care: A prerequisite to action. *Pediatrics* 113(1):185-198.

Forrest, C. B., L. Simpson, and C. Clancy. 1997. Child health services research: Challenges and opportunities. *Journal of the American Medical Association* 277(22):1787-1793.

Homer, C., L. Simpson, K. Adams, K. Streb, A. Charrow, and W. Vernon. 2010. *Promoting alignment: National Priorities and Child Health Measures Conference 2010.*

IOM (Institute of Medicine). 1999. *To err is human: Building a safer health system.* Washington, DC: National Academy Press.

IOM. 2001. *Crossing the quality chasm: A new health system for the 21st century.* Washington, DC: National Academy Press.

IOM. 2006a. Medicare's Quality Improvement Organization Program: Maximizing potential. In *Pathways to quality health care*, edited by the Committee on Redesigning Health Insurance Performance Measures, and Performance Improvement Programs, and Board on Health Care Services. Washington, DC: The National Academies Press.

IOM. 2006b. *Performance measurement: Accelerating improvement.* Washington, DC: The National Academies Press.

IOM. 2006c. Rewarding provider performance: Aligning incentives in Medicare. In *Pathways to quality health care*, edited by Board on Health Care Services. Committee on Redesigning Health Insurance Performance Measures, and Performance Improvement Programs. Washington, DC: The National Academies Press.

Kavanagh, P. L., W. G. Adams, and C. J. Wang. 2009. Quality indicators and quality assessment in child health. *Archives of Disease in Childhood* 94(6):458-463.

Leape, L. L., and D. M. Berwick. 2005. Five years after To Err Is Human: What have we learned? *Journal of the American Medical Association* 293(19):2384-2390.

Mangione-Smith, R., A. H. DeCristofaro, C. M. Setodji, J. Keesey, D. J. Klein, J. L. Adams, M. A. Schuster, and E. A. McGlynn. 2007. The quality of ambulatory care delivered to children in the United States. *New England Journal of Medicine* 357(15):1515-1523.

McGlynn, E. A., S. M. Asch, J. Adams, J. Keesey, J. Hicks, A. DeCristofaro, and E. A. Kerr. 2003. The quality of health care delivered to adults in the United States. *New England Journal of Medicine* 348(26):2635-2645.

Miller, M. R., P. Gergen, M. Honour, and C. Zhan. 2005. Burden of illness for children and where we stand in measuring the quality of this health care. *Ambulatory Pediatrics* 5(5):268-278.

Scanlon, M. C., K. P. Mistry, and H. E. Jeffries. 2007. Determining pediatric intensive care unit quality indicators for measuring pediatric intensive care unit safety. *Pediatric Critical Care Medicine* 8(Suppl. 2):S3-S10.

Schwalenstocker, E., H. Bisarya, S. T. Lawless, L. Simpson, C. Throop, and D. Payne. 2008. Closing the gap in children's quality measures: A collaborative model. *Journal for Healthcare Quality* 30(5):4-11.

Simpson, L., and G. Fairbrother. 2010. *Quality measurement and children: Where have we been? Where do we need to go?* (Prepared as a background paper for NQF/NICHQ meeting, January 2010).

Simpson, L., D. Dougherty, D. Krause, C. M. Ku, and J. M. Perrin. 2007. Measuring children's health care quality. *American Journal of Medical Quality* 22(2):80-84.

D

Overview of Data Sources for Measures of Health Care Quality for Children and Adolescents

This appendix reviews sources of data on the quality of health care services for children and adolescents, including both administrative data sources (claims or claims and encounters) and population health surveys.

There are two key administrative data sources:

- the Medicaid Statistical Information System (MSIS), which contains state-level claims and encounter data; and
- the Healthcare Effectiveness Data and Information System (HEDIS©) data collection for managed care beneficiaries.

Administrative data, primarily from claims, are an important source of information on how the system is performing. A bill is generated to obtain reimbursement whenever a service is provided that requires payment. In contrast to population health surveys, which provide household reports and snapshots of the health of the population and experiences with care, claims-based data tend to provide a more detailed picture of the services received and costs of care for given diagnoses over time (as long as the individual is enrolled in that system). Administrative data therefore serve as a fundamental tool for monitoring the adequacy of care, although they have significant limitations, as noted in an earlier chapter.

In addition to the above two administrative data sources, quality measures can be found in population health surveys, especially in the data sets compiled by the National Health Information Survey (NHIS) for the Centers for Disease Control and Prevention and three surveys conducted by the Maternal and Child Health Bureau (MCHB): the National Survey of Children's Health (NSCH), the National Survey of Children with Special Health Care Needs (NS-CSHCN), and the National Survey of Early Child Health (NSECH). The NSCH is the most far-reaching of the three MCHB surveys in terms of the population covered, the sample size, and the topics covered.

THE MEDICAID STATISTICAL INFORMATION SYSTEM

The MSIS is a national database of Medicaid claims and eligibility data that is maintained by the Centers for Medicare and Medicaid Services (CMS) and consists of an aggregation of individual state-level claims databases. Reporting by states to the MSIS is mandatory for state Medicaid agencies. Thus, the MSIS contains data on all Medicaid children and Children's Health Insurance Program (CHIP) children who are part of Medicaid expansions (although not children in separate CHIP programs). The state-level data reported to CMS for the MSIS provide a base that is useful for some measures, although it has some major limitations.

On the positive side, state-level files contain data on claims and encounters for services, which include data on health insurance, diagnoses, and the services or procedures provided as core data elements. The records contain a state-assigned unique personal identifier; this identifier can be used consistently to identify a given individual across different years and different enrollment periods, making it possible to track Medicaid beneficiaries over time within that state (MacTaggart, 2010).

The major weakness of the state-level data reported to the MSIS lies in its nature as a claims-based system. In most states, claims for services rendered under Medicaid primary care case management and fee-for-service care show a complete record of the services provided and generate a reimbursement for those services. However, contractors with managed care organizations may receive a capitated payment for beneficiaries. In such cases, their claims data may not necessarily describe the actual services provided. Managed care organizations may submit encounters or "shadow claims," which, because they do not actually generate reimbursement, may be incomplete. CMS has indicated it is working with states to improve encounter data (MacTaggart, 2010). Furthermore, the Children's Health Insurance Program Reauthorization Act (CHIPRA) requires the Department of Health and Human Services (HHS) to collect and analyze the MSIS data from states within 6 months. MSIS data have not been used as a source of reporting in the past (MacTaggart, 2010; Simpson et al., 2009), but the new federal reporting requirements, combined with federal efforts to improve state claims/encounter databases, may lead to more usable data in those databases. In the interim, states may combine the use of their claims/encounter databases with chart audits for a sample of children to report on quality measures, using an approach analogous to the HEDIS hybrid methodology (see below).

A second weakness in the current MSIS database is the omission of children who are enrolled in separate (non-Medicaid) CHIP programs. The MSIS also does not include privately insured or uninsured children. Since CHIPRA now requires states to compare the status of children and adolescents served by public plans with that of the general population of children and adolescents on a statewide basis, MSIS data can provide only a partial picture of the services or outcomes of those who are enrolled in Medicaid or Medicaid-expansion CHIP plans.

HEDIS

Currently, administrative data from the HEDIS collection of data from managed care plans are a primary source of information at the state level for reporting on current and new quality-of-care measures. It should be noted that in a managed care environment, the state usually provides a negotiated payment to the managed care organizations (MCOs) for services, and the MCOs pay the providers. In cases where the providers are paid on a fee-for-service basis, claims data will exist. In cases where health plans pay providers through a negotiated payment per member, there is no need for claims, and providers instead generate shadow claims for the encounter.

Developed by the National Committee for Quality Assurance (NCQA), HEDIS is a tool used by more than 90 percent of health plans to report on quality (NCQA, 2010). In its annual *State of Health Care Quality* report, NCQA releases detailed, plan-specific performance information for both commercial and Medicaid plans. NCQA's 2008 report for Medicaid provided information on 52 measures of clinical quality (NCQA, 2008). States also release their own reports. For example, Michigan releases an annual report on its HEDIS results by MCO (MDCH, 2008). New York has long issued annual report cards (Quality Assurance Reporting Requirement) on health plan performance on HEDIS as well as state-level measures (NYDOH, 2010).

Many of the initial core measures published and posted for public comment by the Secretary of HHS are HEDIS measures that health plans currently use to report on quality. The measures on immunization, prenatal care, chlamydia screening, and well-care visits are examples of the HEDIS measures in the core set. This is not surprising given that the AHRQ committee recommending measures and the CHIPRA legislation placed a premium on measures that were grounded and in use. Further, because claims data form the basis for HEDIS measures, these measures generally are limited to whether a service has been delivered, rather than broader care processes across episodes of care or outcomes. For example, there is a measure of whether chlamydia screening took place, but not whether appropriate follow-up occurred if the result was abnormal.

HEDIS protocols for assessing measures specify either methods that use administrative data alone or hybrid methods that combine the use of administrative data with chart reviews for a sample of beneficiaries. These HEDIS protocols form a strong base for CMS to use in guiding the states on reporting, but there are important cautions. First, these measures were designed to be used by managed care plans, and the protocol includes features designed to ensure that members are "continuously" enrolled in health plans long enough to benefit from their quality improvement policies (frequently 11 out of 12 months, but the "continuous enrollment" period can be longer for some measures). As a result, Medicaid children who are not enrolled in a managed care plan for the required amount of time are omitted from the measurement results, even if they have been registered in Medicaid for the designated period. As an example, HEDIS specifications for reporting immunization coverage specify that only children enrolled for 11 or more of the prior 12 months be included in the reporting denominator (NCQA, 1996). In one study, fewer than half of all enrolled Medicaid children (39 percent) were included in the health plan denominator in the 12 state studies, although most (78 percent) had been on Medicaid for the required length of time (Fairbrother et al., 2004). This problem becomes more acute as the continuous enrollment periods increase (asthma measurement, for example, requires 2 years of continuous enrollment).

A second problem is that data are not reported in a standardized manner (Partridge, 2007). Thus, although almost 90 percent of Medicaid programs and 100 percent of CHIP programs reported using HEDIS access and effectiveness measures related to child health in 2009, the data may not be comparable across states (Smith et al., 2009). Standard definitions frequently are not used, with states modifying HEDIS definitions to accommodate a Medicaid population with shorter coverage spells, as well as other local concerns (Partridge, 2007). For example, although the 1997 State Children's Health Insurance Program (SCHIP) statute required each state to file an annual report—including the state objectives for SCHIP, the performance measures used, and progress that year toward meeting the objectives—it did not specify exactly how measures were to be reported. A review of state reports in 2005 on four HEDIS measures showed great variation in the number of states that reported on the measures, from a high of 34 to a low of 10 (Partridge, 2007). Furthermore, states modified the HEDIS specifications to accommodate their priorities, so that even though states reported on the same measures, the data were not strictly comparable. The reviewers concluded that comparable data were sufficient to build a national SCHIP database and generate national averages for two of the four measures (Partridge, 2007). This issue of the level of comparability will need to be addressed in developing the reporting format required by CHIPRA.

The HEDIS protocols are an important starting point for measurement under CHIPRA. But the measures will need to be respecified to be appropriate for the entire Medicaid and CHIP population through inclusion of a denominator that addresses enrollment in these two programs. And with the emphasis in the Affordable Care Act (ACA) on all populations of children, measures may need to be respecified again to include all children, regardless of payer.

NATIONAL SURVEY OF CHILDREN'S HEALTH

The NSCH is a nationally representative household survey of children aged 0–17 that includes state-level estimates. It has been administered twice (in 2003 and 2007); a third fielding is planned for 2011 that is expected to include additional items on child well-being/thriving, health insurance and access to care, and items relevant to life-course research. The third wave of survey data may also include nearest cross-street information to enhance the geocoded linking of these data to other neighborhood-level data systems.

The NSCH represents responses of parents/guardians of a randomly selected child in each household. Survey questions encompass child health status and health conditions, health insurance and medical home, parental health, school engagement, media exposure, youth activities, and neighborhood conditions. The NSCH produces estimates for numerous demographic, socioeconomic, and health status subgroups of children, including whether their health insurance coverage is public or private, whether they have special health care needs, their race/ethnicity, their primary language, whether they are foreign born or adopted, the immigration status of their parents, their household income, and the household's use of public assistance. NSCH national and state-level findings for numerous subgroups are posted at www.childhealthdata.org.

The NSCH includes multiple patient-centered categories of data relevant to the measurement of health care quality for children and adolescents (these data components are in addition to measures of physical and dental health, mental and emotional health, health insurance coverage, and other topics relevant to the child's physical and social environments). The categories include preventive medical care visits, preventive dental care visits, getting needed mental health care, one or more unmet needs for care, medical home, personal doctor or nurse, usual sources for sick and well care, family-centered care, problems in obtaining needed referrals, effective care coordination, access to specialty care or services, receipt of care from specialist doctor, doctor asks about concerns, and developmental screenings.

NATIONAL HEALTH INTERVIEW SURVEY

As described in Chapter 4, the NHIS is an annual household survey conducted by the National Center for Health Statistics that collects information on all household members, including children and adolescents. NHIS data provide the basis for the AHRQ reports on health care disparities, indicating how many children and adolescents have access to health care coverage, as well as a specific source of usual health care, and how many children and adolescents rely on hospital-based services (such as outpatient or emergency departments) for usual or ongoing care. NHIS data also are used in identifying sources of health care disparities, especially in areas that involve access to care or treatment for conditions such as asthma and mental and emotional disorders.

RESOURCES FOR DATA ANALYSIS AND LINKAGE

This section describes four key resources for data analysis and linkage:

- the databases and tools that are part of the AHRQ Healthcare Cost and Utilization Project (HCUP);
- the application forms for public insurance, which contain demographic information on Medicaid and CHIP beneficiaries;
- the Physician Quality Reporting Initiative (PQRI); and
- examples of state-based data warehouse capacities that foster linkage across multiple database systems.

HCUP Databases and Tools

The HCUP databases, supported by AHRQ, represent the largest collection of multiyear, all-payer hospital and emergency room discharge data that can be applied to hospital claims to assess safety events, ambulatory care–sensitive hospitalizations, and other measures of potential interest. More than 40 states provide data as part of the project, collectively representing more than 95 percent of all discharges (AHRQ, 2010). The HCUP databases are constructed using a core set of clinical and nonclinical details found in a typical discharge claim for hospitals and emergency rooms, including data on primary and secondary diagnoses and procedures, admission source and discharge disposition, patient demographics, expected payment source, total charges, length of stay, and hospital characteristics. From this core set of discharge information, several subsets of data can be extracted to create inpatient, ambulatory care, emergency care, and child-specific databases, as shown in Table D-1. Each database in turn can be used to examine quality of care with the AHRQ quality indicators, to

TABLE D-1 HCUP Databases

	Year Started	Years Available	Number of States	Number of Hospitals
National				
Nationwide Inpatient Sample (NIS)	1988	Yearly	42 in 2008	1,056 in 2008
Kids' Inpatient Database (KID)	1997	1997, 2000, 2003, 2006	38 in 2006	3,739 in 2006
Nationwide Emergency Department Sample (NEDS)	2006	Yearly	27 in 2007	966 in 2007
State				
State Inpatient Databases (SID)	1990	Yearly	40	
State Ambulatory Surgery Databases (SASD)	1997	Yearly	28	
State Emergency Department Databases (SEDD)	1999	Yearly	27	

aggregate data using clinical classification codes (the *International Classification of Diseases* [ICD]-9-CM and ICD-10 codes), and to identify and measure coexisting conditions using Comorbidity Software (see Table 2 in Fairbrother et al., 2010).

HCUP also includes software tools and indicators with which to measure quality (see Table D-2). AHRQ first developed three indicator sets: the Inpatient Quality Indicators (IQI), for the quality of care received in hospitals; the Prevention Quality Indicators (PQI), for potentially preventable hospital admissions; and the Patient Safety Indicators (PSI), for preventable complications of care. These measures were constructed based on adult health issues, complications, chronic conditions, and patterns of care and were not adequate to address the complexity of child and adolescent health care needs. Responding to this gap, AHRQ developed a fourth set of indicators focused on the safety and quality of pediatric hospital care—the Pediatric Quality Indicators (PDIs) (see Table D-3). These indicators focus on potentially preventable complications arising from inpatient care and on preventable hospitalizations for pediatric patients. This software could be used, for example, in calculating pediatric catheter-associated blood stream infection rates, one of the initial AHRQ core measures, using a state's inpatient database.

While the HCUP tools and indicators provide important ways to

TABLE D-2 HCUP Software Tools and Indicators

Clinical Classification Systems (CCSs)	
CCS for ICD-9-CM	Provides a means of classifying ICD-9-CM diagnoses or procedures into clinically meaningful categories, which can be used for aggregate statistical reporting.
CCS for ICD-10	Provides a means of classifying ICD-10 diagnoses into clinically meaningful categories. It will be used in 2012 when the tenth revision of the ICD codes is implemented.
CCS-MHSA for Mental Health and Substance Abuse	Defines mental health variables that identify general categories for MHSA diagnoses. Beginning in 2008, the CCS-MHSA was permanently integrated into the CCS tool and is no longer stand-alone.
CCS Tools	
Chronic Condition Indicators	Allows for categorizing conditions as chronic or not chronic.
Comorbidity Software	Assigns variables that identify coexisting conditions on hospital discharge records.
Procedure Classes	Allow for categorizing procedure codes as minor diagnostic, minor therapeutic, major diagnostic, and major therapeutic.
Utilization Flags	Provide a means of assessing use of procedures or services, such as intensive care unit (ICU), critical care unit (CCU), neonatal intensive care unit (NICU), and specific diagnostic tests and therapies.
Supplemental Files	
Cost-to-Charge Ratio	Supplements the data elements in the HCUP Nationwide Inpatient Sample (NIS) and State Inpatient Databases (SID) and permits conversion of hospital total charge data to cost estimates.
Hospital Market Structure	Hospital-level files designed to supplement the data elements in NIS, the Kids' Inpatient Database (KID), and SID.
AHRQ Quality Indicators (QIs)	
Prevention Quality Indicators	Identify hospital admissions that evidence suggests could have been avoided.
Inpatient Quality Indicators	Used for quality of care inside the hospital.
Patient Safety Quality Indicators	Used for quality of care inside the hospital as well as potentially avoidable complications.
Pediatric Quality Indicators	Used for quality of care inside the hospital as well as potentially avoidable complications for children (under age 18).

TABLE D-3 Pediatric Quality Indicators (PDIs)

Provider-Level Indicators

Accidental Puncture or Laceration	Cases of technical difficulty (e.g., accidental cut or laceration during procedure) per 1,000 eligible discharges
Decubitus Ulcer	Number of patients with decubitus ulcer per 1,000 eligible admissions
Foreign Body Left in During Procedure	Number of patients with a foreign body left in during a procedure per 1,000 eligible admissions
Iatrogenic Pneumothorax (in Neonates at Risk)	Number of patients with iatrogenic pneumothorax per 1,000 eligible admissions
Iatrogenic Pneumothorax (in Non-Neonates)	Number of patients with iatrogenic pneumothorax per 1,000 eligible admissions
Postoperative Hemorrhage and Hematoma	Number of patients with postoperative hemorrhage or hematoma requiring a procedure per 1,000 eligible admissions
Postoperative Respiratory Failure	Number of patients with respiratory failure per 1,000 eligible admissions
Postoperative Sepsis	Number of patients with sepsis per 1,000 eligible admissions
Postoperative Wound Dehiscence	Number of abdominopelvic surgery patients with disruption of abdominal wall per 1,000 eligible admissions
Selected Infection Due to Medical Care	Number of patients with specific infection codes per 1,000 eligible admissions
Transfusion Reaction	Number of patients with transfusion reaction per 1,000 eligible admissions
Pediatric Heart Surgery Mortality Rate	Number of in-hospital deaths in patients undergoing surgery for congenital heart disease per 1,000 patients
Pediatric Heart Surgery Volume Rate	Number of patients undergoing surgery for congenital heart disease

Area-Level Indicators

Asthma Admission Rate	Number of patients admitted for asthma per 100,000 population
Diabetes Short-Term Complications Admissions Rate	Number of patients admitted for short-term complications of diabetes (ketoacidosis, hyperosmolarity, coma) per 100,000 population
Gastroenteritis Admission Rate	Number of patients admitted for gastroenteritis per 100,000 population
Perforated Appendix Admission Rate	Number of patients admitted for perforated appendix per 100 admissions for appendicitis within an area
Urinary Tract Infection Admission Rate	Number of patients admitted for urinary tract infection per 100,000 population

measure the quality of care in hospital and emergency room settings, their capacity to measure disparities is limited: more than a quarter of the claims for children do not indicate race/ethnicity (HCUP, 2006). Moreover, the nature of the disparities varies with each measure. Finally, even though the measures reflect the most prominent safety issues, the prevalence of these complications is relative low, limiting the types of analysis that can be performed. Another issue with HCUP is that income data are at the community and not the individual level.

Application Forms for Public Insurance

Application forms for public insurance (Medicaid and CHIP) are a source of demographic information because they ask parents about their child's or adolescent's race, ethnicity, age, gender, income, and in some cases language. A validation study conducted in New York comparing race and ethnicity information collected from applications with information collected directly from parents as part of the Consumer Assessment of Healthcare Providers and Systems (CAHPS) surveys showed high levels of concordance between the two for all races and ethnicities (Fairbrother and Simpson, 2010).

Some states, such as New York, Kentucky, and Georgia, have the capacity to link demographic information from the application forms with claims-based data. This approach enables these states to monitor services and outcomes by selected demographic characteristics that are included on the application form and thus monitor disparities by race, ethnicity, language (if collected), and income. The federal MSIS data set also links claims/encounters data to demographic data from encounters, thus creating the potential to monitor race, ethnicity, language, and income disparities at the federal level. However, the ability to monitor disparities at the national level is restricted because the states do not collect their demographic enrollment data in a systematic manner. A review of application forms from all states (Fairbrother and Simpson, 2010) shows that only 18 states ask for "Hispanic/Latino" ethnicity as a separate category, while 19 states merge ethnicity with racial categories. Of these, 7 allow the applicant to choose more than one "race"; hence, an individual could select both "black" and "Hispanic" in these states but not in the others. Eight states have no race/ethnicity categories, but leave a blank for applicants to fill in. With respect to primary language, 14 states ask for "English," "Spanish," and "other" or list specific languages. However, 21 states have only a blank for applicants to fill in with their primary language. The design of application forms has been left to the states in the past; with the new emphasis on monitoring disparities at both the federal and state levels, standardization will be necessary.

Physician Quality Report Initiative

The Medicare PQRI is a quality reporting system that supports incentive payments for eligible professionals who report data on quality measures based on parameters established by CMS. The American Recovery and Reinvestment Act (ARRA) Health Information Technology for Economic and Clinical Health (HITECH) legislation significantly expanded the significance of the PQRI and the PQRI registry, which now incorporate providers who serve patients enrolled in Medicaid and CHIP plans as well as Medicare. Most of the 179 quality measures in the 2010 PQRI system are specified for adults. However, a significant number of measures are designed explicitly for children (especially those associated with the treatment of asthma, ear infections, childhood cancers, pediatric end-stage renal disease, and HIV/AIDS). Other measures include children and adolescents in the denominator, but the measurement age breaks limit the feasibility of determining how many children are included in certain data sets.

The specifications for the quality measures under PQRI provide the details for the numerator and denominator and therefore support analyses of the percentage of a defined patient population that receives a particular process of care or achieves a particular outcome. For example, PQRI measure 65 focuses on the avoidance of inappropriate use of antibiotic treatment for children with upper respiratory infections.

Examples of Data Warehouses and State-based Linkage Activities

Although states vary in their capabilities to collect, store, and analyze data, some states, such as New York, Georgia, and Kentucky, have strong warehousing capabilities, including in some cases the ability to link state databases. New York, for example, collects member-level data reported by Medicaid managed care plans (for all members) as part of annual HEDIS reporting and has created linkages of quality measurement results with eligibility files and CAHPS surveys. The resulting linked data set is organized at the person level, and includes demographic and service delivery information for Medicaid members in each measure. The resulting data warehouses can be used to monitor quality on a variety of measures and to display results by race/ethnicity, age, gender, and geography, making it possible to monitor performance for the population as a whole and for vulnerable groups.

Furthermore, some states have linked health data sets, giving them the ability to monitor over time and across settings. For example, New York has a linked data set consisting of childbirth and fetal death certificates, maternal and child hospital discharges, and Medicaid claims before and after the birth. Using this linked data set, New York can relate, for example, aspects of prenatal care to subsequent outcomes and health behaviors. Linking data across time can also make it possible to monitor important aspects of chronic care, such as whether a child has filled all prescriptions for medications needed to treat specific conditions, whether there are duplicative or overlapping medications in a regimen, or whether a rehospitalization occurred.

REFERENCES

AHRQ (Agency for Healthcare Research and Quality). 2010. *Healthcare Cost and Utilization Project (HCUP)*. http://hcupnet.ahrq.gov/ (accessed December 2, 2010).

Fairbrother, G., and L. Simpson. 2010 (unpublished). *Measuring and reporting quality of health care for children: CHIPRA and beyond.*

Fairbrother, G., A. Jain, H. L. Park, M. S. Massoudi, A. Haidery, and B. H. Gray. 2004. Churning in Medicaid managed care and its effect on accountability. *Journal of Health Care for the Poor and Underserved* 15(1):30-41.

Fairbrother, G., R. Sebastien, J. McAuliffe, and L. Simpson. 2010 (unpublished). *Monitoring changes in health care for children and families.* Child Policy Research Center.

HCUP (Healthcare Cost and Utilization Project). 2006. *The KIDS' inpatient database.* http://www.hcup-us.ahrq.gov/kidoverview.jsp (accessed November 19, 2010).

MacTaggart, P. 2010 (unpublished). *Overview of development & use of quality measures for children.* George Washington University Medical Center.

MDCH (Michigan Department of Community Health). 2008. *Michigan Medicaid HEDIS Report.* Lansing, MI: MDCH.

NCQA (National Committee for Quality Assurance). 1996. *HEDIS 3.0 Manual.* Rockville, MD: AHRQ.

NCQA. 2008. *The state of health care quality 2008.* http://www.ncqa.org/portals/0/newsroom/sohc/SOHC_08.pdf (accessed March 22, 2011).

NCQA. 2010. *HEDIS & quality measurement.* http://www.ncqa.org/tabid/59/Default.aspx (accessed March 22, 2011).

NYDOH (New York State Department of Health). 2010. *Managed care reports.* http://www.health.state.ny.us/health_care/managed_care/reports/ (accessed December 3, 2010).

Partridge, L. 2007. *Review of access and quality of care in SCHIP using standardized national performance measures.* Washington, DC: National Health Policy Forum.

Simpson, L., G. Fairbrother, J. Touschner, and J. Guyer. 2009. *Implementation choices for the Children's Health Insurance Reauthorization Act of 2009.* New York: The Commonwealth Fund.

Smith, V., J. Edwards, E. Reagan, and D. Roberts. 2009. *Medicaid and CHIP strategies for improving child health.* New York: The Commonwealth Fund.

E

Biographical Sketches of Committee Members and Staff

Gordon H. DeFriese, Ph.D. (*Chair*), holds joint appointments as professor of social medicine, dental ecology, epidemiology, and health policy and administration. He is a former director of the Cecil G. Sheps Center for Health Services Research and the Institute on Aging at the University of North Carolina, Chapel Hill. His primary area of interest is aging, specifically the factors that motivate and enable community-dwelling older adults to learn and practice self-care skills, particularly when faced with functional limitations. In addition to this work, he has been engaged in a number of studies of the problems associated with low levels of childhood immunization in the United States, including evaluation of the national All Kids Count registry system demonstrations funded by The Robert Wood Johnson Foundation. Since the mid-1990s, he has focused most of his work in the area of state-level health policy, serving as president and chief executive officer of the North Carolina Institute of Medicine. This role has included special studies of long-term care, dental care for low-income persons, health insurance for low-income children, the health care safety net, the nursing workforce, and Latino health issues and will soon expand to include work on child abuse, health literacy, and the uninsured. Dr. DeFriese is an elected member of the Institute of Medicine (IOM) and has served on numerous National Research Council (NRC) and IOM committees. He received his Ph.D. in medical sociology from the University of Kentucky.

Paula A. Braveman, M.D., M.P.H., is a professor in the Department of Family and Community Medicine, School of Medicine, and director of the Center on Social Disparities in Health at the University of California,

San Francisco (UCSF). Her areas of interest include documenting and understanding socioeconomic and racial or ethnic disparities in health, particularly in maternal and infant health, and translating research into information to inform policies to reduce health disparities. Dr. Braveman also focuses on methodological and conceptual issues in studying socioeconomic and racial or ethnic inequalities in health in the United States and internationally, particularly the development of measures of experiences of racial discrimination for use in studies of adverse birth outcomes among African American women in the United States, the measurement of socioeconomic factors in U.S. health research, and the concept and measurement of health inequalities in the United States and internationally. During the 1990s, she worked with World Health Organization staff in Geneva to develop and implement a global initiative on equity in health and health care. Throughout her career, Dr. Braveman has collaborated with local, state, federal, and international health agencies to see research translated into practice, with the goal of achieving greater equity in health. She is an elected member of the IOM. She received an M.D. from UCSF and an M.P.H. in epidemiology from the University of California, Berkeley.

Claire D. Brindis, Dr.P.H., M.P.H., is director of the Philip R. Lee Institute for Health Policy Studies and a professor in the Department of Pediatrics, Division of Adolescent Medicine, and the Department of Obstetrics, Gynecology and Reproductive Sciences at UCSF. She is also executive director of the National Adolescent Health Information and Innovation Center and associate director of the Public Policy Analysis and Education Center for Middle Childhood, Adolescent and Young Adult Health, all at UCSF. Dr. Brindis's research interests focus on health disparities and access to health for children, adolescents, and young adults; analyses of child and adolescent health policy; and women's health. She serves as a frequent policy advisor to federal, state, and local policy makers and private foundations. Her writings, publications, and personal consultation in the field of adolescent pregnancy prevention have been extensively utilized in the planning and implementation of various state and federal initiatives. Dr. Brindis has served as chair of the population, reproductive health, and family planning section of the American Public Health Association and participated on the steering committee of the Centers for Disease Control and Prevention's (CDC's) National Health Objectives for the Year 2010. Currently, she serves on the Steering Committee for the National Initiative to Improve Adolescent and Young Adult Health, co-led by the federal Office of Adolescent Health, Maternal and Child Health Bureau, and the Division of Adolescent and School Health, CDC, as well as 30 national organizations. She also is a member of the national advisory committee for the National Campaign to Prevent Teen and Young Adult Pregnancy's National Advisory

Committee-Latino Initiative. In the area of reproductive health, Dr. Brindis has led a multidisciplinary team evaluating California's Office of Family Planning's Family PACT (Planning, Access, Care and Treatment) program, as well as reproductive health programs in Iowa, Colorado, and New York. In addition, she is conducting two evaluations of policy coalitions devoted to asthma and community clinics. Dr. Brindis has served on numerous IOM and NRC committees, most recently the IOM Committee on a Comprehensive Review of the DHHS Office of Family Planning Title X Program. She received a Dr.P.H. from the University of California, Berkeley, and an M.P.H. from the University of California, Los Angeles.

Barbara J. Burns, Ph.D., is professor of medical psychology and director of the Services Effectiveness Research Program in the Department of Psychiatry and Behavioral Sciences at Duke University, School of Medicine. Dr. Burns is a nationally recognized mental health services researcher. She has coauthored more than 250 publications and was lead author for the review of effective treatment for mental disorders in children and adolescents for the 1999 U.S. Surgeon General's Report on Mental Health. Her research career emerged from clinical practice in an integrated health/mental health center and interest in exploring the implications of that model. For nearly a decade at the National Institute of Mental Health, she focused on improving mental health services from primary to tertiary care. She is currently investigating the effectiveness of an enhanced model of long-term treatment foster care, best practices for child trauma, the effectiveness of group homes, and mental health services for children in the child welfare system. Her primary focus is on strategies to increase the diffusion of evidence-based interventions for youth with severe emotional disorders. Throughout her research, teaching, clinical practice, and policy career, Dr. Burns has studied and advocated for responsive and innovative community-based treatment. She received a Ph.D. in psychology from Boston College.

Glenn Flores, M.D., is professor of pediatrics and public health, director of general pediatrics, Judith and Charles Ginsburg chair in pediatrics, and director of the Academic General Pediatrics Fellowship at the University of Texas Southwestern and Children's Medical Center Dallas. He founded and is former codirector of the Pediatric Latino Clinic at Boston Medical Center. Dr. Flores is a former Robert Wood Johnson (RWJ) generalist physician faculty scholar and a former RWJ minority medical faculty scholar. His research focuses on racial/ethnic disparities in health and health care, Latino children's health, access to health care, and culture and clinical care. Dr. Flores chaired the Latino Consortium of the American Academy of Pediatrics Center for Child Health Research and is a member of the Committee on Pediatric Research of the American Academy of Pediatrics. He is chair of the Research Committee of the Academic Pediatric Association and is also a member of the National Advisory Committee of the RWJ Harold Amos Medical Faculty Development Program. He received an M.D. from the University of California, San Francisco School of Medicine.

Gary L. Freed, M.D., is Percy and Mary Murphy professor of pediatrics and community health in the Department of Pediatrics at University of Michigan Health Systems. He has more than 18 years of experience in children's health services research and has published extensively on child health policy and health economics, physician behavior, and interspecialty variation in the provision of preventive services to children. Dr. Freed is immediate past president of the Society for Pediatric Research and immediate past chair of the Department of Health and Human Services (HHS) National Vaccine Advisory Committee. He is a member of the American Board of Pediatrics and a fellow of the American Academy of Pediatrics. He received an M.D. from Baylor College of Medicine.

Deborah A. Gross, R.N., D.N.Sc., is Leonard and Helen Stulman chair in mental health and psychiatric nursing at Johns Hopkins University School of Nursing and in the Department of Psychiatry and Behavioral Sciences in the School of Medicine. Prior to her appointment at the School of Nursing, she served as associate dean for research and as department chair at Rush University College of Nursing. Dr. Gross's research focuses on promoting positive parent child relationships and preventing behavior problems in preschool children from low-income neighborhoods. With colleagues at Rush, she developed the Chicago Parent Program, an innovative parenting program that has been shown to improve parenting behavior and reduce child behavior problems. This program is currently used in a number of settings, including Head Start centers in Chicago and New York City. From 2006 to 2009, Dr. Gross was a Robert Wood Johnson fellow in the Executive Nurse Fellows Program. She has served on numerous National Institutes of Health (NIH) panels and received several awards, including the President's Award for outstanding research from the Friends of the National Institute for Nursing Research.

Maxine Hayes, M.D., M.P.H., is state health officer for the Washington State Department of Health. As the state's top public health physician, her role includes advising the governor and the secretary of health on issues ranging from health promotion and chronic disease prevention to emergency response, including pandemic influenza preparedness. She also works closely with the medical community, local health departments, and community groups. Prior to her appointment as health officer, Dr. Hayes was assistant secretary of community and family health. She is clinical professor of pediatrics at the University of Washington, School of Medicine, and on the Maternal and Child Health faculty of the School of Public Health. Dr. Hayes is an elected member of the IOM and has served as a member of the NRC–IOM Board on Children, Youth and Families and as chair of the Committee on the Impact of Pregnancy Weight on Maternal and Child Health. She received an M.D. from the State University of New York at Buffalo and an M.P.H. from Harvard School of Public Health.

Charles J. Homer, M.D., is president and chief executive officer of the National Initiative for Children's Healthcare Quality (NICHQ). He is also an associate professor in the Department of Society, Human Development and Health at Harvard University School of Public Health and an associate clinical professor of pediatrics at Harvard Medical School. Prior to his position at NICHQ, he was director of the Clinical Effectiveness Program at Children's Hospital Boston and served as program director of the first federally supported fellowship training program in pediatric health services research. Dr. Homer is a frequent speaker on quality measurement and quality improvement for children's health care. He served on the IOM Committee on Crossing the Quality Chasm-Next Steps Summit. He received an M.D. from the University of Pennsylvania.

Kevin B. Johnson, M.D., M.S., is professor and vice chair of biomedical informatics and professor of pediatrics at Vanderbilt University School of Medicine. Dr. Johnson is an internationally respected developer and evaluator of clinical information technology. His research interests have included the development and adoption of clinical information systems to improve patient safety and compliance with practice guidelines; the uses of advanced computer technologies, including the Worldwide Web, personal digital assistants, and pen-based computers, in medicine; and the development of computer-based documentation systems for the point of care. He also directed the development and evaluation of evidence-based pediatric care guidelines for Johns Hopkins Hospital. Dr. Johnson was awarded membership in the American College of Medical Informatics in 2004, is a member of the American Board of Pediatrics' Program for Maintenance of Certification Task Force, and has been actively involved with the program of Maintenance of Certification developed by the Board for all pediatricians. His knowledge of electronic health records and patient safety led to his appointment to the IOM's Committee on Data Standards for Patient Safety and Committee on Identifying and Preventing Medication Errors. He received an M.D. from Johns Hopkins Hospital in Baltimore and an M.S. in medical informatics from Stanford University.

Genevieve M. Kenney, Ph.D., is a senior fellow and health economist at the Urban Institute with more than 20 years of experience in conducting research. She is a nationally renowned expert on health insurance coverage and health issues facing low-income children and families. Dr. Kenney was a lead researcher on two major evaluations of the Children's Health Insurance Program (CHIP): a congressionally mandated evaluation for HHS and an evaluation supported by a number of private foundations. She has published numerous articles on insurance coverage and access to care for low-income children, pregnant women, and parents. In her research, she has examined a range of issues, including family coverage policies and the structure of CHIP financing; participation and barriers to enrollment; access and use differentials among low-income children; the effects of premium increases on enrollment; and the impacts of CHIP expansions on insurance coverage, crowd-out, and access to care. Dr. Kenney has also conducted research on a number of Medicaid and Medicare topics, including the impacts of Medicaid eligibility expansions for pregnant women and children, the adoption of managed care in Medicaid, the use of home health services among the dual-eligible population, and the impacts of Medicare's prospective payment system on postacute services. In her current research, she is examining state-level Medicaid reforms, Medicaid coverage of family planning services, and state efforts to enroll more children in Medicaid and the State Children's Health Insurance Program (SCHIP). She holds a Ph.D. and M.A. in economics and an M.A. in statistics from the University of Michigan.

Marie C. McCormick, M.D., Sc.D., is professor of maternal and child health in the Department of Society, Human Development, and Health and professor of pediatrics at Harvard Medical School. She also serves as senior associate director of the Infant Follow-up Program at the Children's Hospital. Her research involves epidemiologic and health services research investigations in areas related to infant mortality and the outcomes of high-risk neonates. More specifically, she focuses on the following areas: outcomes of infants experiencing neonatal complications such as low birth weight and interventions with the potential to ameliorate adverse outcomes, evaluation of programs designed to improve the health of families and children, and maternal health and prematurity. Dr. McCormick is a member of the IOM and most recently served on the Board on Children, Youth, and Families' Committee on Developmental Outcomes and Assessments for Young Children. She received an M.D. from Johns Hopkins Medical School and an Sc.D. from Johns Hopkins School of Hygiene and Public Health.

Kathryn M. McDonald, M.M./M.B.A., is executive director of the Center for Health Policy (CHP) and the Center for Primary Care and Outcomes

Research (PCOR) at Stanford University. She is also a senior scholar at the centers and associate director of the Stanford UCSF Evidence-based Practice Center (EPC) in collaboration with RAND. Her work focuses on evidence-based medicine, medical technology assessment, health care quality, and patient safety measures and interventions. Her health care quality and patient safety research portfolio includes the publicly released Agency for Healthcare Research and Quality (AHRQ) Quality Indicators; the first comprehensive review of patient safety practices published in 2000 (*Making Healthcare Safer*); and more recently, a series of evidence reports on quality improvement strategies (*Closing the Quality Gap*). She continues to lead the Stanford development team for expansion of the AHRQ Quality Indicators, including the Pediatric Quality Indicators. She is also an active member of the Society for Decision Making and currently serves as its president. In earlier years at the Stanford School of Medicine, Ms. McDonald acquired her health services research training through her role as project director and investigator for a number of research projects, including the Cardiac Arrhythmia Patient Outcomes Research Team. Previously, she worked as a manager for technology optimization and business development at Stanford Hospital and as a research manager for new product development at a medical device company. She received a master of management degree (M.B.A. equivalent) from Northwestern University's Kellogg School of Management, with an emphasis on the health care industry and organizational behavior, and holds a B.S. in chemical engineering from Stanford University.

Michael J. O'Grady, Ph.D., is a senior fellow at the National Opinion Research Center (NORC) at the University of Chicago and principal of O'Grady Health Policy LLC, a private health consulting firm. At NORC, he concentrates on health policy research and analysis for public and private nonprofit organizations. Dr. O'Grady's current research includes serving as principal investigator for the cost-effectiveness component of a multiyear diabetes clinical trial, the formulation of policy options for an expanded federal role in the development of a national health information exchange, and the assessment of new developments in health insurance benefit design and cost sharing. He also serves on the Board of Scientific Counselors at CDC's National Center for Health Statistics. At O'Grady Health Policy LLC, he concentrates on strategic consulting and analysis for a range of for-profit organizations. This research includes the development of new modeling and methods for improving the federal budget process by introducing the latest disease-based epidemiological modeling into budget estimates for interventions for chronic illness, particularly diabetes and obesity. Dr. O'Grady is a veteran health policy expert with 24 years of experience working in Congress and HHS. From 2003 to 2005, he was assistant secretary for planning and evaluation at HHS, where he directed both policy development and policy research across the full array of issues confronting the Department. During his tenure as assistant secretary, he increased the quality and rigor of the Department's research and analysis significantly, providing rapid and critical analyses of legislative and regulatory proposals. Prior to his Senate confirmation as assistant secretary, Dr. O'Grady served as senior health economist on the majority staff of the Joint Economic Committee of the U.S. Congress. Previously, he held senior staff positions with the Senate Finance Committee, the Bipartisan Commission for the Future of Medicare, the Medicare Payment Advisory Commission, and the Congressional Research Service of the Library of Congress. He received a Ph.D. in political science at the University of Rochester.

Alan R. Weil, M.P.P., J.D., is executive director of the National Academy for State Health Policy. Previously, he served for 7 years as director of the Assessing the New Federalism project at the Urban Institute, one of the largest privately funded social policy research projects ever undertaken in the United States. He has also held a cabinet position as executive director of the Colorado Department of Health Care Policy and Financing, was health policy advisor to Colorado Governor Roy Romer, and was assistant general counsel in the Massachusetts Department of Medical Security. He is coeditor of two books—*Welfare Reform: The Next Act* and *Federalism and Health Policy*—and has authored chapters in a number of books and published articles in journals including *Health Affairs* and *Inquiry*. Mr. Weil was an appointed member of President Clinton's Advisory Commission on Consumer Protection and Quality in the Health Care Industry, which drafted the patient's bill of rights. He is a member of the Kaiser Commission on Medicaid and the Uninsured and the Commonwealth Fund Commission on a High Performance Health System. Mr. Weil currently serves on the IOM Board on Health Care Services. He received an M.P.P. from the John F. Kennedy School of Government at Harvard University and a J.D. from Harvard Law School.

Alan M. Zaslavsky, Ph.D., is professor of health care policy in the Department of Health Care Policy at Harvard Medical School. His health services research focuses primarily on developing methodology for quality measurement of health plans and providers and understanding the implications of these quality measurements. An important part of his work concerns the development, implementation, and analysis of the Consumer Assessment of Healthcare Providers and Systems (CAHPS) survey. He has studied individual characteristics affecting responses to the survey, dimensions of quality measured, the contributions of the health plan and geographic location to CAHPS-measured quality, comparisons of traditional Medicare and Medicare Advantage, and risk selection among health plans. He is developing methods for integrating cancer registry data with surveys and medical record reviews to better detect such relationships. Dr. Zaslavsky has served on numerous NRC and IOM committees and currently serves on the Committee on National Statistics and chairs the Panel to Review Alternative Data Sources for the Limited-English Proficiency Allocation Formula under Title III, Part A, Elementary and Secondary Education Act. He received an M.S. in statistics and computer science from Northeastern University and a Ph.D. in applied mathematics, with a specialty in statistics, from the Massachusetts Institute of Technology.

Study Staff

Rosemary Chalk is director of the Board on Children, Youth, and Families, a joint effort of the IOM and NRC. She is a policy analyst who has been a study director at the National Academies since 1987. She has directed or served as a senior staff member for more than a dozen IOM and NRC studies, including studies on vaccine finance, the public health infrastructure for immunization, family violence, child abuse and neglect, research ethics and misconduct in science, and education finance. From 2000 to 2003, Ms. Chalk directed a research project on the development of child well-being indicators for the child welfare system at Child Trends in Washington, DC. She previously served as a consultant for science and society research projects at the Harvard School of Public Health and was an Exxon research fellow in the Program on Science, Technology, and Society at the Massachusetts Institute of Technology. She was program head of the Committee on Scientific Freedom and Responsibility of the American Association for the Advancement of Science from 1976 to 1986. She holds a B.A. in foreign affairs from the University of Cincinnati.

Patti Simon is a program officer for the Board on Children, Youth, and Families at the National Academies. She is currently working on studies for two IOM/NRC committees: the Committee on Pediatric Health and Health Care Quality Measures and the Committee on Oral Health Services: Equity and Access to Care. Prior to joining the National Academies, Ms. Simon worked in the Department of Health Policy at The George Washington University, where she managed a national program focused on health disparities and the social determinants of health. She holds an M.P.H. and a B.S. in psychology, both from the University of Texas.

Pamella Atayi is a senior program assistant for the Board on Children, Youth, and Families. She is currently supporting the Committee on Pediatric Health and Health Care Quality Measures, as well as a project on the science of family research. Ms. Atayi has worked with a number of nonprofit organizations over the past 10 years—most recently with the Evangelical Lutheran Church in America's public policy office on Capitol Hill. She received her B.A. in English from the University of Maryland University College and holds a diploma in computer information systems from Strayer College.

Wendy E. Keenan is a program associate for the Board on Children, Youth, and Families. She helps organize planning meetings and workshops that cover current issues related to children, youth, and families, and provides administrative and research support to the Board's various program committees. Ms. Keenan has been on the National Academies' staff for 10 years and has worked on studies for both the IOM and NRC. As a senior program assistant, she worked with the NRC's Board on Behavioral, Cognitive, and Sensory Sciences. Prior to joining the National Academies, she taught English as a second language for Washington, DC, public schools. She received a B.A. in sociology from The Pennsylvania State University and took graduate courses in liberal studies at Georgetown University.

Yeonwoo Lebovitz is a research associate with the Board on Children, Youth, and Families. Prior to joining the Board in November 2010, she worked as a program associate with IOM's Board on Health Sciences Policy and as a regulatory affairs associate at Amgen. Ms. Lebovitz earned a B.A. in International Affairs and German Language and Literature from the George Washington University, and is an M.S. candidate for the Biomedical Science Policy and Advocacy program at Georgetown University.

Julienne Marie Palbusa is a research assistant for the Board on Children, Youth, and Families. She joined the staff in December 2008. She is a 2007 graduate of The College of William and Mary in Williamsburg, Virginia, where she earned a B.S. in psychology with a minor in kinesiology.

Only Appendixes A-E are printed in this volume. The other appendixes are included on the CD in the back of the report or online. Go to http://www. nap.edu/catalog.php?record_id=13084.

Index